HELPING CHILDREN WITH
AGGRESSION AND CONDUCT PROBLEMS

Helping Children with Aggression and Conduct Problems

Best Practices for Intervention

MICHAEL L. BLOOMQUIST
STEVEN V. SCHNELL

Foreword by John E. Lochman

THE GUILFORD PRESS
New York   London

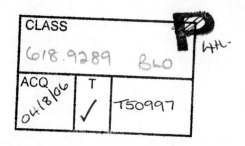
© 2002 The Guilford Press
A Division of Guilford Publications, Inc.
72 Spring Street, New York, NY 10012
www.guilford.com

Paperback edition 2005

Printed in the United States of America

This book is printed on acid-free paper.

Last digit is print number: 9   8   7   6   5   4   3

Library of Congress Cataloging-in-Publication Data

Bloomquist, Michael L.
  Helping children with aggression and conduct problems : best practices
for intervention / by Michael L. Bloomquist, Steven V. Schnell.
     p.   cm.
  Includes bibliographical references (p.) and index.
  ISBN 1-57230-748-X (hc)   ISBN 1-59385-240-1 (pbk)
    1. Agressiveness in children. 2. Conduct disorders in children. 3. Violence
in children. 4. Oppositional defiant disorder in children—Treatment.
I. Schnell, Steven V.   II. Title.

  RJ506.A35 B56 2002
  618.92′89—dc21   2001056869

To my wife, Rebecca Syverts—M. L. B.

To my wife, Mary Mullaney Schnell—S. V. S.

About the Authors

Michael L. Bloomquist, PhD, is a Senior Clinical Psychologist in the Children, Family, and Adult Services Department of Hennepin County and a Research Psychologist/Instructor in the Department of Psychiatry at the University of Minnesota, both in Minneapolis, Minnesota. He has extensive applied and research experience in prevention and treatment activities with children exhibiting behavior problems. Dr. Bloomquist is a coinvestigator on several longitudinal studies examining the development of children with aggression, as well as evaluating the effects of comprehensive prevention programs. He is the author of *Skills Training for Children with Behavior Disorders: A Parent and Therapist Guidebook* (Guilford Press, 1996) and has coauthored articles in peer-reviewed journals.

Steven V. Schnell, PhD, has many years of experience working with children exhibiting aggression and conduct problems as a Clinical Child Psychologist at North Psychology Clinic, Brooklyn Center, Minnesota, and at the North Star Family Resource Center, which is part of Minneapolis Public Schools. Dr. Schnell works closely with schools and has a special interest in integrating mental health and educational services. In addition to providing mental health services for children and families, he has conducted training and consultation to teachers and schools, made numerous presentations to professional groups, and coauthored articles in peer-reviewed journals.

Foreword

This volume arrives at an important time when we are frequently reminded in the popular press, as well as in our professional journals, of the frequency and severe consequences of adolescent violence and serious conduct problems. Longitudinal research clearly indicates that aggressive behavior problems in the elementary school years are significant predictors of later severe problems with antisocial behavior in adolescence. In this book, Michael Bloomquist and Steven Schnell address the extraordinarily important treatment and prevention needs of this preadolescent population and do an extraordinary job.

This book covers the topic of children with aggression and conduct problems in a very comprehensive, broad manner, and is well organized into five sections on the nature of children's aggressive behavior problems, on assessment and identification, on child and family interventions, on school and community interventions, and on integration and challenges for these interventions. Thus, the focus of the book is not only on defining the nature of the problem, and on explaining contemporary thinking about theories that account for the development and maintenance of these patterns of antisocial behavior, but also on how to intervene with these problems in "real-world" settings in schools and in communities. The review of the background literature is quite comprehensive, but also very readable, and it provides many references to the most current research and professional thinking about conduct problems in children.

The authors use an excellent conceptual framework involving a developmental and multisystemic model to organize their approach to practice, and provide richly detailed, integrated coverage of the conceptual models, measurement models, and intervention models for externalizing behavior in children. The review of risk and protective factors is state of the art, provides a firm basis for the conceptual model articulated here, and gives the reader a sophisticated view of the multiple, interacting causes of childhood aggression and conduct problems. It is critically important that our methods for assessment are firmly rooted in our thinking about the developmental model for these behavioral disorders, as this text nicely indicates. It is even more essential that the intervention model be designed to target precisely those processes that we know are deficient or are distorted within these children and their families. Only too often psychologists and counselors resort to using an intervention approach that they have learned at a workshop or from a colleague, but which does not address the proven, specific underlying deficits for the behavioral problems, has no evidence for its effectiveness, and may, in some circumstances, have negative iatrogenic effects. An important strength of this book is that it argues convincingly for this need for developmentally appropriate, well-researched interventions, and then provides a synthesis of empirically supported intervention approaches for children with aggressive behavior problems.

There is useful, thoughtful coverage of related topics throughout the book as well, such as research on the types of aggressive and conduct problem behaviors. This key focus can allow us to begin to think about our research-based models in much more finely discriminating ways, and can allow us to address the real differences we experience clinically among our clients with conduct problems. For example, the nature of the social-cognitive difficulties of reactively aggressive children is clearly different from that of proactively aggressive children, and our approaches to intervention must take these variations among subtypes of aggressive children into account.

Two of the key strengths of this book are (1) provision of the best discussion at this time of the range of empirically supported interventions for aggressive, conduct problem children, and (2) innovative and creative effort to abstract important common content elements from empirically supported intervention programs. This book not only overviews the empirically supported interventions that have been used with aggressive children in outpatient clinics or in counselors' offices, but also explains how other broader interventions, such as interventions provided at the level of a whole classroom or a whole school, can also be quite effective. Excellent examples are given of these various programs, along with references to learn more about them. However, what is most unique about this book is its effort to abstract best practices for intervention from the existing literature on research-supported interventions. This effort to provide a broad intervention, which is a careful synthesis of the best programs currently available, truly sets this book apart from other recent texts on children with aggression and conduct problems. Bloomquist and Schnell have approached this task in a highly systematic and thoughtful manner, and the result is outstanding.

Additional useful features are the book's critical emphasis on multicomponent and coordinated services programs, with excellent examples, and a very useful section on engagement of families into intervention. As emphasized by the authors, the available research data suggest that the most effective interventions for children with high levels of aggressive behaviors and conduct problems are, in fact, multicomponent interventions, which target multiple risk factors within the child, the family, and the peer group. Of course, it is one thing to have an effective intervention program and another thing entirely to entice families to participate in the program, and to receive a large enough "dose" of the intervention to make a difference. Bloomquist and Schnell provide very helpful advice on how to maximize parental involvement in the intervention.

As well as being very useful for practitioners, this book is highly appropriate as a classroom text, especially in advanced undergraduate and graduate student courses on developmental psychopathology, child therapy, and prevention science.

JOHN E. LOCHMAN, PHD
Professor and Saxon Chairholder in Clinical Psychology
University of Alabama

Acknowledgments

*T*his book would not have been possible without the assistance of many individuals. We cannot adequately express our appreciation to our wives, Rebecca Syverts (M. L. B.) and Mary Schnell (S. V. S.), for providing support and assistance. Without their sacrifices and help, this book truly would never have been written. We greatly benefited from the input of Gerald August, Lauren Braswell, William Dikel, Devin Hazenson, Isabella Moreno, Rick Ostrander, Michael Sancilio, and Jason Walker, who read and commented on early drafts of this book. Their valuable and insightful feedback helped shape the book to its present form. Many thanks to Kitty Moore, Senior Editor at The Guilford Press, for her assistance in preparing and producing this volume. Her thoughtful and excellent editing and numerous creative ideas greatly enhanced the book. Janice McClain did a fine job in typing the text. We are thankful for her many hours of work and for putting up with numerous revisions. Finally, we acknowledge our debt to the clients we have had the pleasure of working with through research and applied activities in clinical, school, and community settings. Our clients were the inspiration for this effort and motivated us to learn as much as possible about effective practices.

Contents

PART II. ASSESSMENT AND IDENTIFICATION

PART III. CHILD AND FAMILY INTERVENTIONS

PART IV. CONTEXTUALLY BASED INTERVENTIONS

Introduction

A recent U.S. surgeon general's report (U.S. Department of Health and Human Services, 2001), which reviewed the epidemic of youth violence in the United States, showed that violence and antisocial behavior among youth is occurring at an alarming rate. The surgeon general noted that "the most urgent need is a national resolve to confront the problem of youth violence systematically, using research-based approaches, and to correct the damaging myths and stereotypes that interfere with the task at hand" (p. 3). The report debunked the myth that children with these problems are beyond help and revealed that there are many innovative interventions that can be used to enable these children to lead more productive lives. Specifically, the surgeon general advocated the use of comprehensive intervention approaches with children who are showing early signs of aggression and conduct problems, as well as for children who are engaging in established patterns of violent and antisocial behaviors. To improve the status of these children, interventions need to be employed that reduce risk factors related to problem development and enhance protective factors related to adaptive development.

Children who display aggression and conduct problems at a young age are at risk for developing violent behaviors, mental health problems, school dropout, chemical dependency, occupational difficulties, marital and family problems, and criminal offending outcomes as adolescents and adults. Those children that persist in their problems impact society directly through victimization or indirectly through the financial costs involved in treating and rehabilitating them in mental health, educational, correctional, medical, and other social service delivery systems. Early-onset aggression and conduct problems in children should be considered a public health problem of equal or greater magnitude to smoking, drug abuse, teenage pregnancy, and sedentary lifestyles.

Fortunately there are many effective assessment and interventions methods available to help children with early aggression and conduct problems. It is difficult, however, for practitioners and other professionals to be fully informed about the range of effective practices and keep up with new developments. In this book we synthesize what is known about the best assessment and intervention procedures to better equip professionals who work with these children and their families. In so doing, we hope to assist practitioners in moving toward the comprehensive approach of assessment and intervention that was called for by the surgeon general.

FOCUS OF THIS BOOK

It is our belief that a wide variety of people will benefit from reading this book. Our primary intended audience is practitioners who work in school, community, clinical, and other service delivery systems where children with aggression and conduct problems are often served. We think the book could be used as a resource to facilitate interdisciplinary collaboration and greater coordination across professionals and service systems. The book will also be useful for researchers who are evaluating practice procedures, administrators who are refining and developing services, policymakers who are looking for information pertaining to effective intervention methods, and students learning about child and family services. Parents and teachers will also profit from reading about the many strategies presented here.

The main goal of this book is to provide a description of best practices in assessment and intervention for children up to age 12. Best practices are based on our review of the research and an integration of practice procedures from numerous sources. Although we do not present exhaustive research literature reviews, we do present enough to demonstrate the utility of a particular intervention and to enhance the confidence of practitioners in using them. In other words, the best practices presented are empirically supported. Likewise, when describing specific practices, we do not review every possible practitioner source. Rather, we identify exemplary or promising models of intervention and try to integrate practice information across selected sources to establish best practice parameters. Our decisions pertaining to which research and practice sources to review and integrate are based on our own judgment. Those judgments were made from the vantage point of our combined 30 years of applied practice and research experience with children who exhibit aggression and conduct problems in clinical, school, and community settings.

Throughout the book we use the terms *intervention* to describe what is being done when best practices are implemented and *practitioner* to describe the individual who delivers it. We are aware that interventions range on a continuum from prevention to treatment. Most of the practices in this book, in our opinion, are not specific to prevention or to treatment. Many of the best practices described could be used in either context. On occasion we refer to prevention or treatment when procedures are specific to those endeavors, but for the most part we stick to the broader notion of intervention when describing best practices. We present best practices and rely on practitioners to apply them within the prevention or treatment context. Likewise, many of the best practices we describe can be conducted in different settings by a variety of human services and educational professionals. In our opinion, similar interventions can be applied in different settings as long as well-trained professionals conduct them. To us, the setting or one's credentials are less important than making sure best practices are used. Most of our discussion of various best practices is not bound to any one setting or kind of professional.

There is a lot of information in this book! One practitioner cannot realistically conduct all the interventions described and a single family would not require them. Therefore we recommend that the reader use this book as a handbook and reference source. The detailed Table of Contents can be used to pinpoint topics that are most relevant to a practitioner. The book will enable the practitioner to derive a good understanding of the best practices that relate to his or her work, and make him or her better informed of best practices that children should receive when they seek services in other settings.

DEFINING AGGRESSION
AND CONDUCT PROBLEMS IN CHILDREN

The heterogeneous nature of children with aggression and conduct problems presented us with a challenge concerning what terms should be used throughout the book to describe them. These children may share the common broad characteristic of exhibiting a form of aggression and conduct problems, but there are a variety of narrow characteristics that distinguish one child in this group from another (e.g., reactive aggression, relational aggression, oppositional, etc.). We grappled with the idea of using a broad term to describe these children versus using the many narrow characteristic terms that are defined in Chapter 1. Ultimately, we chose a middle ground. It seemed to us that it would be confusing and cumbersome to continuously go back and forth between the many characteristic definitions. We also recognized, however, that it would be helpful to specify narrow characteristics when they relate to specific practices. Thus throughout the book we use the broad term *aggressive/conduct problem* (ACP) to describe the general population of children with aggression and conduct problems. *The ACP definition denotes children who manifest some form of early-onset aggressive behavior and who also display, or who are at risk for displaying, covert an-*

tisocial actions. This definition simplifies discussion of the material because the book is largely about describing best practices that may be applicable to a wide range of aggressive behaviors and conduct problems in children. We also rely on narrow characteristic terms to relate to specific assessment and/ or intervention methods, where applicable. In other words, we articulate general best practices for the broad group, but also note specific practices when warranted.

A DEVELOPMENTAL–MULTISYSTEMIC MODEL OF PRACTICE

In this book, a developmental perspective (see, e.g., Cummings, Davies, & Campbell, 2000; Luthar, Cicchetti, & Becker, 2000; Masten & Coatsworth, 1998) is blended with the multisystemic intervention approach (see, e.g., Henggeler, Schoenwald, Borduin, Rowland, & Cunningham, 1998). The resulting developmental–multisystemic model of practice is a theoretical and heuristic framework used as a basis for developing and conducting interventions with children manifesting ACP. This model of intervention is utilized to articulate procedures to redirect children who are progressing down a developmental pathway of escalating problems to a resilient developmental course. *The developmental–multisystemic model of practice attempts to promote resilient development by reducing risk factors and promoting protective factors in the child, parent/family, social/peer, and contextual "life domains"* (i.e., areas of influence on children's development). To accomplish this, comprehensive interventions that reach across these four life domains need to be employed. The developmental–multisystemic model of practice is detailed in Chapter 2 and is the basis for the assessment and intervention practices described throughout the book.

ORGANIZATION OF THIS BOOK

The book is organized into five parts. Part I examines the nature of the problem. It contains two chapters that lay the foundation for the book by describing the characteristics, developmental pathways, and associated risk factors that are seen in children with ACP. In addition, information pertaining to protective factors observed in resilient children is also presented. This culminates in a more detailed description of a developmental–multisystemic intervention model that organizes interventions to reduce risk factors and promote protective factors in the child, parent/family, social/ peer, and contextual life domains.

Part II presents information pertaining to assessment and identification. The single chapter in this part reviews basic issues that are important in the assessment of any childhood problem. The discussion then moves toward specific issues for assessing children with ACP. Procedures are suggested to diagnosis children and to evaluate the presence of potential risk factors in the four life domains. This comprehensive approach leads to effective treatment planning to reduce risk factors and to promote protective factors.

Part III, consisting of three chapters, presents child and family interventions that directly influence individual, parent/family, and social/peer factors. Skills training interventions that enhance children's social competencies are described. Interventions focused on parent and family skills development are also presented. Finally, there is a discussion of mental health treatments that deal with entrenched problems. Many or all of these interventions may be necessary when intervening with children exhibiting ACP and their families.

Part IV, with four chapters, presents contextually based (i.e., school and community) interventions. The school-based interventions described in this part make an impact on individual, social/peer, and contextual domains. They include efforts to enhance academic skills, improve school behavior, and teach social and emotional skills in the school setting. The community-based interventions that are discussed improve individual, parent/family, social/peer, and contextual factors to varying degrees. The interventions provide child and family support. The contextually based approaches to intervention are essential for children exhibiting ACP and their families.

Part V deals with integration and challenges. The two chapters in this part attempt to build upon the previously described intervention strategies. University-derived multicomponent interventions and "real-world" coordinated services programs that simultaneously affect two or more life domains are described in one chapter. The underlying assumption is that comprehensive and multifaceted interventions will be the most effective. To effect change, however, it is important to engage families and ensure that systems are set up to offer such comprehensive intervention approaches. Therefore, the last chapter deals with the challenges of effectively engaging families and creating coordinated service delivery systems.

THE AUTHORS' HOPE

We recognize that one practitioner cannot provide all the assessment and intervention procedures described in this book. We do think, however, that practitioners should understand all the different practice options, should conduct their work using best practices, and should provide an opportunity for children and families to participate in a broad array of necessary interventions. We have also observed that truly effective interventions ultimately

require coordination among many practitioners and service systems. Therefore we advocate that all professionals make it a priority to provide such
coordinated services. Being aware of the research and best practices
pertaining to different assessment and interventions methods will make
practitioners more effective in providing services and coordinating with
other service systems. We hope this book will assist practitioners and other
professionals in being able to realize the best approaches to practice. We
further hope that practitioners and other professionals will translate these
best practices into improved lives for children with ACP and their families.

PART I

NATURE OF THE PROBLEM

CHAPTER 1

Characteristics and Developmental Course

*I*n this chapter we will review the basic characteristics and developmental course of children with ACP. The chapter is designed to create a foundation to familiarize the reader with the behaviors, prevalence rates, coexisting problems, developmental pathways, and gender differences found in this population of children. Ultimately this information will assist practitioners in implementing appropriate and effective assessment and intervention procedures. The characteristics and associated problems of these children is the initial target of interventions. Potential differences between boys and girls need to be taken into account. Practitioners also need to understand developmental processes to implement development-enhancing interventions. We will expand upon the relevance of characteristic and developmental information to intervention throughout this chapter.

DIMENSIONS OF AGGRESSION AND CONDUCT PROBLEMS

In this first section we review specific dimensions or characteristics that are commonly observed in children who exhibit ACP. Research has determined that these dimensions are meaningful descriptors that have implications for children's development. These dimensions need to be taken into consideration when conducting interventions with these children.

Overt Aggression

Overt aggression includes harmful verbal and physical acts of aggression that are directed toward others, property, or self (Connor, Melloni, & Harrison, 1998; Hughes, 1988). Overtly aggressive acts also involve fighting and delinquent crimes with direct confrontation (e.g., rape, assault, robbery) (Loeber & Stouthamer-Loeber, 1998). Boys are more likely than girls to display overt aggression. When the generic term *aggression* is used, it usually implies overt aggression.

Children show aggression in home, school, and community settings (Loeber & Stouthamer-Loeber, 1998). Confrontations at home between the aggressive child and his or her parents or other family members can range from severe oppositional behavior to physical aggression. Aggression at school usually stems from disagreements between children, but occasionally involves direct confrontation with teachers. Aggression occurring in community settings can involve violent crimes and/or coexisting covert conduct problems (e.g., stealing, vandalism, firesetting).

Overtly aggressive children are often described as "fighters." Some fight at home only, some at school only, and some in both settings. Those children who fight in both home and school settings have the most entrenched and severe problems in the social, academic, and emotional domains (Loeber & Dishion, 1984). Boys are more likely to fight, but some girls exhibit fighting during the elementary school-age years. The frequency of fighting dissipates somewhat as children grow into adolescence (Loeber & Stouthamer-Loeber, 1998), with boys and girls equaling each other in later adolescence (Achenbach & Edelbrock, 1986). Boys who persist in fighting over many years develop numerous psychiatric diagnoses and display global impairment (Loeber, Green, Lahey, & Kalb, 2000).

Reactive/Proactive Aggression

Whether aggressive behavior is spontaneous or carefully planned further defines overt aggression (Vitiello & Stoff, 1997). One subtype is reactive aggression (similar to affective aggression in animals), an unplanned responsive aggressive behavior to an evoking stimulus. The stimulus may be real or perceived. When the stimulus is present, the individual has an expectation of a negative outcome (e.g., that self will be harmed if not for an aggressive response), becomes physiologically aroused, and responds aggressively. Another subtype is proactive aggression (similar to predatory aggression in animals), when aggressive behavior is planned with a goal in mind. The individual who engages in this type of aggression is typically calm (not physiologically aroused), has high self-confidence, and has positive expectations for the result of the aggression. Different neurological/anatomical and biochemical processes are involved in the activation and maintenance of different forms of aggression (Vitiello & Stoff, 1997).

Reactive and proactive forms of aggression are seen in some children. Reactive aggression is observed when a child exhibits an angry or hostile reaction to a real or perceived threat (Dodge & Coie, 1987). For example, a child gets bumped in the hallway and starts throwing punches in response. Proactive aggression occurs when a child uses intentional and planned aggressive actions to achieve a goal or to dominate another child (Dodge & Coie, 1987). For example, a child believes another child offended him during the school day and deliberately plans to beat up that child after school. Reactive aggression occurs more often than proactive aggression, and boys are more likely than girls to exhibit either form of aggression (Coie & Dodge, 1998; Day, Bream, & Pal, 1992; Dodge & Coie, 1987). In addition, reactively aggressive children are less well liked, have poorer social skills, have problems with inattention/impulsivity, and exhibit more emotion disregulation than proactively aggressive children (Day et al., 1992; Dodge & Coie, 1987; Dodge, Lochman, Harnish, Bates, & Pettit, 1997; Price & Dodge, 1989; Rubin, Coplan, Fox, & Calkins, 1995; Shields & Cicchetti, 1998). Researchers have also determined that many reactively aggressive children come from backgrounds of physical abuse (Dodge et al., 1997).

Even though the reactive and proactive forms of aggression are distinct, they are also highly correlated with overall overt aggression. Both forms of aggression are associated with overall global impairment, classroom behavior problems, and peer adjustment difficulties (Dodge & Coie, 1987; Washbusch, Willoughby, & Pelham, 1998). Some children exhibit both reactive and proactive aggression and can be more accurately classified as "pervasively aggressive."

Relational Aggression

Relational aggression is characterized by the intentional actions of one child toward another that are designed to harm through manipulation and damage to relational status (Crick, 1995). The aggressor withdraws or threatens to withdraw affiliation from another child and excludes that child from a friendship group (Crick & Grotpeter, 1995). Most research suggests relational aggression is more characteristic of preschool- and school-age girls than boys (Crick, Casas, & Mosher, 1997; Crick & Grotpeter, 1995; Rhy & Bear, 1997). Crick and Grotpeter (1995) theorized that relational aggression is more effective in girls harming other girls because it interferes with girls achieving the important goal of maintaining intimate friendships. One study, however, found that both relational and overt aggression were more prevalent in school-age boys than in school-age girls (David & Kistner, 2000). The gender discrepancies across these studies may reflect differences in the samples examined or the experimental procedures used.

Relationally aggressive children have a variety of adjustment problems. These children are more socially and emotionally maladjusted, are more likely to be rejected by peers, and are more likely to be defiant, impulsive, and depressed/anxious compared to normal peers (Crick, 1995, 1997;

Crick et al., 1997; Crick & Grotpeter, 1995). It appears that children who display nonnormative forms of aggression—for example, relationally aggressive boys and overtly aggressive girls—have the most significant adjustment difficulties and peer rejection (Crick, 1997).

Bullying

Bullying involves one child directing aversive behavior to another child that physically or emotionally harms or intimidates (Farrington, 1993; Olweus, 1991, 1994). Bullying is repetitious and characterized by relationships with an asymmetrical power hierarchy (i.e., the bully has more power than the victim does) (Smith & Brain, 2000). The most typical pattern of bullying is a boy bullying another boy or a girl. But some girls will bully other girls. Most bullying takes place during the primary or elementary school years, but it can also occur during the secondary school years. Olweus (1991, 1994) reported that bullying could occur both in and out of school, but is most prevalent in school settings. Bullies are aggressive to their victims but are also aggressive to other children in general and even to adults. Bullies are more likely to exhibit impulsiveness, lower levels of empathy, and lower levels of anxiety than nonbullies. Many bullies are on the trajectory of antisocial behavior development.

Bullies can use a variety of verbal/physical/psychological techniques or behaviors to accomplish their bullying acts. Bullying boys use physical intimidation, while bullying girls use verbal or psychological intimidation. Boys' physically aggressive behaviors decline as they get older, but their verbally aggressive behaviors increase (Craig, 1998); girls' verbal and psychological intimidation stays fairly stable across developmental periods.

Some children end up being both bullies and victims. These children have significant psychological disturbances, exhibit a variety of externalizing and internalizing psychological problems, and are often referred for psychiatric services (Kumpulainen et al., 1998).

Violence

Childhood aggression and acts of violence can be related but are not necessarily synonymous. Loeber and Stouthamer-Loeber (1998) summarized much of the literature on childhood aggression and violence. They discuss a continuum of severity that distinguishes between aggression and violence. Aggression involves a pattern of actions that inflicts mild to moderate physical or mental harm on others. Violence involves an act or pattern of actions that inflicts serious physical harm on others, including assault, rape, robbery, and murder. Not all aggressive children are violent, and not all violent children display long-standing patterns of aggression. It is true, however, that children with early aggression are at risk to commit violence. The more risk factors that a child has (see Chapter 2), the more likely it is that the child will display violence (Loeber & Stouthamer-Loeber, 1998; Verlinden, Hersen, & Thomas, 2000).

Covert Stealing and Firesetting

Covert antisocial behaviors are actions that violate conventional social norms—for example, lying, cheating, smoking, drinking, disobeying, truancy, and so on. In preadolescent children the most common serious forms of covert antisocial behaviors are stealing and firesetting. The incidence rates for these behaviors are less than for forms of aggression. These behaviors are also less well studied than aggression.

Patterson's (1982) research showed that children who steal on a regular and frequent basis are likely to develop later adolescent delinquent behavior. Children who steal and are aggressive have the most problems and are especially at risk for later delinquency. Often the parents of children who steal are ineffective in discipline and do not adequately monitor their children's whereabouts and actions.

Kolko (1996) distinguished between children who set fires with the intent of harming others/destroying property and children who "play" with fire resulting in accidentally harming others/destroying property. The intentional firesetting children are more maladjusted. Firesetting children usually have social interaction difficulties and emotional problems. They commonly come from families who experience multiple problems and adversity. Their parents do not adequately supervise them and have not provided consequences for earlier firesetting behaviors.

Child Delinquency

Delinquency is a legal term applied to children who have committed a crime serious enough to warrant involvement in the juvenile correctional system (Kazdin, 1995). Loeber and Farrington (2000) defined a child delinquent as a child between the ages of 7 and 12 years who has committed a crime. Child delinquents engage in a variety of offenses, including assault, rape, vandalism, firesetting, robbery, theft, and other antisocial acts. About 10% of children who are charged with such offenses are under 12 years of age. Boys are about three times more likely than girls to be designated as child delinquents.

Child delinquents can be further classified as "serious" and "other" (Loeber & Farrington, 2000). The serious child delinquents display a pattern of delinquent actions across time, whereas other child delinquents may engage in an offense but eventually curb that behavior. Obviously, the serious child delinquent is more impaired and is more likely to come from a background with many risk factors.

Psychopathy

Psychopathic children exhibit aggression, as well as risk-taking and sensation-seeking behavior (Lynam, 1996). These children are egocentric and self-centered. They tend to be emotionally shallow, have diminished capacity for empathy, and express little remorse for their misdeeds. Children identified as psychopathic also tend to be hyperactive and impulsive, and have internalizing emotional problems (Lynam, 1997, 1998).

Callous/unemotional traits are likely the most salient characteristics in psychopathic children (Frick, 1998a; Frick, Barry, & Bodin, 2000). They are manipulative, experience minimal guilt, and also manifest low levels of emotional distress or anxiety. Children who exhibit callous/unemotional characteristics typically exhibit higher levels of aggression, and also have contacts with police early on, as compared to children with impulsivity/conduct problems and those without conduct problems (Christian, Frick, Hill, Tyler, & Frazer, 1997). Children exhibiting callous/unemotional traits are more likely to be classified as psychopaths, whereas children with impulsivity/conduct problems are more likely to be classified as exhibiting "traditional" conduct disorder (Frick, O'Brien, Wooton, & McBurnet, 1994). Impaired/ineffective parenting is associated with children who are impulsive and have the more common form of conduct problems. This type of parenting is not, however, associated with children who are callous/unemotional (Wooton, Frick, Shelton, & Silverthorn, 1997).

The overall applicability of the term *psychopathy* to children has not been fully determined at this time (Frick et al., 2000). It has not yet been extensively studied in children. When it has been studied, the samples are primarily comprised of boys. The findings discussed in this section need to be replicated across other studies and research groups. It is also important for researchers to obtain longitudinal information that relates to psychopathy in children. The concept of psychopathy in children, however, may have broad implications for assessment and intervention.

Empirically Derived Subtypes

Loeber and Schmaling (1985) used meta-analysis, a statistical procedure in which the results of many studies are combined, to determine trends across studies pertaining to children with ACP. They examined the data from 28 studies. The meta-analysis revealed one dimension that accounted for most of the statistical variance: a continuum ranging from overt to covert manifestations of conduct problems. The overt end of the continuum described children who exhibited arguing, temper outbursts, fighting, and other forms of overt aggression. The covert end of the continuum described children who engaged in stealing, truancy, firesetting, and the like. The middle of the continuum described children who displayed disobedience/defiance, rule-breaking behavior, and so on. Loeber and Schmaling noted that the overt, covert, and disobedient clusters of behavior were unique in and of themselves, but also highly intercorrelated.

Frick and colleagues (1993) conducted another meta-analysis of 44 studies that comprised a total sample size of more than 28,000 children and adolescents. Frick and colleagues replicated the overt/covert continuum and found another continuum that described destructive versus nondestructive behavior. Table 1.1 summarizes the results of the Frick and colleagues meta-analysis. This table lists the four conduct disturbance subtypes that emerged in the meta-analysis, associated dimensions, and the characteristics of children within the subtypes. Frick and colleagues argued that the oppositional subtype corresponds to the American Psychiatric Association's (1994) diagnostic category of oppositional defiant disorder, while the ag-

TABLE 1.1. Summary of Meta-Analysis Including Subtypes, Associated Dimensions, and Child Characteristics

Oppositional subtype (overt, nondestructive)

- Stubborn
- Annoys
- Angry
- Defies
- Temper
- Touchy

Aggression subtype (overt, destructive)

- Blames others
- Assaults
- Bullies
- Fights
- Cruel
- Spiteful

Property violations subtype (covert, destructive)

- Firesetting
- Stealing
- Lying
- Vandalism
- Cruelty to animals

Status violations subtype (covert, nondestructive)

- Runaway
- Truancy
- Substance use
- Swears
- Breaks rules

Note. Data from Frick et al. (1993).

gressive, property violations, and status violations subtypes correspond to the diagnostics category of conduct disorder.

Summary

Many specific dimensions or characteristics can be used to describe children with ACP. They pertain to forms of aggression, covert conduct problems, and combinations of these difficulties. Although there is overlap, the distinctiveness of the different dimensions are meaningful and relevant to practice. Assessment methods need to be employed that identify the presence of specific characteristics in a child or group of children so that the best intervention can be employed to address them. For example, if a child is exhibiting reactive aggression, then a social competence training intervention might be utilized, or if oppositional behaviors are a concern for another child, then parent and family skills training might be called for. Our later discussion of assessment and intervention methods will suggest different procedures that take these dimensions into account.

DIAGNOSTIC CATEGORIES
OF DISRUPTIVE BEHAVIOR

Diagnostic categories of disruptive behavior provide another perspective in describing the problems of children with ACP. Whereas the dimensions just reviewed relate primarily to unique characteristics, diagnostic categories involve the clustering of symptoms to form broader descriptors of children's functioning. The resulting diagnosis describes broad patterns of maladjustment in children, which are linked to various mental health treatments. The American Psychiatric Association's (1994) *Diagnostic and Statistical Manual of Mental Disorders*, fourth edition (DSM–IV), aids professionals involved in diagnostic and treatment activities with people. It contains disruptive behavior diagnostic categories that relate to patterns of aggression and conduct problems in children, as well as difficulties related to attention deficits/hyperactivity/impulsivity.

According to DSM–IV, several criteria must be met to qualify for a behavior disorder diagnosis. A child must exhibit a cluster of symptoms and behaviors for a specified period of time. These behaviors must be evident at a level that is developmentally inappropriate and must be directly related to the child having functional difficulty in several settings (typically home and school). Children as young as preschool age can be diagnosed reliably as manifesting behavior disorders (Keenan & Wakschlag, 2000; Lahey et al., 1998). Table 1.2 presents Quay's (1999) abridged summary of oppositional defiant disorder (ODD), conduct disorder (CD), and attention-deficit/hyperactivity disorder (ADHD) according to DSM–IV. Although there is overlap between the three behavior disorder diagnostic categories, they are considered to have distinct features that warrant the different diagnostic labels (Loeber, Burke, Lahey, Winters, & Zera, 2000).

Oppositional Defiant Disorder

The DSM–IV diagnostic category of ODD describes children who exhibit persistent developmentally inappropriate levels of anger, irritability, defiance, and oppositionality, which causes functional impairment. A child who qualifies for this diagnosis must exhibit the symptoms persistently for at least 6 months and the symptoms must cause functional impairment. It is noteworthy that elements of verbal aggression are included in the diagnosis of ODD and that some children with ODD also display physically aggressive behavior (Loeber, Burke, et al., 2000). An early history of ODD is often present in children later classified as CD (Kazdin, 1995; Loeber et al., 1993). ODD emerges earlier (average age of onset is 6 years) than childhood-onset CD (average age of onset is 9 years) (Hinshaw & Anderson, 1996). Most children are diagnosed with ODD during the preadolescent years.

Conduct Disorder

The DSM–IV category of CD pertains to children who manifest overt and covert antisocial behavior. Age of onset has been found to predict ultimate outcome (Moffitt, 1993), so DSM–IV reflects this knowledge in distinguishing between the childhood-onset and the adolescent-onset subcategories of CD. To qualify for a diagnosis of either childhood-onset or adolescent-onset CD, a child must exhibit persistent aggressive and/or antisocial behavior for at least 6 months and the behavior must cause functional impairment.

Children manifesting childhood-onset CD are typically more aggressive, exhibit more functional impairments, and have more temperamental, cognitive/neuropsychological, family history, family environment, and social problems than children with adolescent-onset CD (Kazdin, 1995; Lahey et al., 1998; Moffitt & Caspi, 2001). The prognosis for childhood-onset CD is poor. Boys, more than girls, are likely to qualify for a diagnosis of childhood-onset CD. The adolescent-onset CD is less severe, and tends to coincide with family and peer problems emerging during the adolescent years. Aggression may or may not be present in adolescent-onset CD. Adolescent-onset CD has a better prognosis. Girls equal boys for prevalence rates of adolescent-onset CD.

Attention-Deficit/Hyperactivity Disorder

The final behavioral disorder category in DSM–IV is ADHD. Although ADHD does not necessarily involve aggression or conduct problems, it is

TABLE 1.2. Abridged Summary of Symptoms Associated with DSM–IV Oppositional Defiant, Conduct, and Attention-Deficit/Hyperactivity Disorders

Oppositional defiant disorder

Often loses temper
Often argues with adults
Often actively defies or refuses to comply
Often deliberately annoys people
Often blames others
Often touchy or easily annoyed
Often angry or resentful
Often spiteful or vindictive

Conduct disorder

Aggression to people and animals
   Bullies, threatens, or intimidates
   Initiates physical fights
   Has used a weapon
   Physically cruel to people
   Physically cruel to animals
   Has stolen while confronting victim
   Forced sexual activity
Destruction to property
   Firesetting with intent to damage
   Destroys others' property
Deceitfulness or theft
   Breaking into house, building, or car
   "Cons" others
   Stealing without confrontation
Serious violations of rules
   Stays out at night beginning before age 13
   Runs away from home overnight at least twice
   Truant from school before age 13

Attention-deficit/hyperactivity disorder

Inattention
   Fails to give close attention to detail; careless mistakes
   Difficulty sustaining attention
   Does not seem to listen when spoken to
   Does not follow through; fails to finish
   Difficulty organizing
   Avoids, dislikes tasks requiring sustained mental effort
   Often loses things
   Easily distracted
   Forgetful
Hyperactivity
   Fidgets, squirms
   Leaves seat
   Runs about or climbs excessively
   Difficulty playing quietly
   Often "on the go"
Impulsivity
   Blurts out answers
   Difficulty awaiting turn
   Interrupts or intrudes on others

Note. Data from Quay (1999).

commonly diagnosed in individuals with these characteristics, and it relates to increased severity of dysfunction. ADHD indicates persistent developmentally inappropriate levels of inattention, hyperactivity, and impulsivity, which cause functional impairment in the child. Symptoms of ADHD must be manifest and cause functional impairment prior to age 7. DSM–IV makes distinctions between different subtypes of ADHD. The primarily inattentive type is associated with difficulties in sustaining attention, disorganization, carelessness, off-task behavior, distractibility, and forgetfulness. ADHD, primarily inattentive type may not be a disruptive behavioral disorder category (Barkley, 1998; Lahey, Schaughency, Hynd, Carlson, & Nieves, 1987; Lahey, Schaughency, Strauss, & Frame, 1984). ADHD, primarily inattentive type may be associated with sluggish cognitive style and learning disabilities. Another ADHD subtype, primarily hyperactive/impulsive, indicates excessive motor movement and verbal/behavioral indicators of impulsivity. It is the hyperactive/impulsive symptoms that are more indicative of disruptive behavior. A third subtype of ADHD is the combined type where a child exhibits symptoms of inattention and hyperactivity/impulsivity. Although boys are more often diagnosed with ADHD, when girls are diagnosed, they tend to have similar symptoms and severity in overall functional impairment (Silverthorn, Frick, Kuper, & Ott, 1996).

Prevalence Rates of Behavior Disorders

Lahey, Miller, Gordon, and Riley (1999) summarized 34 epidemiology studies of prevalence rates of behavioral disorders in the general population for children ages 4–18 years in the United States and other countries. The research they reviewed was derived from child, peer, parent, and teacher sources and utilized dimensional ratings and diagnostic interview methodologies. Lahey and colleagues organized dimensional and interview data to conform to the diagnostic categories of ODD, CD, and ADHD in order to facilitate and simplify presentation of prevalence rates information. Although they noted methodological problems in these studies, they offered some basic conclusions regarding prevalence rates. For boys and girls combined, the following prevalence rates were observed:

- ODD: range = 3–22.5%; median = 3.2%
- CD: range = 0–11.9%; median = 2.0%
- ADHD: range = 0–16.6%; median = 2.0%

These statistics suggest that a fairly high proportion of the general population of children manifest these behavioral disorders. Lahey and colleagues also found that a majority of studies revealed a high rate of comorbidity across the categories and a higher prevalence rate for boys than for girls. There is no clear pattern of prevalence rates being more or less for different race/ethnic groups. Most studies find no age differences in prevalence rates for ODD. The prevalence of CD increases from elementary school age to adolescence (although children are less overtly aggressive and more covertly antisocial as they get older). Rates of ADHD increase from preschool- to elementary school-age years, and decline somewhat in adolescence.

Lahey et al. also observed different prevalence rates with respect to family and contextual factors. In general, there are higher prevalence rates of all three disruptive behavior disorder categories in families with single parents, frequent change of parental figures, parents who have psychopathology (e.g., depression, antisocial behavior) and/or substance abuse, marital problems, and parents who have poor parenting skills. There is also a higher rate of behavior disorders in economically disadvantaged populations. Higher rates of CD are observed in disadvantaged neighborhoods (e.g., with dilapidated housing, high crime rates, rundown schools). These family and contextual variables, and their association with children's behavior problems, will be expanded on in Chapter 2.

Comorbidity and Behavior Disorders

The comorbidity of ODD/CD with ADHD, as well as overlap between dimensional characteristics of overt/covert antisocial behavior and impulsive/hyperactive behavior, is commonly seen in children reporting for mental health services (Hinshaw & Anderson, 1996). Children with CD/ADHD exhibit greater functional impairment than children with CD only (Walker, Lahey, Hynd, & Frame, 1987). CD/ADHD in children is more difficult to treat and has a poorer long-term prognosis than CD alone or ADHD alone (Hinshaw, Lahey, & Hart, 1993). Comorbidity between ODD/CD and ADHD is somewhat higher in urban areas than in suburban middle-class settings, presumably because fewer social family risk factors are implicated in the suburban population (August, Realmuto, MacDonald, Nugent, & Crosby, 1996). A combination of hyperactive/impulsive/attention deficit symptoms with conduct problems has been associated with very significant social/academic functional problems in children (Gresham, MacMillan, Bochian, Ward, & Forness, 1998). ADHD, CD, and ADHD/CD combined should be considered as three unique entities each requiring different treatment modalities (Schachar & Tannock, 1995).

"Internalizing" emotional problems such as depression and anxiety occurs at a higher rate among children and adolescents with ODD/CD and with ADHD/CD than in the general population of children (Eiraldi, Power, & Nezu, 1997; Loeber, Burke, et al., 2000; Moffitt, 1993). Children with anxiety problems combined with ADHD and/or ADHD/ODD/CD present with more significant problems and are harder to intervene with than children presenting with any of those disorders separately. The relationship between CD and anxiety is moderated by whether or not the child exhibits callous/unemotional traits. Frick, Lilienfeld, Ellis, Loney, and Silverthorn (1999) found that some children with CD also have problems with anxiety; among these children, those with callous/unemotional traits (i.e., psychopathy) displayed lower anxiety. More research is needed to definitively describe the relationship between behavior disorders and internalizing problems and the ramifications of this association.

Recently, much has been written pertaining to bipolar disorder and behavioral disorders in children. Geller and Luby (1997) described childhood-onset bipolar disorder as different than the adulthood-onset type. In children, bipolar disorder is manifested by a rapid, chronic, and continuous cycling of mood between elated and irritable affects. Children with bipolar disorder display erratic behavior that can appear similar to, or be seen in combination with, CD or ADHD (Biederman, Faraone, Chu, & Wozniak, 1999; Biederman et al., 1997). Making an accurate diagnosis of bipolar disorder in children is challenging because the symptoms of bipolar disorder are similar to those seen in the behavior disorders. Unfortunately, some children with bipolar disorder are misdiagnosed as children with CD and/ or ADHD. Other children with bipolar disorder may have comorbid CD and/or ADHD. It should be noted that it is rare to diagnose bipolar disorder as the only disorder in children (Carlson, 1998). According to DSM–IV, the criteria for adult bipolar disorder must be met to make the diagnosis in children. Careful diagnosis is important because bipolar disorder is considered primary to other possible diagnoses (Biederman et al., 1999). Although there are no prevalence rates available for children, only 1–2% of the adult population has bipolar disorder. Therefore bipolar disorder in children is probably rare.

The relationship between CD and intelligence is somewhat controversial. Most researchers have concluded that there are no IQ differences between children with and without CD when socioeconomic status (SES) or presence of ADHD is controlled (Hogan, 1999; Kazdin, 1995). Others have taken a different stance. Loeber, Farrington, Loeber-Stouthamer, Moffitt, and Caspi (1998) summarized several studies from the Pittsburgh Youth Study that examined the link between delinquency (including aggression) and IQ. Loeber and colleagues found an 8-point IQ difference between the delinquent and nondelinquent school-age boys. Even after controlling for social class, race, validity of test administration, neighborhood, and levels of impulsivity, the IQ differences between the delinquent and the nondelinquent groups did not change appreciably. Loeber et al. argued that differences in IQ are real and may account for delinquent behavior to some extent. Loeber et al. suggested that low IQ boys may become frustrated at school due to experiencing academic failure, which then can lead to increased levels of delinquency. The link between CD/delinquency and IQ needs further research.

Mental retardation and aggressive behavior coincide in some children.

Mental retardation is defined as an individual exhibiting an IQ score below 70 with corresponding deficits in adaptive functioning. Self-injurious behavior and physical aggression is related to mental retardation in children and adolescents to some extent (Davidson et al., 1996). Mentally retarded aggressive children are described as more impulsive and as having more social/anxiety problems (Bihm, Poindexter, & Warren, 1998). Certainly the occurrence of both mental retardation and aggressiveness in children presents daunting challenges for intervention efforts.

The combination of reading/academic problems and ADHD or ADHD/CD is frequently observed in children. Research suggests that ADHD symptoms are more strongly related to reading/academic problems than are CD symptoms (Frick et al., 1991; Hinshaw, 1992a; Maguin & Loeber, 1996; Smart, Sanson, & Prior, 1996). Reading problems and CD can overlap, but usually reading problems precede the development of CD. The combination of ADHD/CD/reading problems has a very poor prognosis (Fergusson & Lynskey, 1997; Moffitt, 1993). Among children with reading problems, boys are more likely than girls to have behavior problems (Smart et al., 1996).

The comorbidity of CD and substance abuse is seen in middle school children and adolescents. Early-onset ADHD/CD has been associated with later development of adolescent substance abuse (Thompson, Riggs, Mikulich, & Crowley, 1996). The combination of CD and depression has also been strongly related to substance use and abuse in adolescents (Henry et al., 1993). Conduct problems have emerged as a stronger predictor of adolescence substance abuse than depression (Miller-Johnson, Lochman, Coie, Terry, & Hyman, 1998). ADHD/CD in middle school children is associated with substance use and abuse; impulsive/hyperactive symptoms are primarily responsible for this association (Molina, Smith, & Pelham, 1999).

Practitioners need to understand comorbid conditions to plan and implement effective interventions (Abikoff & Klein, 1992). Generally speaking, the more a child exhibits comorbidity, the more challenging the treatment will be. Children who have severe behavior problems with other comorbid conditions, for example, typically have severe levels of global impairment and present significant intervention challenges (Lambert, Wahler, Andrade, & Bickman, 2001; Shelton et al., 1998; Stormshak, Bierman, & Conduct Problems Prevention Research Group, 1998).

Summary

Some children exhibit multiple behavior problem symptoms, which adversely effects their functioning in several settings, thereby warranting a DSM–IV diagnosis of ODD, CD, and/or ADHD. These children often display other comorbid conditions too. Assessment procedures that derive diagnoses and interventions that lessen symptoms and functional problems must be used. For example, a child diagnosed as CD/ADHD might benefit from a mental health intervention, while a child with comorbid reading deficits might gain from an educational intervention. The relevance of diagnostic considerations and comorbidity to assessment and intervention efforts for these children will be expanded upon later in this book.

HETEROGENEOUS NATURE OF CHILDREN WITH AGGRESSION AND CONDUCT PROBLEMS

Thus far we have described the varied characteristics and diagnostic catagories associated with children who display ACP. Table 1.3 offers a summary of this information. It reveals that this is a heterogeneous population of children, although one with a commonality of broad aggression and conduct problems. This heterogeneity is important to keep in mind because of its implications for interventions. It is necessary to understand the characteristic differences within the group of children who manifest ACP in order to design and implement effective interventions.

The heterogeneity of children with ACP adds to the challenge of intervention. For example, at one elementary school there may be a group of children who display broad aggression and conduct problems. Within this group of children some children may display overt aggression, while others may show relational aggression or stealing, and so on. Within this group of children there may be some who are diagnosed as CD, others who are diagnosed as CD/ADHD, still others who are CD with reading problems, and so on. Interventions at this elementary school will need to address the common characteristic of the group of children who manifest aggression and conduct problems but also take into account their differences. Table 1.3 can assist in pinpointing intervention targets for these children.

DEVELOPMENTAL PROGRESSION OF CHILDREN WITH AGGRESSION AND CONDUCT PROBLEMS

In this section we review the developmental progression for children with persistent ACP. We will discuss normal development, the general development of aggression and conduct problems, and specific pathways within the general model. In addition, we will present information regarding the desistance and persistance of these problems. This information will form a foundation for our later presentation of intervention information.

The concept of a developmental pathway must first be reviewed to serve as a foundation for this discussion. A developmental pathway describes the process of adaptation for a child moving toward a developmental outcome (Cummings et al., 2000; Sroufe, 1997). It has to do with the

TABLE 1.3. Characteristics and Associated Behaviors of Children Manifesting Forms of Aggression and Conduct Problems

Characteristic	Associated behaviors
Dimensions	
Overt aggression	Harmful verbal and physical actions
Reactive aggression	Angry and hostile reactions
Proactive aggression	Intentional and planned actions
Relational aggression	Intentional and manipulative actions to damage relational status
Bullying	Physical and verbal actions that harm and/or intimidate
Violence	Single act or pattern of actions that inflict serious physical harm
Covert stealing and firesetting	Serious stealing and/or firesetting
Psychopathy	Aggressive and/or antisocial actions with callous/unemotional traits
Child delinquency	A pattern of serious criminal behavior
Oppositional empirical subtype	Arguing, defiance, etc.
Aggressive empirical subtype	Verbal and physical aggression
Property violations empirical subtype	Vandalism, stealing, firesetting, etc.
Status violations empirical subtype	Swearing, truancy, substance use, etc.
DSM-IV disruptive behavior disorder categories	
Oppositional defiant disorder	Persistent oppositional/defiant actions
Conduct disorder	Persistent aggressive/antisocial actions
Attention-deficit/hyperactivity disorder	Persistent hyperactivity/impulsivity with or without inattention
Possible comorbid conditions	
ODD/CD/ADHD	One or more disruptive behavior disorders
Anxiety and/or depression	Distressed and/or dysphoric
Bipolar disorder	Rapid, chronic, and continuous cycling of mood
Lower intelligence	Limited adaptive functioning
Reading/academic problems	Academic delays
Substance use/abuse	Use that impairs functioning
Gender differences	
Boys	More overt actions
Girls	More relational actions
Nonnormative	Boys who display high relational actions and girls who display high overt actions

Note. Children with aggression and conduct problems may display one or more of these characteristics.

level of mastery that a child achieves with successive tasks in the social, emotional, cognitive, and physiological domains of functioning. The *early-onset continuous adaptive pathway* is observed when a child is exposed to minimal levels of risk and displays early competence or adjustment that persists over time (e.g., "normal"). The *early-onset continuous maladaptive pathway* is seen when a child is exposed to varying levels of risk (low to high) and displays early maladjustment that persists and intensifies over time (e.g., early-onset ACP). The *resilient pathway* occurs when a child is exposed to varying levels of risk and displays early maladjustment that eventually transitions to adjustment or to an adaptive pathway (e.g., the "resilient child"). The *late-onset maladaptive pathway* is manifested when a child is exposed to varying levels of risk and displays early adjustment that eventually transitions to maladjustment or to a maladaptive pathway (e.g., late-onset CD). There can be many variations of these four main developmental pathways; level of adjustment can also vary across developmental domains (e.g., an individual can be resilient in the social domain and maladjusted in the emotional domain). Specific examples of these types of developmental pathways are provided next. Later we present practice methods that could be used to assist children with ACP in moving from the early-onset maladaptive pathway to the resilient adaptive pathway.

Normal Development

To understand the development of ACP, one must first understand "normal" development. This will enable a comparison between the normal and the ACP developmental pathways. Normal children proceed down an early-onset continuous adaptive developmental pathway and achieve competence. These children acquire mastery of tasks at different stages of development. Table 1.4 from Masten and Coatsworth (1998) summarized a variety of self-control, social, emotional, and academic/career tasks negotiated by most children before adulthood. These tasks are defined by contemporary culture and society. Children master earlier tasks to progress to later tasks. Children eventually go through all stages of development to achieve competence in adolescence and childhood. Competence is defined as effective adaptation and mastery.

General Developmental Model
of Aggression and Conduct Problems

Young children who display early-onset ACP have been characterized as "early starters" (Patterson, Capaldi, & Bank, 1991), "life-course persistent" (Moffit, 1993), or "early-onset/persistent" (Aguilar, Sroufe, Egeland, & Carlson, 2000) because they are developing early maladaptive characteristics that often lead to the continuation and escalation of their problems. These children are not mastering developmental tasks and are traveling

TABLE 1.4. Normal Developmental Progression of Children

Infancy to preschool

- Attachment to caregivers(s)
- Language
- Differentiation of self from environment
- Self-control and compliance

Middle childhood

- School adjustment (attendance, appropriate conduct)
- Academic achievement (learning to read, do arithmetic)
- Getting along with peers (acceptance, making friends)
- Rule-governed conduct (following rules of society for moral behavior and prosocial conduct)

Adolescence

- Successful transition to secondary schooling
- Academic achievement (learning skills needed for higher education work)
- Involvement in extracurricular activities (e.g., athletics, clubs)
- Forming close friendships within and across gender
- Forming a cohesive sense of self-identity

Note. From Masten and Coatsworth (1998). Copyright 1998 by the American Psychological Association. Reprinted by permission.

down the early-onset continuous maladaptive developmental pathway. A tremendous amount of research documents the developmental course of children who manifest early-onset ACP. Numerous longitudinal studies have examined the persistence of this problem and how it can escalate and elaborate over time. These studies include boys (primarily) and girls, from varying ethnic backgrounds, derived from both community and clinical samples. We will rely on contemporary reviews of the literature and summaries of specific research programs to present five stages of general development of ACP in children (Campbell, 1995; Frick & Loney, 1999; Kazdin, 1995; Keenan, Shaw, Delliquadri, Giovannelli, & Walsh, 1998; Loeber & Hay, 1997; Loeber & Stouthamer-Loeber, 1998; Olweus, 1979; Patterson et al., 1991). Although these literature reviews utilize slightly different definitions of problems and review slightly different studies, they arrive at similar conclusions regarding general patterns that emerge across development. Table 1.5 summarizes our interpretation of this information in an effort to present a general developmental progression for children with ACP.

Infancy and toddlerhood (birth–2 years) appears to be a stage of activation for ACP development. Children at this age may manifest a difficult temperament and be characterized as irritable, difficult, angry, and easily frustrated. They likely show early symptoms of tantrums and defiance. Few gender differences exist in the types of aggression seen during this period.

The preschool period (3–5 years) is a stage of acceleration where problems become magnified and more entrenched. Tantrums, argumentativeness, and defiance persist, but now elaborate to include aggressive actions. Differences in the types of aggression emerge at this period. Boys show higher base rates of overt aggression. Relational aggression becomes characteristic of girls. Some girls do, however, show overt aggression during this period. Impulsivity/disinhibition may be seen in some children. Coercive parent–child interactions occur.

The early elementary school years (6–8 years) are a time of stabilization with some elaboration of problems. Overt aggression and defiance persists. Those children who manifest early-onset aggressive behavior are at risk for developing covert antisocial behaviors such as stealing, lying, sneaking, and the like. Some children will show signs of both overt and covert symptoms. Coercive parent–child interactions persist; teacher–child interactions may become coercive at school. It is at this stage that children with ACP may experience rejection from prosocial peers and begin to affiliate with aggressive and antisocial peers. They may have early experiences with school failure and become alienated from the school. Children manifesting overt aggressive symptoms display atypical social information-processing biases and deficits.

The later elementary and middle school years (9–14 years) are a time of continued elaboration. Although the frequency of overt aggressive behavior declines during this period, it remains higher than the norm. When older children do display aggressive behavior, it is often more violent. Covert behaviors appear to increase, including vandalism, skipping school, firesetting, substance use/abuse, and so on. Antisocial peers begin to reinforce each other's overt and covert antisocial behavior, especially during the teen years. Coercive parent–child and teacher–child interactions can persist. Children still require supervision and monitoring during these years, yet their parents may lack these parenting skills. Family conflict may develop as a result of these ongoing problems.

Adolescence and adulthood (15+ years) is a time of crystallization. Children tend to exhibit more covert than overt antisocial actions, but some commit violence. Guns and other weapons may be utilized during violent acts. Organized gangs develop during this period; boys more often than girls are involved in these gangs, but girls do affiliate with them. Covert actions move into the arena of serious crime. Cross-gender aggression emerges with some boys engaging in coercive and/or violent behavior while dating girls. Sexual intercourse base rates are higher for children with ACP at this time, and there is a higher likelihood of teenage pregnancy. Previous experimentation with substance use can magnify into a substance abuse problem. It is estimated that approximately one-third of children with early-onset ACP go on to develop adult antisocial personality disorder. The remaining individuals often have adult functional problems such as unemployment, marital difficulty, violence, psychopathology, and criminal histories.

TABLE 1.5. General Developmental Progression of Children with Aggression and Conduct Problems

Infancy and toddlerhood (0–2 years)

- Difficult temperament, including being irritable, difficult, easily frustrated, angry, and hard to soothe
- Early tantrums and defiance
- Few gender differences in behavior

Preschool (3–5 years)

- Tantrums, defiance persist
- Aggressive actions develop
- Gender differences emerge, including relational aggression for girls
- Impulsivity/disinhibition seen in some children
- Coercive interactions with parent

Early elementary school (6–8 years)

- Overt, covert, or combined behaviors observed
- Coercive interactions with peers and teachers
- Social problems seen in some children
- Negative peer reputation seen in some children
- School problems seen in some children
- Information-processing biases and deficits are manifest in some children

Later elementary and middle school (9–14 years)

- Overt behaviors decline (but remain higher than normal), while covert behaviors increase
- Substance use and/or abuse seen in some children
- Peer, family, and school problems

Adolescence and adulthood (15+ years)

- Covert actions are predominant, except for a subset of violent individuals
- Covert actions involve serious crime
- Cross-gender violence emerges
- High rates of intercourse and pregnancy
- Serious substance abuse problems
- Antisocial personality and/or lifetime functional problems for some adults

Note. "Early starter" boys and girls can follow a similar developmental progression, although girls may display covert conduct problems somewhat later than boys.

Specific Developmental Pathways of Aggression and Conduct Problems

Children with ACP can take one or more pathways to the same developmental destination (i.e., equifinality). What follows is a discussion of specific developmental pathways of children with ACP. The longitudinal research we review in this section examines the subtly different steps children take toward serious forms of ACP and related difficulties.

Proceeding from early overt (primarily aggressive) maladjustment to later covert (delinquency/conduct problems) maladjustment has been observed in boys (Patterson, Forgatch, Yoerger, & Stoolmiller, 1998; Tremblay, Masse, Vitaro, & Dobkin, 1995), and in boys and girls combined (Stanger, Achenbach, & Verlhulst, 1997). Children following this pathway display early aggression, which leads to increased covert conduct problems and delinquency in later years. Although the base rates for aggressive behaviors decline over time, they are still higher than normal for these children throughout development. A subgroup of children continue to display high levels of overt problems along with covert problems in their later years. Although boys exhibit a higher level of overt aggressive behavior and covert conduct problems than do girls, the developmental pattern is similar for both boys and girls (Stanger et al., 1997). Family adversity and parent practices are strongly linked to this developmental trajectory.

Another pathway goes from overt (aggressive) maladjustment to substance abuse. Boys (Dobkin, Tremblay, Masse, & Vitaro, 1995) and boys and girls (Brook, Whiteman, Finch, & Cohen, 1996) who manifest early-onset overt aggressive and hyperactive behaviors are at significant risk to develop into substance-abusing adolescents and young adults. Earlier significant behavioral problems appear to be a strong predictor of later substance abuse outcomes. Association with antisocial peers mediates the relationship between early aggression and adolescent substance use (Brook et al., 1996; Dobkin et al., 1995).

Kokko and Pulkkinen (2000) found that manifestation of aggression at age 8 predicted long-term unemployment at age 36. A developmental pathway emerged, revealing that the aggressive 8-year-olds displayed school maladjustment at age 14, problem drinking and lack of occupational alternatives at age 27, and chronic unemployment at age 36. Poor parenting and self-control problems in children were related to this developmental progression.

The progression from early ADHD to later antisocial behavior has been demonstrated under certain conditions. Generally, "pure" ADHD (without comorbidity) is not related to the development of later conduct problems and antisocial behavior in children (Barkley, 1998; Loeber et al., 2000; Nagin & Tremblay, 1999). Notably, the early presence of ADHD by itself is not a strong predictor of adolescent substance abuse (Loeber, Stouthamer-Loeber, & White, 1999). Comorbid aggression/defiance/antisocial symptoms are better predictors of later maladjustment in individuals with ADHD (Nagin & Tremblay, 1999; Patterson, DeGarmo, & Knutson, 2000). Children with comorbid ADHD and CD generally exhibit an earlier onset of behavioral problems than children with CD only (Loeber, Burke, et al., 2000). Children with ADHD/CD typically have parents who are ineffective and coercive in discipline (Patterson et al., 2000).

Frick and colleagues (1993) found that the four empirically derived subtypes discussed earlier (see Table 1.1) were characteristic of children at different ages. Starting at about age 6, the oppositional subtype was most prevalent. The aggression subtype was most evident at about age 6.75 years. The property violations subtype was observed most often at about 7.25 years. Finally, the status violations subtype was typically observed when children were age 9 years. Although cause and effect cannot be determined, this cross-sectional data suggests that children may progress from oppositional/aggressive overt behaviors to property violations/status violations covert behaviors.

Multiple pathways have been explored as they relate to boys' development. Loeber and colleagues (1998) summarized the Pittsburgh Longitudinal Study, which examined the developmental trajectory of boys across 10 years who began the study during the first, fourth, or seventh grades. Loeber and colleagues found that boys can go down one of three possible developmental pathways, which are summarized in Figure 1.1. In terms of age of onset, the earliest pathway appears to be "authority conflict," where boys move from being stubborn, to defiant, to having authority avoidance difficulties. The second "overt" pathway involves boys moving from minor aggression, to fighting, to more severe levels of aggression. The third "covert" pathway has to do with boys moving from minor covert actions, to property damage, to delinquency. Boys can go down one or more pathways at any one particular point in their development. Family and parenting factors were found to be the strongest predictors of persistence of various forms of behavior in the Pittsburgh Longitudinal Study.

In a similar fashion, Nagin and Tremblay (1999) reported on multiple pathways. They observed that some elementary school-age children with ACP proceeded from being oppositional to exhibiting covert delinquency in adolescence. Another pathway was for elementary school-age children with early-onset ACP to exhibit overt aggression and then move to overt (violent) delinquency in adolescence.

Finally, Frick and colleagues (2000) speculated that there may indeed be two childhood onset pathways in the antisocial trajectory of development. The first pathway is the impulsive conduct problem *without* callous/unemotional traits pathway. It could be that children in this pathway have parenting problems, lower IQ scores, and hostile attributions that develop because of growing up in an abusive family situation. These children may exhibit an overactive/impulsive temperament style. The second pathway is the conduct problem *with* callous/unemotional traits pathway. Biological processes may be implicated as a cause for these children's difficulties. Children going down this pathway are described as disinhibited, fearless (low anxiety), thrill seeking, insensitive to punishment, and unresponsive to parenting efforts. Both of these pathways can lead to conduct problems, but Frick et al. hypothesized that children going down the callous/unemotional pathway have a poorer prognosis.

Earlier we pointed out that there is characteristic heterogeneity among

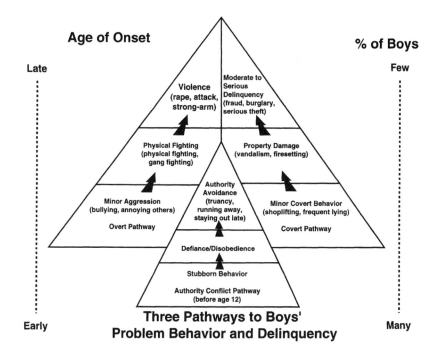

FIGURE 1.1. Model of three developmental pathways toward serious juvenile offending for boys. From Loeber and Hay (1994). Copyright 1994 by Blackwell Publishers. Reprinted by permission.

children with ACP. This section demonstrated that there is also heterogeneity in terms of the developmental pathways these children follow. Practitioners need to take into account these different specific developmental pathways in conceptualizing and conducting interventions

Persistence of Aggression and Conduct Problems

Approximately 42–75% of children with ACP or a behavior disorder will persist in their difficulties through childhood (August, Realmuto, Joyce, & Hektner, 1999; Bennett et al., 1999; Biederman, Mick, Faraone, & Burback, 2001; Campbell, 1995; Kingston & Prior, 1995; Loeber, Burke, et al., 2000; Speltz, McClellan, Deklyen, & Jones, 1999). Frick and Loney (1999) summarized the strongest factors that are associated with persistence of problems. These factors include high initial severity, earlier rather than later onset of problems, comorbid ADHD, lower intelligence levels, and family adversity (e.g., lower SES and family/parenting problems). Some children with early-onset ACP desist or evidence a reduction of their problems, especially when they are in transition from either the preschool to the elementary school or from the late adolescence to the adulthood developmental periods (Loeber & Stouthamer-Loeber, 1998). Children with ACP who desist presumably have fewer risk factors than do children with ACP who persist.

Persistence of ACP in children relates to subsequent mental health diagnosis. Children who exhibit persistent "hard-to-manage" behavior up to age 9 are more likely to be diagnosed as ODD or CD during their later elementary school years than hard-to-manage children who desist prior to age 9 or children who never displayed hard-to-manage behavior (Pierce, Ewing, & Campbell, 1999). In one study, school-age boys who evidenced persistent fighting were three times more likely to have a psychiatric disorder 7 years later than were boys who had desisted (Loeber, Green, et al., 2000).

Summary

The information contrasting normal and ACP developmental pathways is useful in designing and implementing effective practices. The normal continuous adaptive pathway shows how children should be developing when they are achieving competence. The various ACP continuous maladaptive pathways demonstrate that the problems of these children start early and worsen over time. Apparently, multiple risk factors account for the persistence of ACP in some children. Interventions must assist children traveling down a maladaptive ACP pathway to find a more adaptive pathway. Assessment methodologies that identify children with early manifestations of ACP should be used. Interventions need to be delivered early in development to reduce the likelihood of persistence of ACP in children. For example, all children in a preschool setting could be screened for the presence of early-onset ACP, and those that meet an acceptable cutoff score on a screening measure could qualify for an early intervention. We present specific assessment and intervention procedures that conform to this framework later in this book.

GENDER DIFFERENCES

It cannot be assumed that assessment and intervention practices work the same for both boys and girls. It is necessary to understand characteristics and developmental pathways that may be unique to boys or to girls so that gender-specific best practice parameters can be defined. In this section we review what is known regarding gender differences in children with ACP.

The prevalence rates of ACP problems in girls may be higher than what is commonly thought. Girls may be underidentified due to the potential bias of criteria used to define aggression and/or CD (Hartung & Widiger, 1998; Keenan, Loeber, & Green, 1999). An emphasis on overt aggression in previous research has resulted in fewer girls being identified and studied. Indeed, the prevalence rates are higher for boys than girls when overt aggression is assessed; but prevalence rates are actually equal when overt and relational aggression is assessed simultaneously (Crick & Grotpeter, 1995).

Few gender differences exist early in development, but as they grow older boys and girls manifest different forms of ACP. Boy and girl toddlers are similar in displaying types of aggression (Keenan & Shaw, 1994). Aggressive toddlers display object-related aggression (e.g., throwing toys, kicking the door), which could be an early indicator of oppositional behavior. Between the ages of 4 and 7 years, clinically referred boys and girls continue to be similar in levels of defiance, arguing, swearing, and yelling at home (Webster-Stratton, 1996a). Gender differences in child-to-child aggression begin to emerge during the preschool years. At this time boys show more overt aggression and girls show more relational aggression (Crick, 1997). Boys continue to display higher levels of overt aggression than girls throughout childhood (Keenan et al., 1999). Although boys and girls are similar in prevalence rates of adolescent-onset CD, gender differences continue to be evident at that period of development (Kazdin, 1995; Zoccolillo, 1993). Girls are more likely to exhibit comorbid internalizing problems in adolescence. Girls are also more likely to manifest the covert forms of CD rather than the overt forms.

Preliminary developmental research reveals some similarities and some differences for how boys' and girls' problems progress over time. It appears that some girls go down a pathway similar to boys when they are exhibiting *early-onset overt (aggressive)* behavior (Moffitt & Caspi, 2001; Rubin, Chen, McDougall, Bowker, & McKinnon, 1995). It has been suggested, however, that many girls manifest severe levels of *covert/conduct problems/ delinquent* behavior at a somewhat later stage of development than do boys even though they may have been exposed to similar early risk factors (Hinshaw & Anderson, 1996; Silverthorn & Frick, 1999; Zoccolillo, 1993). More research is needed to better understand gender-related developmental differences (Loeber, Burke, et al., 2000).

The person targeted by the aggressive boy or girl also determines the type of aggression and level of maladjustment of the aggressive child. For example, Russell and Owens (1999) found that aggressive girls use more physical aggression with boys and more "indirect" aggression with girls. As we indicated earlier, boys and girls who engage in gender nonnormative aggression (e.g., boys who exhibit relational aggression and girls who exhibit overt aggression) have the most significant social/psychological maladjustment among aggressive children (Crick, 1997).

Gender differences are also seen with ADHD during the elementary school years. Girls are referred for problems related to ADHD at a much lower rate than are boys. When girls are referred, however, they are very similar to boys in exhibiting the primary symptoms of hyperactivity, impulsivity, and inattentiveness (Horn, Wagner, & Ialongo, 1989). Gaub and Carlson (1997) conducted a meta-analysis and review pertaining to gender differences in ADHD. They concluded that there are no differences in terms of impulsivity, academic, social, and family problems between boys and girls with ADHD. Girls, however, are less hyperactive and less likely to develop additional conduct problems.

Summary

Gender differences in the types of ACP most commonly seen in boys and girls begin in preschool and continue throughout development. Preliminary research suggests that boys and girls are similar when they display early-onset overt-aggressive behavior, but girls may develop covert conduct problems somewhat later than boys. Practitioners need to be aware of gender differences and make sure that girls are not underserved. For example, boys are more commonly referred for behavioral difficulties, but this may be a function of the obvious nature of overt aggression, which gets them noticed by parents and teachers. Girls, who are more likely to exhibit relational aggression, as well as to internalize their emotional problems, are less obvious to referral sources. Assessment procedures that identify less visible forms of maladjustment should be used to identify girls who are struggling, and interventions should be administered accordingly. We discuss gender-specific practices more fully later in this book.

CONCLUSION AND IMPLICATIONS FOR INTERVENTION

The literature we reviewed in this chapter shows that the characteristics of children with ACP can be diverse, yet can also overlap considerably. The first step in any intervention is to identify among the full realm of possible characteristics and problems those that are most indicative of a given child or population of children. Table 1.3 can be used to assist practitioners in pinpointing target problems of children who will receive interventions.

The information pertaining to normal development, general ACP development, and specific developmental pathways for ACP is equally important. The problems of children with ACP worsen as they get older. These accumulated problems become additional risk factors that lead to the persistence of ACP. These at-risk children with ACP need to be identified early and provided with effective interventions to steer them toward a more adaptive or resilient developmental pathway. The interventions we describe later in this book are designed to promote resilient development in children with ACP.

The next chapter will examine child (e.g., biological), parent/family, social/peer, and contextual risk factors that serve to cause, maintain, and/or escalate these problems and characteristics. It will also highlight protective factors that buffer children who face these risks and/or who display early signs of ACP. Understanding these risk and protective factors will ultimately inform intervention efforts.

CHAPTER 2

Risk and Protective Factors Targeted in Intervention

*E*ffective interventions for children who exhibit maladjustment increases the odds of them moving toward a resilient developmental pathway by reducing risk factors and promoting protective factors (August, Anderson, & Bloomquist, 1992; Cummings et al., 2000; Masten & Coatsworth, 1998). A *risk factor* is a characteristic within an individual (e.g., ADHD) or a circumstance (e.g., poverty) that increases the probability of a maladjusted developmental outcome. Different risk factors can exert direct or indirect influences on children's development. A *protective factor* is a characteristic within an individual (e.g., intelligence) or a resource (e.g., effective parent) that buffers the effect of risk and increases the probability of a resilient developmental outcome. Different protective factors can exert direct or indirect effects on children's development and are more or less effective as a buffer in the face of varying levels of risk.

Interventions with children who display early-onset ACP attempt to reverse the trend of problems "stacking" on top of problems by promoting developmental competence. To accomplish this, it is first necessary to understand risk factors that potentially cause, maintain, and amplify these children's problems so they can be reduced. Next, protective factors that may serve as a buffer against risk in children need to be identified so they can be increased. In this chapter we review the risk and protective factors associated with the early-onset ACP and resilient developmental pathways in children. Information related to risk and protective factors in children only shows an association with developmental outcomes and cannot necessarily indicate causation (Pettit, 2000). Nonetheless, by contrasting factors associated with the ACP and resilient developmental pathways, our subsequent discussions of interventions will be clearer in terms of what developmental factors are targeted and what procedures are utilized to potentially enhance children's development.

We will present information about risk and protective factors within the context of the child, parent/family, social/peer, and contextual life domains (i.e., areas of influence in children's development). Accordingly, we first discuss potential risk factors such as biologically based child characteristics that may activate ACP problems; parent, parent–child, and family factors that accelerate ACP problems; social and peer factors that elaborate ACP problems; and contextual factors that adversely affect children with ACP and their families. Next we present information about protective factors and organize them according to the four life domains framework. At the end of this chapter we present a developmental–multisystemic model of practice that proposes interventions to reduce risk and enhance protection within the four life domains.

CHILD BIOLOGICAL RISK FACTORS

In this section we review factors attributed to biologically based characteristics and/or processes implicated in children with ACP. This line of inquiry investigates whether or not the central nervous system (CNS) of children with ACP is different than the CNS of normal children. In Chapter 1 we noted that ADHD coexists in many children who have ACP and that ADHD may be a catalyst for the development of more significant psychopathology in these children. Here we offer an overview of biological factors, including genetic vulnerability, neurological processes, and biological markers associated with ACP and ADHD in children.

These biologically based child factors are important to consider in practice with children exhibiting ACP because they may be related to the initial activation of the early-onset ACP developmental trajectory. Although practitioners cannot change the structure of a child's CNS, they need to understand the biological processes that may be implicated in a child's problems. This understanding should lead to more compassionate and effective interventions.

Genetic Vulnerability

Genetic predisposition to atypical CNS functioning plays a role in the initial expression of ACP in many children (Cadoret, Leve, & Devor, 1997; Cadoret, Yates, Troughton, Woodsworth, & Stewart, 1995; Deater-Deckard & Plomin, 1999; Miles & Carey, 1997; Simonoff, Pickles, Meyer, Silberg, & Maes, 1998). In a comprehensive study, Hudziak, Rudiger, Neale, Heath, and Todd (2000) examined genetic contributions to predicting attention problems and aggression in a large sample of male and female twins. They found that both attention problems and aggression were highly influenced by genetic factors for both boys and girls. Although genetics does appear to play a causal role, research suggests that genetic predispositions are more likely to be expressed in certain environmental circumstances. For example, Miles and Carey (1997) conducted a meta-analysis of 24 genetically informative studies on human aggression. They found that genetic factors accounted for about 50% of the statistical variance, but that more variance was explained when genetic and environmental factors were considered simultaneously. In other words, it appears that genetic factors operate as a vulnerability for the possible expression of ACP, but that environmental risk factors and stressors increase the likelihood of expression of these problems.

Tannock's (1998) comprehensive review provided evidence concerning the heritability of ADHD. Genetic factors are implicated in the development of ADHD in both boys and girls. Other researchers have determined that the genetic contribution to ADHD is stronger than the genetic contribution to other behavioral disorder categories (Levy et al., 1997; Plomin, Owen, & McGuffin, 1994). Pure environmental causes of ADHD are not supported. Environmental factors may be influential in the development of comorbid conditions such as oppositional defiant disorder/conduct disorder/aggression (Barkley, 1998; Goodman & Stevenson, 1989; Tannock, 1998).

Neurological Processes and Biological Markers

Quay (1993, 1997) put forth a theory of disinhibition, which he argued is descriptive of CNS problems underlying aggressive conduct disorder and ADHD in children. Quay relied on Gray's model of self-regulation. Gray (1985) suggested that the flight/fight system in the brain activates arousal in response to environmental cues. According to Gray, the behavioral activation system (BAS) is responsible for initiating behavior when it is needed. Gray also argued that the behavioral inhibition system (BIS) is responsible for inhibiting behavior when that response would be adaptive. The BAS and BIS systems are regulated by the frontal lobes. Quay (1993) argued that aggressive children have an underactive BIS and an overactive BAS. Therefore aggressive children do not inhibit aggressive behavior and are prone to emit aggressive behavioral responses. Quay (1997) argued that children with ADHD have only an underactive BIS, and therefore have problems inhibiting responses.

"Executive functioning," which is largely controlled by the frontal lobe, has been implicated in the problems of aggressive and disinhibited children (Barkley, 1998; Moffitt, 1993; Quay, 1993, 1997). Executive functioning refers to the cognitive processes used to maintain attention and effort, inhibit inappropriate responses, and regulate emotional and behavioral responses. Children who exhibit aggressive and disinhibited behavior (including ADHD) perform poorly on neuropsychological tests measuring aspects of executive functioning (Giancola, Martin, Tarter, Pelham, & Moss, 1996; Giancola, Moss, Martin, Kirisci, & Tarter, 1996; Halperin et al., 1995; Oosterlaan, Logan, & Sergeant, 1998; Oosterlaan & Sergeant, 1996; Seguin, Pihl, Harden, Tremblay, & Boulerice, 1995). It is noteworthy that one study found executive function problems were stronger for boys than for girls (Seidman et al., 1997). Finally, Morgan and Lilienfeld (2000) conducted a meta-analysis of 39 studies of adolescents and adults displaying antisocial behavior. They found a medium to large effect size, suggesting that these individuals perform worse than controls on various measures of executive functioning.

Additional biological processes, some of which may be genetically transmitted and/or indicative of frontal lobe dysfunction, have also been implicated in ACP and ADHD. One such indicator is lower levels of or lower neural receptivity to serotonin metabolite (5-HT) neurotransmitters in aggressive children (Halperin, Newcorn, Kopstein, et al., 1997; Halperin, Newcorn, Schwartz, et al., 1997; Moss & Yao, 1996). Lower levels of catecholamine and dopamine neurotransmitters have also been implicated in ADHD (Tannock, 1998; Zametkin & Rapoport, 1987). There is mixed evidence that aggressive children may have higher levels of the hormone testosterone (Scerbo & Kolko, 1994; Schaal, Tremblay, Soussignan, & Susman, 1996). Finally, miscellaneous biological indicators such as an abnormal electroencephalograph (EEG), neurological "soft signs," and minor physical anomalies have been associated with childhood aggression and ADHD (Barkley, 1998; Pincus, 1991).

CNS assaults may cause ACP and/or ADHD in some children. This area of inquiry has produced mixed results, so caution is needed in interpreting these findings. Elevated blood lead levels (Thomson et al., 1989) and elevated blood copper/zinc levels (Walsh, Isaacson, Rehman, & Hall, 1997) have been found in some samples of children with ACP. Children who are born prematurely (before 29 weeks gestation) have been found to be at elevated risk for behavior problems at age 5 (Girouard et al., 1998). Behavior problems in adolescence have been associated with poor maternal health during pregnancy and birth complications (Allen, Lewensohn, & Seely, 1998). Mothers' smoking of cigarettes during pregnancy predicts CD and substance abuse in later life (Weissman, Warner, Wickramaratne, & Kandel, 1999). Being born with a very low birth weight has been associated with ADHD (Botting, Powls, Cooke, & Marlow, 1997). There is some evidence to suggest that pregnancy and birth complications, elevated lead levels, and prenatal exposure to alcohol and tobacco may be associated with ADHD (Barkley, 1998). Finally, the abuse of alcohol by mothers during pregnancy has been associated with increased incidents of antisocial behavior and learning problems in adolescence (Olson et al., 1997).

Physiological underreactivity is observed in some children with ACP. This is indicated in studies that show that some children with ACP have lower sensitivity to pain (Seguin, Pihl, Boulerice, Tremblay, & Harden, 1996) and lower resting heart rates (Raine, Venables, & Mednick, 1997). There is also evidence of lower levels of cortisol in the implicated areas of the CNS of some children with ACP (McBurnett, Lahey, Rathouz, & Loeber, 2000; Moss, Vanyukov, & Martin, 1995; Vanyukov et al., 1993). Cortisol has been described as the adrenal "stress hormone." Lower levels of it may suggest an underaroused CNS. Perhaps physiological under-reactivity relates to different subtypes of ACP in children.

Summary

Biologically based processes are vulnerability and risk factors that are associated with increased probability of initial expression of early-onset ACP and ADHD. They may be inherited in some children, and may possibly be derived from CNS assaults in others. It appears that the frontal lobe area of the CNS is implicated in the executive functioning deficits and related disinhibition problems in some children with ACP and/or ADHD. Biological processes indicating underarousal may be important to consider with other children with ACP. Child biological factors need to be considered to facilitate a greater understanding of children with ACP and to inform intervention efforts. For example, children with early and significant disinhibition (likely influenced by CNS functioning) may profit from interventions designed to "manage" behaviors, such as medications or behavioral contingency strategies. Additional intervention approaches for children with potential biologically based behavior problems are discussed later in this text.

There are limitations to this information that should be noted. Much of the research on biological processes and children relates to overt aggression and ADHD. Therefore not all of the preceding discussion may apply to other subtypes of ACP such as relational aggression, covert behavior problems, and so on. Although girls are represented in the research described here, boys are more likely to be studied than girls. More research is needed to investigate the biological basis for the problems of children exhibiting differing subtypes of ACP and more research needs to include girls.

PARENT, PARENT–CHILD RELATIONSHIP, AND FAMILY RISK FACTORS

Environmental factors can initiate ACP in some children and serve to escalate or stabilize it in others. Parent, parent–child, and family difficulties are the most widely studied set of environmentally based variables in this regard. In this section we review characteristics of the parent, parent–child relationship, and family that have been associated with childhood ACP.

As this review indicates, parent, parent–child, and family risk factors exert considerable influence on the worsening of problems for children with ACP. Therefore, it is imperative to fully understand the impact of these risk factors so that interventions can be utilized to address them.

Parent Characteristics

Incidence rates of depression are higher in mothers of aggressive, conduct problem, oppositional, and ADHD children than in the general population (Boyle & Pickles, 1997; Dumas & Serketich, 1994; Lahey et al., 1998; Nigg & Hinshaw, 1998; Webster-Stratton & Hammond, 1998). Depressed and "distressed" mothers do evidence parenting difficulties and problematic interactions with their children (Gelfand & Teti, 1990; Harnish, Dodge, & Valente, 1995; Jouriles, Murphy, & O'Leary, 1989; Webster-Stratton & Hammond, 1988). Lovejoy, Graczyk, O'Hare, and Neuman (2000) conducted a meta-analysis of 46 observational studies. They found that depression in mothers was associated with negative/coercive behaviors, with disengaged behaviors, and, to some extent, with lower positive interactions with their children. In addition, maternal insularity (i.e., low levels of social support), which could be related to maternal depression, is also fairly common in the mothers of children with ACP (Dumas & Serketich, 1994; Webster-Stratton, 1990a). Maternal depression and child behavior problems are correlated, but we do not know which is the cause and which is the effect (Griest, Wells, & Forehand, 1979).

Higher levels of antisocial behavior and substance use/abuse have been found in parents, especially fathers, of children with ACP (Frick, 1994). Specifically, parents who have antisocial personality disorder have been found to have more children with ACP (Frick et al., 1992). Sons of substance-abusing fathers are more likely to exhibit higher levels of aggression than sons of non-substance-abusing fathers (Malo & Tremblay, 1997; Moss, Mezzich, Yao, Gavaler, & Martin, 1995). Having a disturbed father increases the likelihood of a child with ADHD exhibiting comorbid oppositional behavioral problems (Johnston, 1996).

Negative cognitions are often found in parents, especially mothers, of children exhibiting ACP (Dix & Lochman, 1990; Kendziora & O'Leary, 1998; Morrissey-Kane & Prinz, 1999). Parents of children with ACP are prone to negative irrational beliefs about their children and/or themselves (Sobel, Ashbourne, Earn, & Cunningham, 1989; Vincent Roehling & Robin, 1986), to an external locus of control regarding their children's misbehavior (i.e., perceiving themselves as ineffective) (Campis, Lynam, & Prentice-Dunn, 1986), and to inattentiveness regarding their children's behavior (Holleran, Littman, Freund, & Schmaling, 1982; Wahler & Dumas, 1989). These same parents are likely to appraise their children's behavior as more problematic than it actually is (Greist, Forehand, Wells, & McMahon, 1980; Middlebrook & Forehand, 1985). Finally, when children with ACP do act up, their parents often attribute that behavior to intentional, negative, internal, stable, dispositional traits that the child could control (e.g., "She's a brat.") (Baden & Howe, 1992; Bickett, Milich, & Brown, 1996; Dix & Lochman, 1990; Miller, 1995; Sobel et al., 1989).

Parents' degrees of depression, stress, and distress relate to how they process information regarding their children. Highly distressed mothers are less able to attend to their children's behavior than are nondistressed mothers (Dumas & Wekerle, 1995). Levels of distress and depression have also been related to maternal negative appraisals and attributions for children's behavior (Geller & Johnston, 1995; Johnston & Freeman, 1997). It remains a topic of debate whether depressed mothers actually "distort" their perceptions of their children or if in fact they may be more accurate than other people in evaluating their children's misbehavior (Conrad & Hammen, 1989; Richters, 1992). In any event, there does appear to be a relationship between parental emotional state, parental cognition, and parenting behavior.

It is assumed that parental cognition (accurate or not) corresponds with parental responses and reactions to children (Johnston & Freeman, 1997; Mash & Johnston, 1990). Presumably, if parents think of their children in negative ways, they will respond to them in a negative fashion. These negative parental responses may exacerbate and continue the escalation of the parent–child interaction difficulties and child behavioral problems. For example, it has been found that mothers who make hostile attributions regarding their children's ambiguous behavior exhibit harsher discipline styles, which in turn relates to their children later developing behavior problems (Nix et al., 1999).

Parent–Child Attachment

Attachment is the quality of the parent–child relationship as seen from the child's perspective. It has to do with how available and how responsive the parent is to meet the child's emotional and physical needs. Internal representational models of relationships form during the first year of life, depending on the quality of attachment (Greenberg, Speltz, & Deklyen, 1993). These internal working models can affect the child's future relationships and how the child "sees" the world. Four types of attachment have been defined: secure, insecure-avoidant, insecure-ambivalent/resistant, and insecure-disorganized/disoriented. Secure attachments develop in the context of responsive caretaking, while insecure attachments develop within the context of unresponsive and/or inconsistent caretaking. Attachment status is fairly stable, especially throughout the preschool- and school-age years (Greenberg et al., 1993).

Attachment classification in childhood is linked to childhood ACP. Insecure attachments in preschool- and school-age children predict difficult peer relationships and anger/irritability/noncompliance problems (Greenberg et al., 1993). In particular, the insecure-ambivalent/resistant and insecure-disorganized/disorientated attachment subtypes have been demonstrated to have the strongest link to ACP in children (Fagot & Pears, 1997; Lyons-Ruth, 1996). The effects of attachment have been found to have long-term implications. Attachment difficulties in infancy predict behavior problems in middle childhood. For example, mothers who are unresponsive to their infants have been found to have children with more significant levels of disruptive behavior during the middle school years relative to mothers who are initially responsive to their infants (Wakschlag & Hans, 1999). The relationship between attachment and ACP in children is stronger for high-risk populations (e.g., low SES, young mothers, etc.) than for low-risk populations (e.g., middle-class, older mothers, etc.) (Greenberg et al., 1993).

Although most attachment research has studied mother–child relationships, some research is available studying father–child relationships. The results of this research are similar to what is found in mother–child relationships. Insecure father–child attachments are associated with early-onset ACP in children (Deklyen, Speltz, & Greenberg, 1998).

Parent–Child Interactions and Parent Practices

Coercive parent–child interactions exist in many of the families of children with ACP (Dansforth, Barkley, & Stokes, 1991; Dumas, Lafreniere, & Serketich, 1995; DuPaul & Barkley, 1992; Moffitt, Caspi, Dickson, Silva, & Stanton, 1996; G. R. Patterson et al., 1991; Patterson, Forgatch, Yoerger, & Stoolmiller, 1998). Coercive interactions are comprised of reciprocal negative parent and child behaviors. The parent behaviors include inconsistent/harsh discipline, poor monitoring/supervision, low levels of warmth/nurturance, and high numbers of negative verbalizations directed toward the child. Child noncompliance/aggression is also often observed in coercive parent–child interactions. Negative reinforcement, or escape conditioning, is the central feature of coercive parent–child interactions. This occurs when either the parent or the child is behaving aversively, causing the other to withdraw and give in to that behavior. For example, the parent directs the child to clean up, the child has a tantrum, and the parent withdraws the original directive. These interactions can become habitual over time. Most research in this area has been conducted with Caucasian boys and their mothers. Recent research, however, has documented that coercive interactions do exist between African American boys and girls with ACP and their parents (Kilgore, Snyder, & Lentz, 2000), as well as between children with ACP and their fathers (Deklyen et al., 1998). Coercive interactions are remarkably stable: parent–child dyads who are classified as coercive during the elementary school years continue to be classified as coercive during the adolescent years (Barkley, Fischer, Edelbrock, & Smallish, 1991; Fletcher, Fischer, Barkley, & Smallish, 1996).

Coercive parent–child interactions are strongly linked to ACP and related DSM–IV categories of child disturbance. Coercive parent–child interactions are associated with ACP in preschool, elementary school, and adolescent populations (Barkley, 1998; Kilgore et al., 2000; G. R. Patterson et al., 1991, 1998; Stormshak, Bierman, McMahon, Lengua, & Conduct Problems Prevention Research Group, 2000). Coercive parent–child relationships during the preschool-/school-age development periods predict aggressive peer relationships and affiliation with antisocial peers in adolescence (G. R. Patterson et al., 1991, 1998). Severity of coercion varies across DSM–IV diagnostic categories in school-age children and adolescents. For example, higher levels of parent–child coercion are associated with children exhibiting comorbid ADHD/ODD than in children with ADHD alone or normal functioning (Fletcher et al., 1996; Gomez & Sanson, 1994; Johnston, 1996). Negative and coercive parenting behavior has been related to children's noncompliance and stealing (Anderson, Hinshaw, & Simmel, 1996). Coercive parenting has been linked to aggression in both boys and girls (McFadyen-Ketchum, Bates, Dodge, & Pettit, 1996). Finally, parents who do a poor job of monitoring their children during the elementary school years (poor monitoring is an element of coercive parenting) are more likely to have adolescents who engage in covert conduct problem behavior and substance abuse (Chilcoat & Anthony, 1996; Dishion & McMahon, 1998).

The longer term effects of coercive parent–child relationships may be different for boys than for girls. For example, McFayden-Ketchum and colleagues (1996) studied boys and girls from preschool to school age. They found that early coercive parent–child relationships predicted continued aggression for boys, but not for girls. They theorized that boys are more likely to resist their parents and to engage in aversive/aggressive behaviors in response to their parents' coercive behavior, whereas girls may be more compliant and withdraw from their parents' aversive behavior. Therefore boys receive more "training" from their parents than girls do. More research is needed to understand the differential effects of coercive parenting on boys versus girls.

Physical abuse, an extreme form of coercive parent–child interaction, has been linked to childhood ACP in both cross-sectional and longitudinal research. Physical abuse is defined as parental actions resulting in injury. It is often due to parental anger and often coexists with psychological (emotional/verbal) abuse (Wekerle & Wolf, 1996). Physical abuse of young children has been found to predict ACP behavior, bullying, and negative peer relationships in children (Dodge, Pettit, & Bates, 1994a; Manly, Cicchetti, & Barnett, 1994; Shields & Cicchetti, 2001). Early physical abuse of children also predicts emotion regulation problems and social cognitive distortion/deficits (see Social and Peer Risk Factors section below), which in turn often leads to later ACP (Dodge, 1993; Dodge, Pettit, Bates, & Valente, 1995; Shields & Cicchetti, 2001).

Spanking or other types of corporal punishment can be conducted in a nonabusive manner (e.g., not hitting hard enough to leave marks and done only with the intent to discipline) or in an abusive manner (e.g., hitting hard enough to leave marks and done out of parental anger). Spanking or corporal punishment has been linked to the development of varying levels of childhood aggression in longitudinal studies. For example, Strassberg, Dodge, Pettit, and Bates (1994) followed children who were either physically abused, spanked but not abused, or nonspanked from preschool to kindergarten. They found that kindergarten children in the physically abused group exhibited the highest level of aggression, followed by the nonabused spanked group who exhibited moderate aggression, and the nonspanked group who exhibited low aggression. Other longitudinal studies have shown a relationship between spanking early in life and subsequent development of aggressive/antisocial behavior in children (see Straus & Steward, 1999). Some literature, however, suggests that physical discipline may not have detrimental effects on all children. This research suggests that nonabusive physical punishment actually reduces the behavioral problems of preschool children (Larzelere, 2000). There may also be differences in how physical punishment affects children from different cultural groups. Early spanking or "punitive" parenting is related to subsequent development of aggression in European American children, but not in African American children (Deater-Deckard, Dodge, Bates, & Pettit, 1996; Stormshak, Bierman, McMahon, Lengua, & Conduct Problems Prevention Research Group, 2000). More research is needed to determine the relationship between physical punishment and the development of ACP in children of different ages and from different cultures.

Different developmental processes appear to be affected by problematic parent–child interactions in children with ACP. First, it is likely that the coercive parent–child interactions disrupt parent–child bonding, resulting in insecure attachment relationships (Greenberg et al., 1993). Second, coercive parent–child relationships in younger children appear to negatively effect the development of self-regulation capabilities that can result in reactive aggression (Shields & Cicchetti, 1998; Shields, Cicchetti, & Ryan, 1994). Third, problematic parent–child interactions are related to social information-processing difficulties (discussed later in this chapter) that are characteristic of overtly aggressive, reactively aggressive, and proactively aggressive children (Crick & Dodge, 1994). Fourth, boys and girls who engage in coercive interchanges with parents are also very likely to engage in similar interactions with peers (Dishion, Duncan, Eddy, Fagot, & Fetrow, 1994; Webster-Stratton & Hammond, 1998), suggesting that early coercive parent–child interactions create a template for social behavior that is applied with later peer–child interactions. Finally, Wolfe (1999) explained that physical abuse and other forms of child maltreatment interferes with normative development, resulting in impaired relational representation, disregulation of emotions, deficits in social awareness, and peer problems, which are related to children developing a variety of emotional and behavioral problems.

Family Interactions and Family Status

Certain characteristics of the family unit as a whole relate to negative developmental outcomes in children. One such characteristic frequently observed in children with ACP is sibling relationship problems. Patterson (1984) found that both older siblings and parents tended to be aversive with clinically referred aggressive children. Garcia, Shaw, Winslow, and Yaggi (2000) discovered that young boys who are involved in conflictual sibling relationships, and who experience parental rejection, tend to be aggressive at both home and school. They further noted that sibling conflict predicted mothers' reports of child delinquency longitudinally. The addition of sibling conflict to the broader array of family interactions may contribute to the "training" of ACP behavior in children.

A broad association has been established between marital problems and a variety of childhood difficulties, including ACP (Crockenberg & Covey, 1991; Kazdin, 1995). Marital problems can include conflict and other dimensions of marital functioning. Marital problems have been related to level of behavior problems in toddlers and preschool children, as well as to negativity in parent behavior while interacting with those same children (Jouriles, Pfiffner, & O'Leary, 1988; Webster-Stratton & Hammond, 1999). A high level of marital disagreement about child rearing has also been linked to behavior problems in children, with the effects stronger for younger children than for older children (Mahoney, Jouriles, & Scavone, 1997). Marital problems also relate to school-age children's level of problem behavior, especially in low SES families and clinic-referred children (Jouriles, Bourg, & Farris, 1991). High levels of marital problems can disrupt or adversely affect parenting; the combination of marital problems with parenting problems is related to the development of ACP in children (Crockenberg & Covey, 1991; Mann & Mackenzie, 1996).

Interparental and family violence contributes to the development of ACP in children. Parental conflicts (e.g., shouting, swearing, throwing objects, etc.) are the strongest marital variable, among a wide variety of marital variables, to be associated with childhood behavior problems in school-age children (Jenkins & Smith, 1991). Researchers have demonstrated a linear relationship between severity of interparental violence and child ACP problems. The higher the level of combined verbal/physical violence between parents, the more aggressive and socially/emotionally maladjusted are preschool- and school-age children (Fantuzzo et al., 1991; Grych, Jouriles, Swank, McDonald, & Norwood, 2000). In school-age children, interparental violence has been linked to a wide variety of childhood disorders, including ACP (McCloskey, Figueredo, & Koss, 1995). Apparently children adapt differently to domestic violence, with some exhibiting externalizing symptoms, some exhibiting internalizing symptoms, and some exhibiting combined externalizing/internalizing symptoms (Grych et al., 2000). Witnessing interparental violence by itself has a significant impact on children and may be associated with other factors related to negative outcomes in children.

It is reasonable to hypothesize that single mothers would be at a disadvantage, when compared to dual parents, in providing adequate parenting. Several studies find that children in mother-led families exhibit higher levels of aggression than children in mother–father or mother–partner families (Pearson, Ialongo, Hunter, & Kellam, 1994; Vanden-Kierman, Ialongo, Pearson, & Kellam, 1995). This relationship is not observed, however, when SES is considered. Both mother-led and mother–father-led low-income households have the same level of aggression in their children (Pearson et al., 1994). It may be that factors associated with low SES are more important contributors to development of ACP than single-mother status. More research is needed regarding the relationship between single-parent status and childhood ACP.

Divorce/separation or other parental transitions can disrupt childhood development and may relate to development of ACP. Boys and girls who experience parental divorce or separation often experience peer rejection (C. J. Patterson, Vaden, & Kupersmidt, 1991). Boys who experience two or more transitions have been found to be more aggressive than boys who experience fewer than two transitions (Capaldi & Patterson, 1991). The effects appear to be indirect because parental transitions likely impact other family processes that influence the development of ACP in children.

Family instability refers to the number of moves a family makes, the number of relationships the primary caretaker has, the number of individuals moving in and out of a home, homelessness, and so on. If family instability is chronic, it likely indicates a chaotic and unstable life for the children in those families. Family instability has been linked to the development of child externalizing behaviors and internalizing symptoms (Ackerman, Kogos, Youngstrom, Schoff, & Izard, 1999). Homelessness may be the most extreme form of family instability because homeless children do not experience a stable or constant residence. It turns out that homeless preschool- and school-age children are prone to higher rates of externalizing behavior problems (Schteingart, Molnar, Klein, Lowe, & Hartmann, 1995) and internalizing symptoms (Buckner, Bassuk, Weinreb, & Brooks, 1999). The instability of the external family environment may negatively effect children's own internal stability, resulting in the manifestation of behavioral and emotional problems.

Even the size of the family and birth order have been linked to childhood ACP. Kazdin (1995) noted that larger families are associated with more children exhibiting aggression and conduct problems, especially in the low SES context. The effect is more pronounced if there are many brothers. Kazdin also noted that middle children in the birth order are more likely to exhibit ACP. It could be that children in large families do not get their emotional needs met, or they are not closely monitored, or they are not provided as much opportunity to bond with their parents, or there may be the increased likelihood of negative role models in the family.

Summary

Parent functioning, parent–child relationships, and family interactions are strongly related to the development of ACP in children. It appears that parent characteristics, such as parental psychopathology and negative cognitions about child/self, likely influence parenting. Children who experience unresponsive parenting, coercive parenting, and inconsistent/ ineffective parent discipline are at heightened risk for the development of ACP. Parenting problems associated with the development of ACP begin as early as infancy and toddlerhood (Shaw, Owens, Giovannelli, & Winslow, 2001). Family variables such as sibling conflicts, marital problems, family violence, single motherhood (combined with low SES), family transitions, family instability, and large family size also contribute to this childhood problem. These parent–child relationship and family variables function as risk factors that have the potential to interfere with normative development in children and amplify the maladjusted early-onset ACP developmental trajectory.

Practitioners need to be able to assess and alter the parent, parent–child, and family factors discussed here. For example, if it is determined that a coercive parent–child relationship exists, it is necessary to provide parent and family skills training and forms of support for the parent and family. Later in this book we suggest ways to identify these problems and to teach parents and family members skills to enhance family relations, as well as methods to provide family support. If successful, these interventions can exert a powerful positive influence on the development of children with ACP.

SOCIAL AND PEER RISK FACTORS

The sphere of influence on children's development widens as they get older to include the peer group. Social and peer factors can exacerbate the problems of children with ACP, sending them further down the maladjusted trajectory of development. In this section we review peer interaction behavior, the emotion processes that affect social behavior, social information-processing factors that affect social behavior, peer status, and peer affiliations that are common in children with ACP. Most of this information pertains to children who manifest forms of early-onset aggression as a primary concern.

The social problems seen in children with ACP operate as a risk factor because they increase the probability of escalating adjustment problems. In other words, social and peer factors have much to do with the worsening of problems for children with ACP. It is important to understand social and peer risk factors so that assessment and intervention practices can focus on them.

Peer Interaction Behaviors

As might be expected, aggressive children exhibit more physical aggression, more reactive aggression, and a higher level of activity (including prosocial and antisocial behaviors) in playgroups and on playgrounds (Coie, Dodge, Terry, & Wright, 1991; Pepler, Craig, & Roberts, 1998). When engaged in structured/cooperative tasks, aggressive children are ineffective in their communication behaviors (Dumas, Blechman, & Prinz, 1994). Aggressive children are less able to ask questions, to elicit information, and to show interest in others. They are more likely to interrupt, be inattentive, make critical comments, and exhibit disapproving behavior toward peers. Reactive aggressive children exhibit social skills deficits in their ability to solve problems, share, and negotiate (Day et al., 1992).

Similarly, children with ADHD are generally more off-task, aggressive, and active in both structured and unstructured situations (DuPaul & Barkley, 1992; Madan-Swain & Zentall, 1990). These children also talk more and ignore others who are talking to them more. Boys with ADHD have also been found to be lacking in communication skills when handling conflict and when engaged in cooperative tasks (Grenell, Glass, & Katz, 1987). Peers end up giving them more commands and saying more negative things to them. Apparently, children with ADHD bother and annoy their peers.

Emotion Processes and Social Behavior

The capacity to understand and regulate emotions influences the social interactions of children with ACP. It has been determined, for example, that children with behavior problems are deficient in emotional understanding of both self and others, so that it is difficult for them to discuss feelings (Cook, Greenberg, & Kusche, 1994). These children also have difficulty identifying adult facial expressions and children's voice tones (Strand & Nowicki, 1999). Finally, hard-to-manage preschool children (Hughes, White, Sharpen, & Dunn, 2000), school-age children with ADHD, combined type/aggressive (Wheeler Maedgen, & Carlson, 2000), and school-age boys with ADHD/aggressive (Melnick & Hinshaw, 2000) manifest poor emotion regulation. These children are prone to emotional lability (overarousal) and lack the capacities to regulate these strong emotions. Their problems with emotion regulation negatively affects these children's social interactions. The aggressive behavior that interferes with social interactions seems to be closely associated with emotion regulation problems in these children (Melnick & Hinshaw, 2000). These research findings suggest that the emotional functioning of children with ACP likely exerts a negative impact on their social relationships.

Social Information Processing and Social Behavior

An association has been demonstrated between aggressive child behavior, peer status, and how children process information about social interactions. Crick and Dodge (1994) summarized theory and research examining the social information-processing characteristics of aggressive and socially maladjusted children. The six-stage Crick and Dodge model is presented in Figure 2.1. Encoding is attending to and receiving information. Interpretation is the process of establishing the meaning of that information. Clarifying goals is about determining an outcome for the situation at hand. Response access is thinking of all the possible responses one could use in a given situation. Response decision pertains to choosing one of the solutions and determining a course of action. Enactment is the implementation of the chosen behavior. Children process this social information sequentially and simultaneously. Information is processed by children through a store of memories or schema they have developed through their previous experiences throughout their lives. Recently, Lemerise and Arsenio (2000) updated the Crick and Dodge model to emphasize how emotion processes are influential for how social information is processed. They argued that social information will be processed differently when a child is emotionally aroused (e.g., angry, anxious, upset) than when he or she is calm. Children with emotion regulation problems are therefore more likely to display social information-processing difficulties.

Aggressive children process information differently than nonaggressive children. During social interactions, aggressive children fail to attend to others' prosocial cues, pay too much attention to others' aggressive cues,

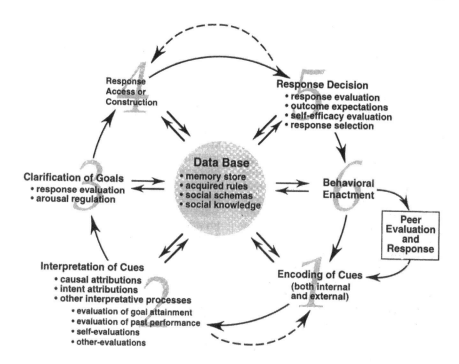

FIGURE 2.1. A reformulated social information-processing model of children's social adjustment. From Crick and Dodge (1994). Copyright 1994 by the American Psychological Association. Reprinted by permission.

interpret others' benign behavior as having a "hostile intent," generate fewer prosocial and more aggressive solutions to solve interpersonal problems, anticipate fewer consequences for their actions, and expect more positive outcomes from employing aggressive solutions to solve their social problems than other children (see Crick & Dodge, 1994, 1996; Dodge, 1993; Pepler, Byrd, & King, 1991). It is noteworthy that reactively aggressive children are most prone to make hostile intent attributions, and that proactively aggressive children are most likely to expect positive outcomes from aggressive solutions. It is also noteworthy that children diagnosed as ODD/CD with or without ADHD are prone to exhibit similar social information processes (Matthys, Cuperus, & Van Engeland, 1999). In short, aggressive children exhibit both cognitive deficiencies and distortions in how they process information (Kendall & MacDonald, 1993).

This pattern of social information processing is entrenched in aggressive children. Aggressive children process information in the manner described above as young as 4 to 7 years of age (Webster-Stratton &

Lindsay, 1999). Social information processing also varies as a function of severity of aggression. Severely violent youth exhibit more extreme social information-processing deficits and distortions than moderately aggressive children, who, in turn, exhibit more social information-processing difficulties than nonaggressive children (Lochman & Dodge, 1994). Even when aggressive children are required to stop and think about their choices, they still choose qualitatively more aggressive responses to solve social problems than normal children (Bloomquist, August, Cohen, Doyle, & Everhart, 1997).

Aggressive children also hold distorted or erroneous beliefs about themselves and their world. They have inflated self-perceptions of their own competence and degree of social acceptance (i.e., they rate themselves better than other adults/children do), as compared to nonaggressive children (David & Kistner, 2000; Hughes, Cavell, & Grossman, 1997; Webster-Stratton & Lindsay, 1999). Aggressive children with inflated self-perceptions are more aggressive than children whose self-perceptions are not inflated (Edens, Cavell, & Hughes, 1999). Finally, aggressive children are likely to believe that aggressive solutions are the best way to solve problems (Erdly & Asher, 1998; Huesmann & Guerra, 1997).

Concern for others is the social–cognitive and behavioral process of thinking of others' perspectives and then demonstrating that concern (if warranted). Hastings, Zahn-Waxler, Robinson, Usher, and Bridges (2000) measured concern for others in children with low, moderate, and severe aggression and behavior problems. The children did not show differences in concern for others during the preschool years. The highly aggressive children, however, decreased significantly in concern for others later during the elementary school-age years. This lack of concern for others was more pronounced in boys than in girls.

Relationally aggressive children also display problematic social information-processing patterns. These children exhibit distorted attributions similar to those of overtly aggressive children, but their attributions are contextually different. Relationally aggressive children assume others have hostile intent for perceived relational provocations (Crick, 1995). Relationally aggressive children assume that others have the intent to shun or slight them, which causes them to feel distressed. Distress in turn may elicit a relationally aggressive behavior. It also has been determined that aggressive boys prefer overtly aggressive solutions to solve interpersonal problems, whereas aggressive girls prefer relationally aggressive solutions to solve interpersonal problems (Crick & Werner, 1998).

Peer Status

Children who are overtly aggressive are often disliked and rejected by their peers (Coie, Dodge, & Kupersmidt, 1990; Coie, Terry, Lenox,

Lochman, & Hyman, 1995; Erhardt & Hinshaw, 1994). Within a population of peer-rejected children, those who are aggressive are usually the most rejected (French, 1988). Aggressive/rejected children have been found to have higher levels of aggression and lower levels of prosocial behaviors compared to aggressive/nonrejected, rejected/nonaggressive, and accepted children (Bierman, Smoot, & Aumiller, 1993). Aggressive children who are liked by some and rejected by others are termed controversial children. These controversial children are most likely to be perceived by their peers as "athletic" and "attractive" (Johnstone, Frame, & Bouman, 1992).

Children with different types of aggression evidence different patterns of peer status. Reactive aggressive children are disliked more than proactive aggressive children (Poulin & Boivin, 1999, 2000), probably because the former are more aversive to others. Even though proactive aggressive children are sometimes classified as being liked, recent research suggests that this status may not be stable. Proactive aggressive children are initially liked, but over time conflicts do develop between proactive aggressive children and their friends (Poulin & Boivin, 1999). Therefore the ability of proactive aggressive children to be able to make friends initially is not necessarily long-lasting. Gender can also affect peer status among aggressive children. For boys, overt aggression is the strongest predictor of rejection, whereas for girls, relational aggression is the strongest predictor of rejection (Crick, 1997).

Similar findings regarding peer status have been found with school-age children with ADHD. These children are often rated lower on sociometric measures, suggesting a rejected status among peers (Carlson, Lahey, Frame, Walker, & Hynd, 1987; Erhardt & Hinshaw, 1994). The combination of ACP with ADHD in school-age children relates strongly to rejected peer status (Pope, Bierman, & Mumma, 1989, 1991).

Aggression and peer rejection in childhood predicts adolescent antisocial behavior (Miller-Johnson et al., 1999). The long-term effects may vary according to the gender of the child. Boys' adolescent antisocial behavior is best predicted by early aggression and peer rejection, whereas girls' antisocial behavior is best predicted by early aggression only (Miller-Johnson et al., 1999). Peer status variables seem to propel the child with early-onset ACP further along the maladaptive ACP developmental pathway.

Peer Affiliations

Peer affiliation is another dimension of peer behavior that is often problematic among children with ACP. Even during the preschool years, aggressive children tend to affiliate with other aggressive peers (Farver, 1996; Synder, Horsch, & Childs, 1997). It has been determined that many proactive aggressive children are liked by, and affiliate with, other proactive aggressive peers (Poulin & Boivin, 2000). Research has shown that aggressive children are rejected by prosocial peers, which causes them to seek out other aggressive children with whom to affiliate (Hektner, August, & Realmuto, 2000).

As children grow up, their peer group associations can increase their risk of developing conduct problems. Those children who manifest early aggression are prone to associate with antisocial children as they get older, which leads to increasing rates of conduct difficulty (Dishion et al., 1994; Fergusson, Woodward, & Horwood, 1999; Vitaro, Tremblay, Kerr, Pagani, & Bukowski, 1997). Over time, affiliation with deviant peers can lead to increased levels of delinquency and conduct problems (violence, theft, vandalism, drug use) in the middle school and adolescent years (Vitaro, Gendreau, Tremblay, & Oligny, 1998). Aggressive or antisocial children apparently reinforce each other for their aggressive and antisocial behavior (Dishion, Andrews, & Crosby, 1995; Dishion, McCord, & Poulin, 1999). Deviancy training, in which peers reinforce each other's antisocial behavior (e.g., by their laughter, encouragement, etc.), has been directly linked to the escalation of aggression and the eventual "metamorphosis" of conduct problems such as substance abuse, delinquency, increased numbers of sexual partners, and violence in boys (Dishion et al., 1999; Patterson, Dishion, & Yoerger, 2000).

Summary

Social and peer factors are implicated in the development and acceleration of ACP in children. Perhaps because of biological predispositions that make children with ACP prone to aggression, and earlier experiences within the family, these children tend to be aversive with other children. Atypical emotion processes and social information distortions/deficiencies in these children exacerbate peer interaction problems. Eventually, many children with ACP end up being rejected by prosocial children and affiliate with other children with ACP. These affiliations appear to accelerate and elaborate the early-onset ACP developmental pathway.

Interventions must address peer and social factors to effect change in children with ACP and to prevent them from developing more problems. For example, assessment may reveal that a child with ACP has social interaction and social information-processing difficulties. That child may improve with a social competence training intervention, along with enrollment in a community-based program that fosters affiliations with prosocial peers. Our subsequent discussions of interventions will provide information pertaining to child-focused social competence training, family interventions, and community supports that facilitate social development in children with ACP.

CONTEXTUAL RISK FACTORS

To fully understand the influences on children's development, it is necessary to examine the individual within an ecological context (Bronfenbrenner, 1979). The sphere of influence of problem development for children with ACP includes broader contextual factors such as SES, neighborhood/community, stressful events, school factors, and broader societal variables. These factors may exert a direct or an indirect influence and relate to the stabilization and elaboration of ACP over time.

In our view, interventions are incomplete unless they address these important contextual issues. This section will enable practitioners to better understand the contextual risk factors implicated in the development of children with ACP so that practices can address them accordingly.

Socioeconomic Disadvantage/Poverty

Socioeconomic disadvantage increases the risk for aggression and antisocial behaviors in children, adolescents, and adults (Guerra, Huesmann, Tolan, Van Acker, & Eron, 1995; Kazdin, 1995; McLoyd, 1998). Children who develop ACP most often live in urban, low SES settings (Kazdin, 1995; Lahey et al., 1999). Low SES predicts lower school achievement and lower cognitive functioning in children living in both urban and rural settings (Dubow & Ippolito, 1994; Felner et al., 1995; McLoyd, 1998; Stipek & Ryan, 1997). There is a linear relationship between SES and ACP in children. As the magnitude of poverty increases, so too does the severity of ACP in children (Bolger, Patterson, Thompson, & Kupersmidt, 1995; Dodge, Pettit, & Bates, 1994b). The association of SES and ACP behavior in children is more pronounced for boys than for girls, and is not directly associated with race or ethnicity (Bolger et al., 1995; Patterson, Kupersmidt, & Vaden, 1990). Race/ethnicity is implicated indirectly, however, because minority youth are disproportionately represented in low socioeconomic and poverty environments.

The relationship between SES and ACP in children is indirect. It affects parents and their parenting, which in turn affects their children. For example, depression is often observed in mothers who have socioeconomic difficulties (Brody & Flor, 1997; Webster-Stratton & Hammond, 1988). In addition, the stress associated with socioeconomic disadvantage negatively effects parent behavior and parenting practices which, in turn, promotes the development of ACP in children (Bank, Forgatch, Patterson, & Fetrow, 1993; Bolger et al., 1995; Dodge et al., 1994b; Kilgore et al., 2000; Larzelere & Patterson, 1990; McLoyd, 1998). Other factors that are commonly associated with low SES that may indirectly affect the development of children with ACP include exposure to aggressive adult models, maternal values reflecting acceptance of aggression, family life stressors, low maternal social support, peer group instability, and lack of cognitive stimulation (Dodge et al., 1994b).

Disadvantaged Neighborhoods

Disadvantaged neighborhoods are characterized by dilapidated housing, high crime rates, isolation, lack of economic resources, concentration of poverty, and generally unsafe conditions. These types of neighborhoods are directly and indirectly associated with increased rates of aggression, violence, crime, and risk taking in children and adolescents (Greenberg, Lengua, Coie, Pinderhughes, & Conduct Problems Prevention Research Group, 1999; Kupersmidt, Griesler, DeRosier, Patterson, & Davis, 1995; Leventhal & Brooks-Gunn, 2000; Paschall & Hubbard, 1998; Peeples & Loeber, 1994). Kupersmidt et al. (1995) found that low SES/single-parent African American families living in disadvantaged neighborhoods had children with higher levels of aggression than families with the same attributes living in middle-class neighborhoods. This finding suggests that a neighborhood exerts powerful influences on the expression of aggressive behavior. Race/ethnicity by itself does not correlate with ACP behavior in children when the effects of disadvantaged neighborhoods are controlled (Greenberg et al., 1999; Peeples & Loeber, 1994). As with poverty, however, minority youth are disproportionately represented in disadvantaged neighborhoods and therefore may be at greater risk for that reason.

It could be that stressors and other problems related to living in disadvantaged neighborhoods are the actual influence impacting children. This includes families having less access to resources (e.g., effective schools, quality child care, mental health services), parents being stressed out, lack of social connections, increased opportunity for negative peer influences, and limited community supports for children and families (see Leventhal & Brooks-Gunn, 2000, for more details).

Community Violence

Community violence includes crimes such as assault, robbery, and murder/attempted murder, as well as crime-related events such as hearing gunshots and seeing a dead body. The rates of child exposure to community violence, which occurs primarily in disadvantaged neighborhoods, are increasing (Osofsky, 1995). Exposure to violence has a negative impact on children and is directly associated with children developing aggression, depression, and posttraumatic stress disorder (i.e., "reliving" bad experiences, anxiety, intrusive thoughts, avoidance) (Fitzpatrick, 1997a; Gorman-Smith & Tolan, 1998; Lynch & Cicchetti, 1998; Miller, Wasserman, Neugebauer, Gorman-Smith, & Kamboukos, 1999). Children who witness violence are also more likely to experience violence and/or physical abuse themselves (Fitzpatrick, 1997a; Lynch & Cicchetti, 1998). It may also be the case that aggressive youth are drawn to environments in which violence regularly occurs, that exposure to violence or the experience of violence changes their normative beliefs about the acceptability of aggression, and that they are exposed to aggressive role models (Gorman-Smith & Tolan, 1998).

Witnessing violence or being the victim of violence seems to affect children in different ways. For example, Schwartz and Proctor (2000) found that school-age children who witness violence exhibit social–cognitive distortions/deficiencies and are prone to aggression. They also found that school-age children who are victims of violence exhibit emotion dysregulation and are prone to social difficulties.

Stressful Life Events

Stressful life events include such negative things as parental separation, exposure to violence, and daily hassles such as arguments with teachers, transportation problems, and so on. School-age children from low-income, disadvantaged neighborhoods experience more negative events and daily hassles than do children from advantaged neighborhoods (Attar, Guerra, & Tolan, 1994; Dubow, Edwards, & Ippolito, 1997). Children who experience high levels of stressful events are at risk to develop ACP regardless of their gender, ethnicity, or grade level (Attar et al., 1994). The combination of high stressful life events and a belief in aggression to cope with problems predicts ACP in children; this is true regardless of ethnicity (Guerra et al., 1995). Stressful life events are also frequently seen in mothers who are depressed (Pianta & Egeland, 1994). Perhaps experiencing stressful events reduces the coping capabilities of children and parents and makes them more vulnerable.

School Factors

Walker, Colvin, and Ramsey (1995) reviewed school factors that appear to be associated with children who display ACP behaviors in school. These school factors could be related to the exacerbation of problems for children with ACP. First, schools react to "unprepared" children. Schools traditionally do not provide proactive programs that prevent children from developing problems; instead, they wait until children cross a line or threshold indicating significant/entrenched problems, and then they try to remediate the difficulty. Unfortunately, children with ACP often have very significant and entrenched problems by the time they are identified by schools. Second, schools often use punishment/exclusion methods to deter children's behavioral problems—for example, suspensions and segregation into special classrooms. Although these procedures may help to maintain order in school, their effect on children with ACP is mixed. Children with ACP who experience these events may end up feeling more alienated and discouraged, causing them to pull away from the prosocial school institution as a source of reinforcement and belonging. In particular, the common practice of aggregating problem children or adolescents together in classrooms could be more detrimental than helpful to them (see Peer Affiliations, above, and Dishion et al., 1999). Third, schools label children to determine their eligibility for services. This may help the school system make orderly decisions about allocating limited resources, but ultimately could have a negative effect on children with ACP. Labels may further alienate these children and create a self-fulfilling prophecy. Fourth, parents of children with ACP are often reluctant to become involved in the school process since school officials often focus on their child's negative behavior, which makes them feel blamed and/or defensive. Walker and colleagues (1995) argued that school factors likely pose additional risks and/or stresses that accelerate the problems of children with ACP.

The quality of the relationship between a child with ACP and his or her teacher can also be a risk factor. In an innovative study, Hughes, Cavell, and Jackson (1999) assessed teacher–child relationship quality in second- and third-grade aggressive children and subsequently followed them for several years. Hughes and colleagues reviewed research that revealed teachers are often negative in their interactions with children with ACP. Perhaps these negative teacher–child interactions are related to the persistence of ACP symptoms. Hughes and colleagues found that those children with ACP who had a poor relationship with their teacher were more likely to maintain aggression, while the opposite was true of children with ACP who experienced a positive teacher–child relationship. The Hughes and colleagues study does not provide evidence of causation. It could be that poor teacher–child relationships cause persistence in children with ACP, or that these children tend to have more negative teacher–child relationships because of their persistent ACP. The influence of teacher–child relationships on children with ACP merits further study.

Other Societywide Influences

Our discussion of larger societal influences on children with ACP begins with mass media, in particular, the effects of television. Reviews by Donnerstein, Slaby, and Eron (1994), Hughes and Hasbrouck (1996), and Villani (2001) have summarized decades of available laboratory, experimental, and correlational research on this topic. A variety of conclusions can be reached about the effects of television. First, children frequently watch violent television, especially if they are left unsupervised. They are therefore exposed to a large amount of observed violence. Second, television violence is directly related to aggressive attitudes and aggressive behaviors in children. Children who watch violent television view violence as normative and are prone to be aggressive. Third, aggressive children are attracted to violent television. This likely reinforces already present attitudes and beliefs about violence, and may serve to maintain or accelerate aggression in these children. Television violence is a risk factor that can influence aggression in children. Other violent media (e.g., video games, music, etc.) could also exert a similar influence.

The availability of guns and other weapons in our society has been implicated in the violent behavior of children. Berkowitz (1994) summarized the literature pertaining to guns and youth. He concluded that guns are readily available in our society and access to them increases the likelihood of violence and/or suicide among youth. Guns and other weapons obviously contribute to the lethality of aggression and violent acts.

Summary

Contextual factors are linked to early-onset ACP in children. These factors may provide a direct or indirect influence on their development. Low SES, disadvantaged neighborhoods, community violence, and associated life stressors make children and families more vulnerable. The school system response, media influences, and accessibility of guns and other weapons add to the risk equation.

Interventions must deal with the full realm of potential influences on the development of ACP in children. This includes the more distal and elusive effects of contextual risk factors. For example, if the family of a child with ACP is poor, and the child is experiencing violence at school, then these factors need to be attended to in intervention efforts. That family may benefit from involvement in supportive community-based programming, and that child may profit from a schoolwide conflict mediation intervention. Our later descriptions of interventions include community- and school-based interventions that address contextual problems.

CUMULATIVE RISK FACTORS

Table 2.1 summarizes the child biological risk factors; parent, parent–child interaction, and family risk factors; social interaction and peer risk factors; and contextual risk factors discussed in this chapter. Simple linear cause-and-effect relationships among risk factors with ACP outcomes in children cannot be assumed (Hinshaw & Anderson, 1996). It is likely that transactional and interactional relationships among these risk factors predict outcome. Some of these risk factors may be direct in their influence on outcome, while others may be indirect. Caution is also advised because most of the research summarized in this chapter pertains to boys who are overtly aggressive. Although exceptions were noted, more information regarding girls and ACP subtypes is needed. This summary is offered as a heuristic framework to focus intervention efforts in pertinent areas. Each risk factor listed in Table 2.1, if present, increases the probability of initial expression of maladjustment and escalation of ACP-related problems in children.

It is intuitive that the more risk factors from Table 2.1 that are present, the more likely the expression of ACP in children. Indeed, research does exist pertaining to the cumulative effects of risk on outcome for children

TABLE 2.1. Summary of Risk Factors Associated with Early-Onset Aggression and Conduct Problems in Children

Child biological risk factors

- Genetic predisposition
- CNS abnormalities, including possible frontal lobe dysfunction, biochemical differences, underarousal, and/or CNS assaults are implicated in different forms of aggression and ADHD

Parent, parent–child interaction, and family risk factors

- Parent characteristics including psychopathology (e.g., depression, antisocial behavior, and substance use/abuse), distorted cognitions, and stress
- Parent–child attachment problems
- Coercive parenting and family interactions
- Physical abuse and other forms of maltreatment
- Family problems, including marital difficulties, family violence, single parenthood, divorce/separation, and family instability

Social and peer risk factors

- Negative peer–child interactions
- Atypical emotion process
- Social information-processing deficiencies and distortions
- Rejection by prosocial peers
- Affiliation with aggressive/antisocial peers

Contextual risk factors

- Socioeconomic status/poverty
- Neighborhood problems
- Community violence
- Stressful life events
- Harmful school responses
- Violent media (television)
- Access to guns and weapons

Note. Simple linear cause-and-effect relationships among variables and child outcomes cannot be assumed. These variables likely interact and cumulate in their association with the development of aggression and conduct problems in children (see text for discussion).

with ACP. Deater-Deckard, Dodge, Bates, and Pettit (1998) studied European American and African American boys and girls in a community sample to examine influences of multiple risk factors on development of ACP. Twenty separate risk factors within the child, parent/family, peer, and social/cultural (contextual) domains were examined. They identified behavioral status and corresponding risk factors in children at ages 5 and 10. Looking at the entire sample, 18 of the 20 risk factors correlated with the ACP (externalizing) outcome at age 10. Each risk domain added incrementally to the expression of ACP so as to support a cumulative risk model. No gender differences were observed. There were ethnic differences, however, in that cumulative risk was a better predictor of ACP for European American than for African American children. The parent/family variables did not predict as strongly for African American children as for European American children. The Deater-Deckard and colleagues (1998) data did not support any one particular pathway to ACP outcomes or any one risk factor as the strongest predictor. Other studies have also shown that cumulative risk is a stronger predictor of maladjustment than single risk factors (Fitzpatrick, 1997b; Greenberg et al., 1999; Shaw et al., 2001). More research is needed to replicate these findings and further examine ethnicity as a moderating variable for outcome.

DEVELOPMENT OF RESILIENCE IN CHILDREN

Resilience is positive adjustment occurring under circumstances of risk and/ or stress (Cummings et al., 2000; Masten & Coatsworth, 1998). It is observed when the adaptive capacity of a child exceeds the level of risk and stress to which he or she is exposed. It involves a child utilizing available internal and external resources to master developmental tasks at different stages of development. Resilience seems to result from a combination of internal and external resources that function as protective factors, buffering or insulating the child in the face of risk.

Interventions will be more successful if they not only reduce the risk factors associated with maladjustment, but also promote the protective factors observed in resilient children. In this section we review research illuminating which factors promote adaptive development in at-risk children. We begin by reviewing several studies that identify protective factors in children faced with known risk factors related to ACP development (e.g., being an aggressive child, having substance-abusing parents, living in a harsh home environment or a disadvantaged neighborhood, facing multiple risks). We conclude with Masten and Coatsworth's (1998) summary of characteristics of resilient children. Once these protective factors are identified, interventions can be developed to promote them in children.

Protection from the Aggressive Child Characteristic

The aggressive child characteristic is a risk indicator for additional maladjustment. Several studies have found that certain protective factors can buffer the effects of the aggressive child characteristic. A study by Morrison, Robertson, and Harding (1998) examined low-income Latino children who were identified as aggressive. In this study, half of the aggressive children were showing good school and academic adjustment (e.g., they were resilient), and half were showing poor school and academic adjustment (e.g., they were maladjusted). The resilient group of children had high self-concept, had good support systems, and was closely supervised by parents when not in school. Supervision by parents turned out to be the strongest variable in its relationship to good school/academic adjustment in aggressive children. Another study by Hastings et al. (2000) followed aggressive children from preschool through later elementary school. They found that those children who exhibited concern for others (i.e., empathy) evidenced reductions in aggression across time. The authors concluded that showing concern for others is a protective factor in these children. Finally, a study by Kokko and Pulkkinen (2000) followed aggressive children into adulthood. They found that aggressive children whose parents utilized "child-centered parenting" and who had higher levels of prosocial behavior had better adult outcomes (e.g., less unemployment and fewer adjustment problems) than those aggressive children without those protective factors.

Protection from Substance-Abusing Parents

Earlier we pointed out that having parents who abuse substances is a risk factor for the development of ACP. Brook and colleagues (Brook, Balka, Brook, Win, & Gursen, 1998a; Brook, Whiteman, Balka, Win, & Gursen, 1998b) examined the role of ethnic identification as a protective factor with adolescents who are at risk for delinquency and substance abuse. Brook et al. found that adolescents who lived with parents who use drugs or who associated with peers who use drugs were at risk. African American (Brook et al., 1998a) and Puerto Rican (Brook et al., 1998b) adolescents living in an urban setting were less likely to use drugs if they had a strong ethnic identification. The adolescents who had a strong sense of and attachment to their communities and cultures were less likely to engage in delinquent behavior and drug use. Brook and colleagues argued that ethnic identification serves as a protective factor.

Vitaro, Dobkin, Carbonneau, and Tremblay (1996) studied resilient boys within a population of sons of male alcoholics (SOMAs). These SOMAs were studied longitudinally from age 6 to age 14. Resilient SOMAs, compared to maladjusted SOMAs (i.e., children who later developed delinquency, substance abuse, school problems), had better educated mothers, were more closely supervised/monitored in early adolescence, and had parents who did not use punishment methods during late adolescence. The resilient SOMAs exhibited better school and social adjustment.

Protection from Harsh Home Environment

The negative effects of difficult and stressful home environments on children's development are well known. Schwartz, Dodge, Pettit, Bates, and the Conduct Problems Prevention Research Group (2000) examined the role of friendship in possibly influencing the relationship between early "harsh home environment" (characterized by harsh discipline, child abuse, marital conflict, and daily hassles) and later peer victimization (being teased and bullied by other children) in aggressive and nonaggressive children using a longitudinal design. Harsh home environment predicted later peer victimization in both aggressive and nonaggressive children who did not have friends. It was not related to later peer victimization for either aggressive or nonaggressive children if they did have friends. Schwartz and colleagues argued that friendship serves as a protective factor that reduces the potentially negative effects of early harsh home environment, even among aggressive children.

Protection from Neighborhood Disadvantage

In the preceding discussions of risk, we observed that neighborhood factors do relate to the development of ACP in children. Kupersmidt and colleagues (1995) studied the influence of neighborhood on elementary-age children who came from low-income, single-parent, African American families. These researchers determined that children who were living in middle socioeconomic neighborhoods were less aggressive than children living in disadvantaged neighborhoods. Kupersmidt and colleagues hypothesized that middle socioeconomic neighborhoods serve as a protective factor against developing aggressive behavior.

Protection from Multiple Risks

Researchers affiliated with the Rochester Child Resiliency Project (Wyman, Cowen, Work, & Parker, 1991; Wyman et al., 1999) have conducted several studies with children who are experiencing major life stressors while living in poor urban environments. They studied one group of 9- to 12-year-old children using a cross-sectional research design and one group of 7- to 9-year-old children using a longitudinal design. The researchers replicated certain child and parent protective factors for both groups of children. Child protective factors included having an easy temperament and having positive psychological characteristics such as perceived competence, positive self-view, empathy, and realistic control attributions. Parental protective factors included responsive parenting attitude, positive parent mental health, and competent parenting characterized by involvement, discipline consistency, and authoritative practices. Parents who were able to provide these parental protective factors for their children had good social support systems themselves within and outside of the family. No differences were found between black and white children as to the benefits of these protective factors (Magnus, Cowen, Wyman, Fagen, & Work, 1999a, 1999b).

Pettit, Bates, and Dodge (1997) determined the protective factors that can reduce the deleterious impact of the "family adversity" risk factor. Family adversity is defined as low SES, single parenthood, and other family stressors. Pettit and colleagues found that supportive parenting predicted long-term adjustment from kindergarten to sixth grade in children who experienced high family adversity. Supportive parenting included proactive teaching, calm discussions during discipline, warm parent–child relationships, and parents who were interested in and involved with their children's activities. Children who received supportive parenting achieved developmental competence in the behavioral, social, and academic areas.

Masten and colleagues (1999) studied children from elementary school age to late adolescence who faced severe and chronic adversity using a long-term longitudinal design. These children lived in urban settings, endorsed high frequency of stress, and experienced many traumas over their childhood. Masten et al. found that children who had a higher IQ and who received high-quality parenting (in terms of warmth, expectations, and structure) were protected against this adversity. Protective factors were associated with resilient developmental outcomes in the areas of academic, behavioral (conduct), and social domains. These resilient children evidenced developmental mastery and competence across time and in a wide variety of different developmental domains.

Benson, Scales, Leffert, and Roehlkepartain (1999) summarized a large survey study of adolescents across the United States, investigating the power of "developmental assets" as protective factors in the face of multiple risks. These researchers defined developmental assets as four external and four internal factors that are associated with positive development in youth. The four external factors include "support" (e.g., supportive families, adults, neighborhoods, and schools), "empowerment" (e.g., safe and facilitative community organizations and individuals within the community), "boundaries and expectations" (e.g., clear rules, clear consequences for breaking them, and clear expectations from families, schools, neighborhoods, and adult role models), and "constructive use of time" (e.g., useful and creative activities in youth, religious, and home environments). The four internal assets include "commitment to learning" (e.g., engaged and motivated at school, bonding to the school institution, and academic achievement), "positive values" (e.g., prosocial values), "social competencies" (e.g., interpersonal and cultural skills), and "positive identify" (e.g., self-esteem and a sense of accomplishment). These researchers administered the Search Institute Profiles of Student Life attitudes and behaviors survey during the 1996–1997 school year to approximately 99,000 sixth- through 12th-grade students in 212 U.S. communities across 25 states. The Search Institute survey measures the 40 development assets and various dimensions of risk, maladjustment, and adjustment in adolescence. As part of a larger study, Benson and colleagues (1999) also examined a subset of the larger sample that were exposed to high levels of risk to see if assets function as protective factors. Approximately 4,000 of the originally screened 99,000 students reported being exposed to five risk factors, including being alone at home a lot, television overexposure, experiencing physical abuse, having been the victim of violence, and being exposed to drinking parties in the home. The researchers found a linear relationship between the number of developmental assets that the youth reported and their level of adjustment within the context of adversity. The more developmental assets the at-risk children had, the less likely they were to manifest developmental or psychological problems, including antisocial behavior. In other words, the external and internal developmental assets served as protective factors for the at-risk adolescents.

Many studies have defined risk in terms of children experiencing stressful life events. Children who experience stressful life events are protected from developing ACP and other forms of maladjustment if they have family support (Dubow et al., 1997), family cohesion and closeness (Kliewer & Kung, 1998), and positive child dispositional characteristics (e.g., higher IQ, easy temperament) with positive family attributes (e.g., positive parent–child relationships and the opportunity for personal growth within the family) (Jackson & Frick, 1998).

Characteristics of Resilient Children

Masten and Coatsworth (1998) summarized 25 years of resilience research with school-age and adolescent children. The research examined focused on children who were confronted with a wide variety of risks and/or stressors. Masten and Coatsworth summarized those characteristics that essentially served as protective factors in deflecting at-risk children away from internalizing and externalizing maladjustment outcomes. Table 2.2 describes the individual, family, and extrafamilial (contextual) protective factors that have been replicated across studies reviewed by Masten and Coatsworth. The most often replicated protective factors for resilient children are high intelligence and having a good supportive relationship with a parenting figure. Masten and Coatsworth rightly pointed out that

TABLE 2.2. Characteristics of Resilient Children and Adolescents

Child

- Good intellectual functioning
- Appealing, sociable, easygoing disposition
- Self-efficacy, self-confidence, high self-esteem
- Talents
- Faith

Family

- Close relationship to caring parent figure
- Authoritative parenting: warmth, structure, high expectations
- Socioeconomic advantages
- Connections to extended supportive family networks

Extrafamilial context

- Bonds to prosocial adults outside the family
- Connections to prosocial organizations
- Attending effective schools

Note. From Masten and Coatsworth (1998). Copyright 1998 by the American Psychological Association. Reprinted by permission.

protective factors do not necessarily give evidence of cause and effect, but these protective factors are associated with resilient outcomes in at-risk children.

Summary

Protective factors reduce the likelihood of maladaptive development among children who are confronted with risk factors, thereby leading to resilient developmental outcomes. Certain protective factors guard against the risk factors that have been implicated in the development of ACP in children. These protective factors fall within the child, parent–child, social/peer, and contextual life domains (see Table 2.3).

Protective factors need to be enhanced in intervention efforts focused on children with ACP. Accordingly, interventions must build competencies within children and parents, arrange opportunities for positive development and prosocial peer influences, and promote community and school support for families. For example, a practitioner may be assisting a peer-rejected child with ACP who comes from a context of family adversity. Interventions that enhance the child's social competencies, teach parents effective discipline strategies, and provide support through school and community programs could potentially enable that child to divert to the resilient developmental pathway.

CONCLUSION AND IMPLICATIONS
FOR INTERVENTION

Developmental Focus

Chapters 1 and 2 describe developmental processes, as well as risk and protective factors, that are associated with ACP and resilient developmental outcomes in children. Effective interventions must reduce risk and promote protection to enhance children's development (Cummings et al., 2000; Reid, 1993; Yoshikawa, 1994). Information regarding risk and protective factors, along with characteristic and developmental information about ACP, can be used to conceptually focus interventions for ACP children.

We offer Table 2.3 as a summary of risk and protective factors according to life domain. We include child characteristics (reviewed in Chapter 1) as risk factors because those characteristics place the child at heightened risk for escalation of problems (i.e., child characteristics are risk indicators). In truth, we do not understand the complex interactions of risk and protective factors. Therefore the summary offered in Table 2.3 is only a heuristic framework to suggest what should be targeted in interventions. If interventions are successful, children should evidence risk reduction and accumulate protection, which would increase the likelihood of them following a resilient developmental pathway (Cummings et al., 2000; Yoshikawa, 1994).

Multisystemic Interventions

An intensive model of intervention will be needed to accomplish the goal of reducing risk factors and increasing protective factors to enhance the developmental status of children with ACP. A multisystemic model of intervention (e.g., Henggeler et al., 1998) will serve as the framework for the remainder of this book in conducting assessment and intervention with children with ACP. Systems and social ecology theories inform the multisystemic model. In this model, the "system" includes all the internal and external factors that influence a child. The multisystemic model views the behaviors of children as a function of the interaction among subsystems of the larger system, and takes into account how child and environmental factors influence each other in a transactional manner over time. This includes the reciprocal influences of child, family, peers, school, neighborhood, and society. Interventions conducted within one subsystem will have direct and indirect influences on other subsystems. For example, by intervening at the neighborhood level, the practitioner will promote changes that will occur in other areas of influence that affect the child. Multisystemic interventions therefore simultaneously address multiple subsystems to effect change.

In view of the literature summarized in Chapters 1 and 2, we agree

TABLE 2.3. A Summary of Risk and Protective Factors According to Life Domain

Life domain	Risk factors related to aggression and conduct problems[a]	Protective factors related to resilience[b]
Child	• Manifestation of an early form of aggression and/or conduct problems • Disinhibition • Callous/unemotional traits • Comorbid ADHD • Comorbid anxiety, depression, substance abuse, etc. • Comorbid academic problem (reading)	• Social, emotional, and self-regulation capacities and skills • High self-esteem and self-efficacy • Prosocial values • Academic skills and success
Parent/family	• Parent personal problems • Parent–child attachment problems • Parent–child coercive interactions • Physical abuse or maltreatment • Family problems	• Functioning parent • Close relationship with parental figure • Supportive and authoritative parenting • Adaptive parent–child interactions • Functional family relationships
Social/peer	• Deficient social skills • Atypical emotion processes • Social information-processing deficiencies/distortions • Rejection by prosocial peers • Affiliation with "deviant" peers	• Association with prosocial peers • Adaptive social interaction skills
Contextual	• Socioeconomic disadvantage • Neighborhood problems • Community violence • Stressful life events • Ineffective or harmful school responses • Violent media influences • Access to guns/weapons	• Bond with prosocial school and community institutions • Attend effective schools • Safe and organized neighborhoods • Opportunities for prosocial school and community activities • Access to effective community services (mental health, social services, etc.) • Prosocial media influences

[a]See review of characteristics (Chapter 1) and risk factors (Chapter 2) of this volume.

[b]See review of protective factors (Chapter 2) of this volume.

with Henggeler and colleagues' (1998) statement that interventions "must have the flexibility to address the multiple known determinants of antisocial behavior, . . . and intervene comprehensively at individual, family, peer, school, and possibly even neighborhood levels" (p. 8). Accordingly, we advocate that assessment and intervention activities for children with ACP must address the interplay of risk and protective factors in the child, parent/family, social/peer, and contextual life domains as summarized in Table 2.3 through a multisystemic intervention approach.

A Developmental–Multisystemic Model of Practice

Table 2.4 summarizes the hypothesized relationship between multisystemic interventions and risk and protective factors according to life domains. This table presents the "big picture" of the model that will be discussed in detail throughout the book. In Table 2.4 we hypothesize the relationships

TABLE 2.4. Summary of Interventions and Hypothesized Risk Factors That Are Reduced and Protective Factors That Are Promoted in Life Domains

Intervention	Child life domain		Parent/family life domain		Social/peer life domain		Contextual life domain	
	Reduce risk	Promote protection	Reduce risk	Promote protection	Reduce risk	Promote protection	Reduce risk	Promote protection
Social competence training (Chapter 4)	X	X			X	X		
Parent and family skills training (Chapter 5)	X	X	X	X	X	X		
Medications and restrictive treatments (Chapter 6)	X	X	X	X	X	X		
Academic engagement and skills building (Chapter 7)	X	X					X	X
Schoolwide interventions and peer mediation (Chapter 8)	X	X			X	X	X	X
Classroom interventions (Chapter 9)	X	X			X	X	X	X
Mentoring and after-school programs (Chapter 10)	X	X			X	X	X	X
Family support and therapeutic foster care programs (Chapter 10)	X	X	X	X			X	X
Multicomponent and coordinated service models (Chapter 11)	X	X	X	X	X	X	X	X

between interventions and global risk and protective factors. We do not address all of the specific risk and protective factors (e.g., Table 2.3). We reasoned that not enough is known about how interventions affect each specific risk and protective factor. We assume, however, that many of the specific risk and protective factors summarized in Table 2.3 are addressed by the interventions depicted in Table 2.4. We describe the specific interventions mentioned in Table 2.4, along with research and best practice parameters, in subsequent chapters.

In keeping with a multisystemic perspective, we think that interventions likely exert direct and indirect influences on risk and protective factors. Table 2.4 only summarizes what we believe are the direct effects. This model is offered simply as an organizational framework to guide interventions, for all the proposed relations among interventions and risk and protective factors have not been empirically tested. Furthermore, we recognize that most children with ACP will not need all these interventions, and that one practitioner could not possibly provide them all. Table 2.4 is a starting point in determining the many intervention options available according to the hypothesized risk and protective factors addressed.

Subsequent chapters will articulate the details of such a model of practice for children with ACP. Chapters 3 through 10 will describe assessment and intervention procedures that could be used to address risk and protective factors in the four life domains. Chapters 11 and 12 will attempt to integrate these practices into comprehensive, intensive, and engaging models of intervention.

PART II

ASSESSMENT AND IDENTIFICATION

CHAPTER 3

Assessment Procedures

The previous chapters discussed the characteristics, risk and protective factors, and developmental pathways of children with ACP. This discussion makes clear that there are multiple factors involved in the genesis, maintenance, and exacerbation of ACP behaviors and that children with ACP can differ from each other along multiple dimensions (e.g., developmental pathway, type of ACP behaviors, severity, and comorbidity). The characteristic heterogeneity of children with ACP makes the matching of interventions to the specific needs of an individual child with ACP a challenging task. Assessment is the process by which the characteristics of a child with ACP and his or her environment are delineated, generally for the purpose of designing an effective intervention.

This chapter is divided into five sections. In the first section we address the different sources of information and methods used for assessment of children with ACP. We also discuss factors related to the selection of assessment methods. The second section discusses the effect of culture on assessments and how culture should be taken into account when assessing nonmajority children. In the next three sections we describe different types of assessments commonly used with children who exhibit ACP: comprehensive assessments of behavior, functioning, and risk/protective factors; functional behavioral assessments in schools; and screening for ACP. These sections discuss the purpose, information obtained, and procedures for each type of assessment. The information presented is useful for all practitioners working with children who manifest ACP. Even if not conducting assessments, practitioners need to be knowledgeable concerning assessment procedures to utilize assessment data in an accurate and productive manner.

SOURCES OF INFORMATION
AND METHODS OF ASSESSMENT

To obtain a thorough assessment of children with ACP, practitioners need to utilize multiple sources of information and methods. In this section we describe the various sources and methods, present their advantages and limitations, and discuss factors affecting the selection of assessment methods. The information presented is summarized from reviews of research and assessment procedures by Anastasi and Urbina (1997), Frauenglass and Routh (1999), Groth-Marnat (1998), Hinshaw and Nigg (1999), Hinshaw and Zupan (1997), Kamphaus and Frick (1996), Kazdin (1995), Mash and Terdal (1997), and McMahon and Estes (1997).

Sources of Information

Obtaining information from multiple individuals in a child's life is necessary for several reasons. Whether you talk to a child, parent, or teacher, each will offer information that is unique and useful but also limited. The information provided by any one individual is likely to be influenced by multiple factors other than the child's actual behavior. So, for example, a mother's report will be tempered by her mood, beliefs, and amount of contact with the child. Also, a child's behavior varies depending on location or context (e.g., home or school). By talking to a range of people who experience the child in different contexts, the practitioner can better hone in on an accurate, detailed picture of the child's behavior.

Children

Children provide information for assessments through interviews, checklists, and tests that measure numerous factors, including cognitive ability, academic achievement, and emotional functioning. Self-report is utilized less with children than with adolescents and adults. There are fewer self-report measures for externalizing behaviors for children. Children provide information on their behavior; family, peer, and contextual factors; and their perceptions of the evaluation process, treatment, and expectations for improvement.

The accuracy and utility of information reported by children in interviews and on checklists varies by age, type of information sought, and the manner in which the information is obtained. Unfortunately, these variables have not been well studied. It has been found that compared to adults, children tend to underreport externalizing symptoms. In contrast, children are important sources for information on covert antisocial behavior and internalizing symptoms. There tends to be a low level of agreement between child ratings and those of parents and teachers. The reliability of child self-reports tends to increase with age.

Parents/Caregivers

For obvious reasons, parents are the most frequently used source of information for evaluating children with ACP. They provide information through interviews, checklists, and questionnaires on demographics, behavioral concerns, child and family history, family functioning, peer relations, and contextual factors. Parents tend to be better reporters of overt child behaviors than of covert behaviors, anxiety, and depression. Factors influencing the accuracy of parental reports include stress, psychopathology, marital discord, and self-esteem.

Parent judgments have been found to correlate with clinicians' judgments. There is often a high level of agreement between mother and father ratings. This level of agreement is lowered by family distress. Parents tend to agree with each other more on the number of problem behaviors than on the specific behaviors. The reliability of parent ratings tends to decrease as their child grows older. There is a common belief that maternal depression results in mothers overreporting behavior problems. However, a review by Richters (1992) questioned the accuracy of this belief. He pointed out that many studies supporting the overreporting hypothesis did not include independent ratings of child behavior and those that did failed to find the negative bias. Yet more recent studies have found a negative bias in depressed mothers' reports (see Boyle & Pickles, 1997; Youngstrom, Izard, & Ackerman, 1999; Youngstrom, Loeber, & Stouthamer-Loeber, 2000).

Teachers

Teachers can be very helpful in assessing children with ACP. Teachers provide information through checklists and interviews; for clinic-based assessments, the interviews are commonly completed over the phone. Teachers are not only the best source of information on children's academic functioning, they can also offer a unique perspective on behavioral and social functioning. Since teachers have extensive contact with many children, they can easily compare a child's behavioral and social functioning with that of his or her peers. In addition, the behavioral, social, and emotional challenges and expectations a child faces are different at school than at home. Consequently, a teacher's information is very helpful in identifying factors affecting ACP behavior. Teachers are able to provide information on the frequency, intensity, and duration of behaviors, along with the effect of peer and school contextual factors.

The agreement between teachers' and parents' ratings is somewhat low. The different ratings may reflect the effect of contextual factors on the child's behavior rather than indicating invalid or unreliable ratings. There is greater agreement between teachers and parents on global ratings (ratings at the diagnostic level) than on ratings of individual symptoms. Teachers and parents tend to agree more on externalizing behavior than on internalizing behavior. The reliability of teacher ratings tends to decrease with older children. Teacher estimates of children's peer status correlate at a low level with peer sociometric ratings. Teachers also display a negative halo effect when children engage in oppositional behavior: teachers tend to inaccurately rate oppositional children as also exhibiting inattention/hyperactive behavior. A recent study found that using a well-operationalized rating scale reduces this effect (Stevens, Quittner, & Abikoff, 1998).

Peers

Peer-referenced assessment strategies involve evaluating how a child's peers perceive the child's functioning. Peer nomination is the most commonly used form of peer-referenced assessment. This procedure requires children in a classroom to select one or more peers who display a certain characteristic or behavior (e.g., helps other children). How many times a particular child is selected is then compared to norms for the procedure. Sociometric techniques are peer nominations focused on social status. Peers are asked to select a child who is liked most (e.g., most like to have as a friend) or liked least (e. g., least like to have as a friend). Peer ratings correlate with independent evaluations of adjustment and predict future conduct problems. Yet, information from peers is generally not available in clinical practice due to ethical considerations and logistical constraints. Another limiting factor is the lack of availability of standardized, well-normed peer-referenced assessment procedures.

Records

School, court, and medical records have long been used as indictors of the existence and severity of ACP; they have also been used as outcome measures to evaluate interventions. The data obtained from these records include school attendance, grades, suspensions, school discipline referrals, police contacts, arrests, medical history, illnesses and injuries, and medications. Many of these factors represent socially significant measures of the impact of ACP and interventions. This data provides information on current and past functioning in different settings. One limitation of records is that most antisocial behavior is not observed or recorded. Therefore what appears in records may offer an incomplete representation of actual behavior. Also, records, like observations and rating scales, are subject to bias. Table 3.1 summarizes sources of information used in the assessment of children with ACP.

Interviews

Interviews are the most widely used method for assessment. Parents, children, and teachers can all be interviewed, as well as any individual who has

TABLE 3.1. Sources of Information for Assessments of Children with Aggression and Conduct Problems

Children

- Information obtained with interviews, rating scales, and tests of cognitive and emotional functioning
- Good source of information on internalizing symptoms, covert behaviors, child's perceptions of problems, and family, peer, and contextual factors
- Low level of agreement with parent and teacher ratings

Parents/caregivers

- Information obtained with interviews and rating scales
- Good source of information on externalizing behaviors, developmental and medical history, and family, peer, and contextual factors
- Accuracy influenced by stress, psychopathology, marital discord, and possibly maternal depression

Teachers

- Information obtained with interviews and rating scales
- Good source of information on academic performance, school behavior, and peer and school contextual factors
- Tendency to inaccurately rate children with oppositional behavior as also exhibiting inattentive/hyperactive behavior

Peers

- Information obtained with peer nomination and sociometric ratings
- Good source of information on peer status
- Peer ratings correlate positively with independent evaluation of adjustment
- Information often unavailable due to practical constraints

Records

- Information obtained by reviewing school, medical, and legal records
- Good source of information on socially significant indicators of ACP such as school discipline referrals and police contacts
- Accuracy is limited because much antisocial behavior is not observed/recorded

significant contact with the child, such as day care providers or relatives. Interviews vary in the amount of flexibility afforded the practitioner and are categorized as unstructured, semistructured, or structured.

Unstructured Interviews

The unstructured interview is most frequently used and relies on the practitioner to use clinical judgment to determine the topics covered, the wording of questions, and the diagnosis given. As a result, the information obtained by different practitioners varies. The main advantage of the unstructured interview is the flexibility it allows the assessor in obtaining information judged to be relevant. This permits exploration of specific family, peer, and contextual factors that may be of vital importance. It also allows the practitioner to respond to the informant's needs and goals in order to maximize rapport and cooperation.

Like other methods of gathering information, unstructured interviews are susceptible to biased or inaccurate information being provided by the informant, as well as bias and judgment error on the part of the practitioner. The effective use of unstructured interviews requires much skill. Studies of both interinterviewer agreement and interview validity report results ranging from poor to excellent. Potential problems with reliability and validity suggest that information from interviews should be used to form hypotheses that are best supported with other data.

UNSTRUCTURED INTERVIEWS WITH PARENTS/CARETAKERS

The unstructured interview with a parent is an extremely important component of most assessments of children with ACP. It involves balancing the goal of obtaining a large amount of information with the need to establish rapport and attend to the parent's goals for the interview. The practitioner should be aware of and sensitive to the expectations, motivations, and affective responses of the parent. Some practitioners find it helpful to have parents complete checklists and questionnaires prior to the interview; the information so gathered can then be used to guide parts of the interview and to utilize the interview time efficiently.

In two-parent families it can be helpful to have both parents present. This allows the practitioner to obtain information on the child's interactions with both parents, observe the level of agreement/disagreement between parents on issues related to the child, and see the marital interaction *in vivo*. A clinician could opt to include members of the extended family if they play a major role in the child's life. Some practitioners prefer to have the child present during the interview to observe parent–child interactions. Others deliberately exclude the child so that parents can discuss issues more freely and/or to prevent the child's ACP behaviors from interrupting the interview. A third option is to have the child present for only part of the interview.

The interview begins with an explanation of the purpose and format of the interview and assessment process. Telling the parents why certain information is needed and how it will be helpful can increase parents' cooperation and the amount of information they provide. Parents are next asked to present their concerns and what they hope to achieve with the assessment and intervention process. Following this, parents are questioned about the child's current and past behaviors; the child's family, medical, and development history; and family, peer, and contextual factors. Details on the information elicited are presented in the section on assessment of behavior, functioning, and risk/protective factors.

UNSTRUCTURED INTERVIEWS WITH CHILDREN

The child's developmental level determines how the unstructured interview is conducted (Bierman, 1983). It can be made more developmentally appropriate for younger children by simplifying questions and the responses required. For example, open-ended questions, especially "how" or "why" questions, can be difficult for younger children. Providing options for the child to select from can be a more productive way to elicit information. Putting the child at ease and establishing rapport are essential if the practitioner is to elicit clinically significant information. Depending on the age of the child, this may involve an initial play period or even allowing the child to play while responding to questions. Questions concerning what the child enjoys and finds rewarding can serve the dual purpose of establishing rapport and identifying potential reinforcements for use in interventions.

The practitioner will commonly elicit the child's degree of awareness and perception of the presenting problems, emotional functioning, family and peer relationships, and school issues. It is helpful to assess whether the child is motivated to make changes and what the child would want to change. Information is obtained not only from the child's verbal responses, but also from observing the child's behavior during the interview. The practitioner should note how well the child attends, follows directions, interacts with the practitioner, and provides information. Based on observations, the practitioner forms initial impressions of the child's level of receptive and expressive language skills, general cognitive level, understanding of relationships and emotions, and ability to take part in interventions.

UNSTRUCTURED INTERVIEWS WITH TEACHERS

Teacher interviews are frequently conducted over the phone after checklists have been completed and reviewed. The information requested focuses on school behavior, factors affecting that behavior, academic functioning, and options available for school interventions. Further details on the information obtained are presented in Table 3.6.

Semistructured Interviews

Semistructured interviews are somewhat more standardized than unstructured interviews. They provide the practitioner with content areas and sometimes with specific questions. This increases the standardization of the process and assures that important content areas are covered. By specifying content, it reduces the demand for practitioner skill, but does not eliminate it. Skill is still required to establish rapport, recognize and respond to informants' needs and goals, and formulate follow-up questions. Scoring criteria may or may not be included. An example of this type of interview is the

Semistructured Clinical Interview for Children and Adolescents (McConaughy & Achenbach, 1994), a protocol of open-ended questions used with children and adolescents ages 6 to 18. It is scored in a manner similar to the Child Behavior Checklist, with scales for observed behavior and self-reported problems.

Structured Interviews

Structured interviews specify the content areas covered and the wording of questions and probes; some even provide algorithms for determining a diagnosis. Trained practitioners are required to conduct some structured interviews. Most structured interviews have both a child and a parent version. They tend to focus on gathering information for the purpose of making categorical diagnoses.

The advantages of structured interviews include their ability to generate a more consistent set of information, specify onset and duration of symptoms, elicit information useful for diagnosis, and provide information on a broad range of symptoms and comorbidity. In addition, some provide standardized methods for scoring, integrating data, and determining diagnoses. The disadvantages of structured interviews include the time involved in training and monitoring of cross-interviewer agreement, the tendency to overdiagnosis (this is reduced if level of impairment or functional level is assessed), and questionable reliability with children under age 9. Additionally, structured interviews tend to generate limited information on family, peer, and contextual factors.

Though essential for research, the clinical utility of structured interviews is not clear, in large part due to the limited attention to contextual factors. The reliability and validity of structured interviews varies by instrument and by diagnosis. A test–retest attenuation effect has been found: informants, especially children ages 6 to 9, report fewer symptoms on repeat administration of the interviews. Hodges (1993) concluded that more research is needed before it can be assumed that structured interviews are reliable and valid.

Structured interviews used to assess children with ACP include the Diagnostic Interview for Children and Adolescents (DISC) and its revisions (Shaffer, Fisher, Lucas, Dulcan, & Schwab-Stone, 2000), as well as the Diagnostic Interview for Children and Adolescents (DICA; Reich, 2000).

Behavior Rating Scales

Behavior rating scales or checklists require informants to judge behaviors in terms of their presence or absence (yes or no) or their severity/frequency (Likert-type ratings). The informant is required to recall and combine memories of behaviors. They provide a quantitative index of the informant's global impression of the child's behavior. Rating scales lend themselves to dimensional classification more so than to categorical classification. Children, parents, and teachers commonly complete rating scales. They are typically used as a first step in an assessment to provide an overview of symptoms, to guide questioning during a clinical interview, and as measures of intervention outcomes.

Due to their many advantages, rating scales are considered a necessary part of assessments for children with ACP. They can cover a broad range of behaviors and are easily quantifiable to allow for normative comparisons. Many rating scales, especially broad rating scales, have very good psychometric properties and strong research support. They are easy and inexpensive to administer and to score, and they allow for the perceptions of others in the child's life to be incorporated into the assessment.

But rating scales also have a number of limitations that need to be taken into consideration. While necessary, they are not sufficient for assessments of children with ACP. Rating scales provide global impressions, not situation-specific information. This can be an advantage or a disadvantage, depending on the purpose of the evaluation. The items on rating scales generally do not parallel diagnostic criteria and they do not generate sufficient information from which to make diagnoses. Rating scales commonly provide limited information on the onset and duration of symptoms. Moreover, there is generally only modest agreement between different informants' ratings of the same child. It is not known whether this is due to differences in the child's behavior in different settings or to other factors.

Rating scales are open to biased reporting by the informant. Hinshaw and Zupan (1997) listed four potential biasing factors: (1) informants' subjective interpretations of specific items; (2) informants' high level of distress; (3) informant's beliefs about disruptive behaviors; and (4) the halo effect (i.e., systematic high or low ratings). Due to potential bias, the use of rating scales as outcome measures for interventions is problematic when the informant (child, parent, or teacher) is involved in the intervention. The informant's motivation and potential biasing factors need to be taken into account when interpreting rating scale information.

Broad Rating Scales

There are two general categories of rating scales: broad/comprehensive and narrow. Broad or comprehensive rating scales survey a wide range of behaviors and are helpful in screening for behavior problems and for identifying comorbidity. Broad rating scales commonly have well-established reliability, validity, and norms. The specific scales on broad rating scales often lack the differentiation present on narrow rating scales. For example, the Attention Problems scale of the Child Behavior Checklist (CBCL) includes items related to inattention, impulsivity, and hyperactivity. These dimensions are not assessed separately as they are on the ADHD Rating Scale–IV (DuPaul, Power, & Anastopoulos, 1998), a narrow rating scale. Broad rating scales commonly used in assessing children with ACP include parent, teacher, and child forms of the CBCL (Achenbach & McConaughy, 1997), Behavioral Assessment System for Children (Reynolds & Kamphaus, 1992), and Conners Rating Scales—Revised (Conners, 2000), as well as the Revised Behavior Problem Checklist (Quay & Peterson, 1987) that can be completed by parents or teachers.

Narrow Rating Scales

These measures focus on one dimension or diagnosis and provide greater specificity in that area. Narrow rating scales generally are shorter, can be repeatedly completed to monitor the effects of interventions, and commonly do not have well-established reliability, validity, and norms. The norms are often not representative of the population, which can limit their utility, especially with minority groups. Narrow rating scales have been developed for evaluating ACP behaviors and many factors related to ACP. Rating scales limited to ACP behaviors with children have not been widely used clinically. Examples of narrow rating scales include the Eyberg Child Behavior Inventory (Eyberg, 1992) and the ADHD Rating Scale–IV (DuPaul et al., 1998).

Direct Observation

In large part due to the potential for bias in child and adult reports of behavior, direct observation is used as a source of information in evaluating children with ACP. Direct observation generally involves recording behavior as it occurs, the use of trained and impartial observers who follow clearly defined rules and procedures, and the coding of behaviors using categories that require minimal inference. This type of data can be collected or measured using five methods: (1) narrative recording (describing what happens); (2) frequency/event recording (recording how often a specific behavior occurs in a given time period); (3) interval recording/time sampling (recording whether a behavior occurs in a given time period); (4) duration or latency recording (recording the length of a behavioral occurrence); and (5) permanent products (recording the lasting products of a behavior—e.g., broken pencils) (Stein & Karno, 1994). Direct observation can take place in the clinic, school, or home. Each setting has its own properties that affect the information obtained (see McMahon & Estes, 1997, pp. 153–164). Direct observation is most commonly used in research and by practitioners working in school settings. Though desirable in clinical practice, it is often impractical.

Direct observation in the clinic generally involves use of a one-way window and is focused on parent–child interactions. A number of complex, microanalytic observation procedures have been developed for research. One example is the system developed by Forehand and colleagues (Forehand & McMahon, 1981). The parent and child are observed through a one-way window in a playroom. A 5-minute free-play situation is followed by a 5-minute parent-directed situation, during which six parent behaviors and three child behaviors are recorded. Clinic observation systems tend to use complex coding systems and require lengthy training of observers. However, many of the clinic observation procedures have modifications that allow for their use in the home.

Some of the complex systems have been adapted for use in schools, but schools tend to use simpler forms. One example is the Direct Observation Form of the CBCL (Achenbach, 1991). Three to six 10-minute observations are made covering different days and different times of the day. The observer writes a narrative description of the child's general behavior and records on-task behavior. Following the period of observation, the observer rates the child's behavior on the Direct Observation Form. This process yields scores similar to those on the CBCL. Another example of a school direct observation procedure is described in the section on functional behavioral assessments.

Direct observation has many advantages. It allows for greater objectivity by attempting to reduce the effects of judgment and memory. It can provide information on the frequency and duration of behaviors, along with data concerning environmental factors related to the maintenance and exacerbation of the problem behavior. Direct observation is especially helpful for the practitioner when he or she questions the reliability of informants or is faced with discrepancies among informants.

Nonetheless, it cannot be assumed that direct observation is necessarily more accurate than rating forms and interviews. Observation is often limited because it does not sample broadly across multiple behaviors or multiple settings. The coding system used may not accurately reflect the salience or significance of behaviors or environmental factors. The observation of brief units of behavior may not accurately reflect the context or meaning of the behavior. Moreover, the act of being observed will often change an individual's or a family's behavior. Observation only allows for evaluation of observable and immediate controlling events and not factors more remote in time or not observable. Direct observation is not helpful with infrequent or covert behaviors. It is time-consuming and costly due to the need for training of observers, the need to evaluate and maintain interobserver agreement, and in most cases the need to travel to the child's school or home. Studies have shown that even when a high level of interobserver reliability can be demonstrated, the level of agreement can drop when observers are not aware they are being monitored.

Projective Methods

Research shows most projective tests to have poor psychometric qualities, yet they remain popular in clinical practice. Projective methods involve a child completing unstructured tasks for which there are no right or wrong solutions. It is hypothesized that how the child perceives and organizes test stimuli reflects basic aspects of that child's psychological functioning. Projective methods have a long history in the assessment of children and include tasks such as drawing (e.g., human figure drawing, Koppitz, 1968; House–Tree–Person [Buck, 1948]), storytelling (e.g., Children's Apperception Test [Bellak & Bellak, 1966]; Roberts Apperception Test for Children [McArthur & Roberts, 1982]), completing sentences (e.g., Rotter Incomplete Sentence Blank [Rotter & Rafferty, 1950]), and describing what they see in ambiguous forms (e.g., Rorschach [Exner, 1993]).

In the hands of skilled practitioners, projective methods can provide useful clinical information related to a child's motivations, desires, conflicts, and perceptions. They can be helpful in developing clinical impressions and in generating hypotheses about a child's functioning. Projective methods can provide information not available with more behaviorally oriented methods. They are not helpful in defining current externalizing behavior, but may be helpful in exploring comorbidity and internalizing symptoms.

Projective methods have historically been limited by concerns with reliability and validity. Progress has been made in regards to reliability and validity with some projective methods, such as the Rorschach using Exner's Comprehensive System (Exner, 1993). Many projective methods lack adequate standardization and are not used in clinical practice in a standard manner. There is generally a lack of objective scoring and interpretation, and most lack adequate norms. Another concern is the time and expense involved in their administration and interpretation.

Anastasi and Urbina (1997) concluded that with few exceptions (e.g., the Rorschach using Exner's system) projective methods are more properly considered "clinical tools" rather than tests. Their value depends to a great extent on the skills of the clinician using them. Anastasi and Urbina see similarities between projective methods and interviewing and view projective methods as serving as qualitative interviewing aids. Factors influencing the decision regarding whether to include projective measures in an assessment of a children with ACP include the purpose of the evaluation, the type of information needed, the skills of the assessor, and the incremental utility provided by the projective method.

Tests of Intelligence, Academic Achievement, and Neuropsychological Functioning

Academic and learning problems are associated with negative outcomes for children with ACP and as a result are potential targets for interventions. If information from interviews or rating scales reveals concerns with academic functioning, further assessment is indicated. Assessments will commonly consist of tests of intellectual ability and academic achievement. Tests of intelligence measure various skills such as reasoning, planning, problem solving, abstract thinking, and speed of learning and processing of information. Scores on these tests correlate positively with school success. Commonly used tests of intellectual ability include the Wechsler Intelligence Scale for Children–III (Wechsler, 1991), the Stanford–Binet Intelligence Scale, Fourth Edition (Thorndike, Hagen, & Sattler, 1996), and the Kaufman Assessment Battery for Children (Kaufman & Kaufman, 1983). Tests of academic achievement measure knowledge of subjects taught in school. Frequently used tests include the Woodcock–Johnson—III Tests of Achievement (Woodcock, McGrew, & Mather, 2001), the Wechsler Individual Achievement Test (Psychological Corporation, 1992), and the Wide Range Achievement Test—Revision 3 (Wilkinson, 1993). These tests generally have high levels of reliability and validity.

Tests of intellectual ability have a number of limitations. Scores can be affected by numerous child and setting variables such as motivation, impulsivity, confidence, and comfort with the examiner. As a result, they must be interpreted in light of these factors and compared to other measures and indicators of ability and achievement to determine their accuracy. Most commonly used tests of intellectual ability assess a limited number of abilities and thus do not provide a comprehensive view of a child's intelligence. These tests have also been criticized for their failure to inform decisions concerning educational interventions, group differences among racial and cultural groups, and their role in the overrepresentation of minority students in special education (Canter, 1997; Frisby, 1999; Reschly, 1997).

If intellectual and academic achievement testing has not adequately defined deficits and targets for interventions, more fine-grained learning disabilities or neuropsychological testing is warranted. Neuropsychological testing assesses a wide range of abilities, including intellectual, academic, memory, language, attention, executive functioning, visuospatial, and sensorimotor (Bengtson & Boll, 2001). It has not been found effective in diagnosing ADHD (Doyle, Biederman, Seidman, Weber, & Faraone, 2000), but is useful for identifying cognitive processes that can be targeted with interventions. Table 3.2 summarizes the instruments and methods used to assess children with ACP.

Selecting Assessment Instruments and Methods

There is no one set of ideal instruments and methods to assess children with ACP. The best approach to use with a particular child will vary depending on the purpose of the assessment (e.g., screening, determining a diagnosis, developing interventions), characteristics of the child (e.g., age, ethnicity, level of cooperation), and practical concerns (e.g., time and resources available, skills of the practitioner, availability of informants). In addition to these factors, the selection of assessment instruments and methods should be informed by the need for multiple methods and multiple informants, the psychometric qualities of the measures, and the type of classification desired.

Multiple Sources and Methods

Each source of information and method of assessment has its strengths and limitations. In addition, ACP behavior varies significantly from one setting and context to another. As a result of these two factors, it is recommended that multiple sources and methods be used when assessing children with ACP.

Multiple informants or sources of information are recommended for two reasons. First, there is a potential for bias and inaccuracy in any one source of information. Efforts can be made to limit the effects of bias by identifying factors that potentially influence an informant's report (e.g., motivation, beliefs about diagnosing children, stress level) and interpreting the data accordingly. However, combining the identification of factors affecting the accuracy of reports with information from multiple informants will produce the most complete and accurate assessment. The second reason for utilizing multiple informants is that ACP behavior varies greatly depending on the setting and the context. As a result, information from

TABLE 3.2. Methods Used in Assessment of Children with Aggression and Conduct Problems

Unstructured interviews

- Practitioner determines content and questions; should be used to form hypotheses that are best supported with other data
- Advantages: flexibility to explore relevant family, peer, and contextual factors and to attend to informant's needs and goals
- Limitations: potential for practitioner bias and judgment error; requires a high level of skill

Semistructured interviews

- Specifies content and sometimes questions
- Advantages: more consistent coverage of important content areas and reduced need for practitioner judgment
- Limitations: the need for practitioner skill and judgment

Structured interviews

- Specifies wording of questions and probes; some provide algorithms for determining diagnoses; focus on making categorical diagnoses
- Advantages: producing consistent data, specifying onset and duration of symptoms, and providing information on a wide range of symptoms and diagnoses

- Limitations: time involved in training and monitoring cross-interviewer agreement, questionable reliability with children under age 9, and limited information on family, peer, and contextual factors

Behavior rating scales

- Behavior is rated in terms of presence/absence or severity/frequency; provides quantitative index of informant's global impression of child's behavior
- Advantages: ability to cover a broad range of behaviors, easily quantifiable to allow for normative comparison, and easy and inexpensive to administer and score
- Limitations: data consists of global impressions and not situation-specific information, limited information on onset and duration of symptoms, modest agreement among different informants, and ratings are open to biased reporting

Broad behavior rating scales

- Survey a wide range of behaviors
- Advantages: ability to screen for behavior problems and comorbidity; generally have better established reliability, validity, and norms than narrow rating scales
- Limitations: specific scales lack the differentiation present on narrow checklists

Narrow behavior rating scales

- Focus on one dimension or diagnosis
- Advantages: greater specificity than broad rating scales; shorter length, which allows for repeated administration for monitoring progress
- Limitations: generally limited established reliability, validity, and norms

Direct observation

- Generally involves recording behavior as it occurs; uses trained and impartial observers; clearly defines rules and procedures; and uses behavioral categories that require minimal inference
- Advantages: allowance for greater objectivity; provides information on frequency, duration, and sometimes environmental factors; helpful when there are discrepancies among informants or concerns with informant reliability
- Limitations: often not sampling multiple behaviors or settings; failure to capture context and saliency of behaviors; behavior can change when observed; not helpful with infrequent or covert behaviors; can be time-consuming and costly

Projective methods

- Child completes an unstructured task for which there are no right or wrong answers
- Advantages: potential to provide information on motivation, desires, conflicts, and perceptions
- Limitations: generally poor standardization, reliability, validity, and norms; lack of objective scoring and interpretation; can be time-consuming and expensive

Tests of intelligence, academic ability, and neuropsychological functioning

- Measure multiple cognitive skills and knowledge of school subjects
- Advantages: high levels of reliability and validity; intelligence tests correlate positively with school success
- Limitations: scores are affected by multiple factors such as motivation, impulsivity, and variables that differ by culture; intelligence tests have limited value for guiding academic interventions

multiple settings is required (e.g., home, school, day care). Information from different settings more accurately defines the extent of ACP behavior, as well as aids in the identification of factors affecting behavior.

In addition to multiple informants, it is recommended that the assessment use multiple instruments or methods. If only one method is utilized, the result is likely to be an inaccurate or incomplete assessment. For example, broad behavior checklists provide useful information on a wide range of behaviors, but limited information on family, peer, and contextual issues and on risk/protective factors. They provide limited information regarding the onset, duration, and intensity of behaviors. Also, the accuracy of ratings is affected by numerous factors. As a result, other methods, such as interviews, narrow checklists, and direct observation, are needed to obtain an accurate and complete impression of a child's functioning.

Psychometric Qualities

There are many unstandardized instruments and methods with unknown reliability and validity that are used for assessing children (Mash & Terdal, 1997). Whether a measure will provide consistent data that assesses the construct it claims to measure should be a major factor in selecting an instrument or method and interpreting its data.

All attempts to measure a behavior or construct are susceptible to error or inaccurate measurement. Measurement error refers to any variation in a score from the "true" score. Errors can be introduced by factors related to the individual, the environment, the behavior/construct being tested, or the test itself. One strategy for reducing measurement error is standardization. Standardization refers to a uniform set of procedures for administrating and scoring a particular test. Without standardization, variations in administration and scoring can seriously reduce a test's reliability and validity.

Reliability refers to the consistency of the data generated. There are a number of different types of reliability to consider when evaluating a test. These include test–retest reliability (i.e., how similar scores are from two different administrations of a test), alternate-from reliability (i.e., how well scores from two different forms of a test correlate with each other), internal consistency (i.e., the homogeneity of the behavioral domain sampled), and interrater reliability (i.e., correlation of scores obtained by two different scorers scoring the same data).

Validity refers to how well a test measures what it claims to measure. Two important types of validity are concurrent/predictive validity and construct validity. Concurrent/predictive validity refers to how well a test predicts performance on other activities. It relates to the practical utility of the test and is measured by correlations. Construct validity utilizes all other types of validity and refers to how well a test measures a theoretical construct or trait. It generally requires the gradual accumulation of data from different sources. Construct validity requires that a test have both convergent and discriminant validity. Convergent validity indicates that a test correlates positively with tests measuring similar concepts and discriminant validity indicates it correlates poorly with tests measuring different concepts.

How to interpret reliability and validity scores varies by the behavior/construct being measured and the purpose for using the test. Some behaviors are very much influenced by contextual factors and variations are expected in different situations and over time. For example, children commonly have more difficulty maintaining attention in school settings than in home settings. This is in part a result of different task demands in the different settings. A low correlation between parent and teacher ratings of attention (interrater reliability) may reflect an accurate measure of the behavior in the different settings rather than errors in measurement due to different raters. The same issue can be present with concurrent and predictive validity. A low correlation between two forms of assessment (e.g., a behavior rating scale and direct observation) may indicate an invalid score/measure or the expected variation in the behavior over different settings and times. It must be remembered that tests are not valid in general; they are valid only for specific purposes and only under specific circumstances.

Classification

Behavioral disorders are commonly classified in categorical or dimensional terms. Categorical classification results in behaviors or functioning being placed in a distinct group or category: a determination is made concerning the presence or absence of a label or diagnosis. Dimensional classification results in behaviors or functioning being placed on a continuum of a characteristic or dimension: a determination is made concerning the degree to which a characteristic applies to a child. Both categorical and dimensional classifications are useful when describing children with ACP. They provide different types of information and each has limitations that are important to understand. As suggested by Hinshaw and Zupan (1997), the most productive approach may be to utilize both systems of classification when assessing children with ACP.

With categorical classification, it is assumed that there is a qualitative difference between those who exceed a certain threshold of severity or number of symptoms and those who do not. The diagnostic categories in DSM–IV, such as ODD, CD, and ADHD, are categorical classifications. Problems associated with this system include the somewhat arbitrary nature of the number of symptoms and how long the symptoms need to be present to qualify for a diagnosis, the suggested discontinuity in functioning once a certain number of symptoms is reached, the large amount of variation within diagnostic categories, and the overlap among the disruptive behavior disorders. This approach to classification also fails to take into account contextual and systemic factors, and includes age and gender in only a limited way.

Behavior rating scales produce dimensional classifications. Ratings of the child's behavior are compared to a normative sample and this determines where on the continuum a score falls. Rather than being in or out of a category, a score is higher or lower on the continuum. For example, on the CBCL, one child's score may place him at the 90th percentile on the Aggressive Behavior Scale while another child's score may place him at the 60th percentile. This approach can easily take age and gender into account with separate norms. Problems with this system include potential bias based on the normative sample, the failure to take contextual and systemic factors into account, the large amount of variation within children at similar levels on the dimensions, and the arbitrary nature of cutoffs for "clinical significance." Table 3.3 summarizes factors to consider in selecting methods for assessing children with ACP.

TABLE 3.3. Factors to Consider in Selecting Assessment Instruments and Methods

Multiple sources and methods

- Allows for increased accuracy of information
- Provides information from different settings
- Allows for the collection of a wide range of information related to ACP behavior and individual, family, peer, and contextual issues

Psychometric qualities

- Standardization refers to uniform procedures for administration and scoring
- Reliability refers to the consistency of the data generated
- Validity refers to how well a test assesses what it is intended to measure
- The selection of reliable and valid instruments and methods increases the accuracy of the information obtained

Classification

- Categorical classification results in behavior or functioning being placed in a distinct group or category
- Dimensional classification results in behavior or functioning being placed on a continuum of a characteristic or dimension
- The use of both approaches is recommended for children with ACP

Summary

This section presented information on the different sources of information for assessments of children with ACP (summarized in Table 3.1), different assessment instruments and methods (summarized in Table 3.2), and factors to consider in selecting methods of assessment (summarized in Table 3.3). Due to the limitations of the various sources and methods, and the variability of behavior over different settings and contexts, the assessment of children with ACP should include multiple methods and multiple sources of information. Information on the strengths and weaknesses of different sources and methods is necessary for all practitioners working with children with ACP to allow for accurate and productive use of assessment data.

ASSESSMENT AND CULTURE

To use assessment instruments and methods in an effective manner, the practitioner must consider the role of culture. The cultures of the child, of the practitioner, and of the informant can affect the assessment process and interpretation of the data. As a result, practitioners need to be aware of the potential influence of culture and take steps to manage and interpret it appropriately.

Cultural Group Differences on Behavior Rating Scales and Tests of Intelligence

The available evidence suggests that teachers tend to rate African Americans higher on behaviors related to ADHD and conduct problems (Epstein, March, Conners, & Jackson, 1998; Reid, 1995; Reid et al., 1998, 2000). Puerto Rican teachers and parents report significantly more behavior problems than do U.S. teachers and parents (Achenbach et al., 1990). Group differences on tests of intellectual ability are well established (Neisser et al., 1996). Asian Americans as a group score similar to white Americans, Hispanic Americans and Native Americans score somewhat below white Americans, and African Americans score one standard deviation below white Americans. Both Native Americans and Hispanic Americans score lower on the verbal portions than on the nonverbal portions of ability tests.

There is little agreement about why these cultural group differences exist. It is not known whether they accurately reflect real behavioral and skill differences among the groups or whether they result from biased measurement. Factors related to the child and his or her culture, the test, or the informant could contribute to group differences. Child factors include variables differentially distributed among cultural groups—for example, prenatal risk factors, psychosocial stressors, access to or denial of academic opportunity, and economic advantages or disadvantages (Reid et al., 1998). Different cultural groups may place more or less value on doing well on tests, speed of performance, and the constructs measured by the tests. Other factors include the cultural similarity or difference between the practitioner and the child, as well as the child's own expectations concerning how well he or she will perform.

Characteristics of the tests or behavior rating scales that could affect group differences include the constructs measured, the content of the test or rating scale, and the quality of the norms. For example, even if a particular cultural group is included in the normative sample, its low numbers in the sample may limit its impact on the overall norms (Reid, 1995).

Rater bias is another potential source of error on behavior rating scales (Hinshaw & Park, 1999; Reid, 1995). The culture of the child being rated, the culture of the rater, and the similarity or difference in culture between the child and the rater may all affect behavioral ratings.

Approaches for Managing Cultural Effects

The use of separate norms for different cultural groups is one option for addressing these concerns (Lindsey, 1998; Nicolosi & Stavrou, 2000; Reid et al., 2000). With separate norms, individuals can be accurately compared to others within their own cultural group. One difficulty with group-specific norms, however, is determining the appropriate normative group. For example, there could be one Hispanic normative group or different norms for Hispanics from Mexico, from Puerto Rico, from Central and South America, and from Cuba. Also, it may be less helpful to use separate norms if the purpose of the evaluation is to determine or predict functioning in the majority culture. A productive approach is to use both group-specific and general population norm scores so that the child's functioning can be assessed in relation to both populations.

In many cases, the discussion of what norms are most appropriate is purely academic: separate culture-specific norms are not available. Regardless of the norms used, providers need to use informed judgment in interpreting normative results. The information should be supplemented with data from other assessment methods and sources of information. When assessing nonmajority children with behavior rating scales, the practitioner should give special consideration to the use of direct observation to supplement the results. With tests of intellectual ability, other sources of information should be used to evaluate the accuracy of the scores.

Other proposed solutions for responding to group differences on tests of intelligence include the use of culture-specific tests (Dana, 1993, 1998) or the use of culture-free tests (Anastasi & Urbina, 1997). Culture-specific tests are designed, validated, and normed within a culture and are only used within that culture. Only within-culture comparisons are made. This approach reduces the concern with the cross-cultural validity and relevance of constructs and works well if the criteria to be predicted remain within the culture. Culture-free, or culture-fair, tests utilize content that is common to multiple cultures in an attempt to minimize group differences. This is often accomplished by limiting the verbal and language demands of the test, as in the Leiter International Performance Scale—Revised (Roid & Miller, 1997) and the Comprehensive Test of Nonverbal Intelligence (Hammill, Pearson, & Wiederholt, 1996). Culture-free tests appear to reduce the impact of culture, but have not been successful at eliminating cultural group differences (Anastasi & Urbina, 1997; Satttler, 1992).

Currently, no agreement exists on the optimal way to use tests with children of different cultural backgrounds (Esters, Ittenbach, & Han, 1997). Anastasi and Urbina (1997) noted that multicultural assessment is moving away from designing special tests to attending more to the role of the assessor. The assessor can introduce bias in his or her choice of tests, by the amount and type of information he or she elicits from the child and adult informant, and through his or her interpretation of the data. Anastasi and Urbina (1997) suggested that the assessor do the following:

1. Obtain information about the examinee's cultural background.
2. Choose tests that are best suited for the purpose for which they will be used.
3. Administer the test effectively for the particular individual.
4. Interpret the results in light of both the individual's background and the context for which the individual is being assessed.

They point out that gathering information about an individual's history to assist in the interpretation and proper use of test scores is a desirable practice when assessing anyone, regardless of cultural differences.

Important factors in understanding a child's cultural background include understanding the child and parent's worldview and group identity. Dana (1993) asserted that practitioners should be aware and accepting of underlying differences in cultural values and the organization of reality that are responsible for some of the observed differences among cultural and racial groups. The practitioner needs to take into account that his or her worldview may differ from that of the individual being assessed and may result in a different view of personal control and responsibility, what constitutes problematic behavior, and appropriate methods of intervention. Dana viewed it as imperative for the practitioner who wishes to provide culturally competent services to explore an individual's group identity. This allows the practitioner to provide the individual with a meaningful context for the assessment and to conduct the assessment and treatment planning in a productive manner.

Summary

Table 3.4 summarizes potential cultural effects on the assessment of children with ACP and approaches for managing them. Awareness and management of cultural effects are important for generating effective treatment recommendations.

ASSESSING BEHAVIOR, FUNCTIONING, AND RISK/PROTECTIVE FACTORS

Assessments of children with ACP are conducted in many settings, including mental health clinics, schools, and community programs. The purpose of the assessments vary, but may include generation of a diagnosis, identification of areas of need, determination of eligibility for a program, the ruling out of significant problems, or development of a comprehensive intervention. The focus and depth of assessments differ significantly: some consist of a brief interview, while others are long and involved. For example, the assessment for a mentoring or after-school program is likely to be relatively brief. It may attempt to identify the child's interests and concerns to help in program selection. It may also rule out significant problems that the program would not have the resources to manage. In contrast, the assessment for a child referred for a day treatment or for a therapeutic foster care program will be much more comprehensive. It may involve detailed descriptions of behaviors and functioning; identification of individual, family, peer, and contextual risk and protective factors; the determination of a diagnosis, and the design of a comprehensive program of interventions targeting multiple behaviors and risk factors.

TABLE 3.4. Assessment and Culture

Cultural group differences on behavior rating scales and test of intelligence

- African Americans as a group are rated higher on measures of ADHD and conduct problems.
- Mean scores on tests of intelligence for African Americans are one standard deviation lower than for white Americans, with mean scores for Native Americans and Hispanic Americans being between these two groups.

Approaches for managing cultural effects

- Use of both culture-specific and general population norms allows for assessment in relation to both populations.
- Normative data should be supplemented with information from other assessment methods.
- Impact of culture should be minimized by considering the child's cultural background and group identity in test selection, administration, and interpretation.

Clinical assessments often result in determination of a diagnosis. This involves establishing the existence of a sufficient number of symptoms and level of impairment or distress. Some diagnoses also require information on the duration of the symptoms, age at which the symptoms began, the ability to rule out other factors, and the presence of symptoms in multiple settings. Due to the heterogeneity of children within diagnostic categories, their failure to incorporate contextual factors, and the multiple pathways hypothesized for the development of ACP behaviors, diagnostic information is generally not sufficient for intervention planning. Level of functioning and risk/protective factors in the child, family, peer, and contextual domains (see Chapter 2) need to be specified to effectively design interventions.

A focus on defining problem behavior, functioning in multiple areas, and risk/protective factors is appropriate for all assessments of children with ACP. The following authors have written on assessing children with ACP; their works have generated the information and practices discussed in this section: (1) Frick's (1998) presentation on assessment of children with conduct disorders and antisocial behavior; (2) Hinshaw and Zupan's (1997) description of the assessment of antisocial behavior in children and adolescents; (3) Huberty and Eaken's (1994) discussion of the assessment of anger and hostility in children and adolescents; (4) Frauenglass and Routh's (1999) presentation on assessment of disruptive behavior disorders; (5) Kamphaus and Frick's (1996) procedures for assessment of child and adolescent personality and behavior; (6) McMahon and Estes's (1997) discussion of the assessment of conduct problems; and (7) Mash and Terdal's (1997) behavioral-systemic approach to the assessment of child and family disturbance. We begin this section by presenting content areas that are addressed in assessments of children with ACP, along with the instruments and methods used. Following this we describe procedures for combining information from different methods and sources, determining level of impairment, organizing risk information, and planning interventions.

Defining Problem Behavior

Detailed information on the problem behaviors is needed to establish the existence of ACP, make the diagnosis, identify targets for intervention, and begin to identify factors associated with the problem behavior. The specific information obtained on the problem behavior is contained in Table 3.5.

The best sources of information on externalizing behaviors are interviews (structured, semistructured, or unstructured) and behavior rating scales (broad and narrow) completed by parents and teachers. Narrow rating scales for identifying ACP behaviors include the Eyberg Child Behavior Inventory and the Sutter–Eyberg Student Behavior Inventory (Eyberg,

1992). The Home Situation Questionnaire and the School Situation Questionnaire (Barkley & Edelbrock, 1987) are used to identify problem situations and the severity of the problem. There are a number of narrow rating scales for identifying subtypes of ACP. These include the Psychopathy Screening Device (Frick & Hare, in press, described in Frick, 1998a; Fisher & Blair, 1998), teacher-rating forms to assess reactive and proactive aggression (Brown, Atkins, Osborne, & Milnamow, 1996; Dodge & Coie, 1987), and teacher rating forms to assess relational and overt aggression (Crick, 1996; Crick et al., 1997).

School, medical, and court records can also be useful sources of information. They not only provide historical and current information on behavior, but also help practitioners to assess the accuracy of information provided by informants. If practical, direct observation procedures can be used. Direct observation is especially helpful if adults are not able to provide sufficient information, there are discrepancies among informants that are not explained by contextual factors, or there are reasons to question the accuracy of reports. If behavior problems occur outside of the home and school (e.g., at day care, a relative's home, an after-school program), information is needed from adults in these settings.

Defining Child Risk/Protective Factors

This category of risk/protective factors includes variables such as comorbid disorders, biological factors, and individual skills. As described in Chapter 1, it is common for children with ACP to have other disorders that impact the ACP and responses to interventions. These comorbid conditions include

TABLE 3.5. Information Obtained on Problem Behaviors

1. Type of behavior
2. Frequency of the behavior
3. Intensity of the behavior
4. Age of onset
5. Course of the behavior (e.g., intermittent, chronic)
6. Changes in the frequency and intensity of the behavior over time (e.g., the behavior is gradually worsening or has remained constant)
7. Setting in which the behavior typically occurs
8. With whom the behavior typically occurs
9. Antecedents of the behavior
10. Consequences of the behavior
11. Impact of the behavior on the child's functioning
12. Previous attempts to manage/change the behavior

ADHD, depression (major depression, bipolar disorder, and dysthymia), anxiety, learning disabilities/low academic ability/low academic achievement, adjustment reactions, and reactions to trauma (posttraumatic stress disorder). Though far less common with children than with adolescents, substance abuse also needs to be ruled out. Child characteristics can also serve as protective factors. A sense of self-efficacy, prosocial values, and adequate levels of intellectual and academic skills serve a protective function for children. Parent, child, and teacher interviews and rating scales are helpful in identifying possible child risk and protective factors. If the data from these methods suggest problems, further information should be obtained via narrow rating scales, projective methods, and tests of intellectual skills.

If problems with hyperactivity, attention, and impulsivity are present, assessment of ADHD should be conducted. Assuming parents and teachers have already completed broad rating scales, they should complete narrow rating scales focused specifically on ADHD symptoms, such as the ADHD Rating Scale–IV (DuPaul et al., 1997, 1998). Other possible explanations for the attention problems—for example, anxiety, boredom, and learning problems—need to be ruled out. Computerized continuous performance tests may be helpful if the information available is inconsistent or there are reasons to question its accuracy. High false-negative rates (children with ADHD scoring in the normal range) need to be kept in mind when using these tests (Gordon & Barkley, 1998).

Further exploration of learning problems and the protective factor of strong intellectual skills involve assessment of intellectual ability and academic achievement. This information is sometimes supplemented with neuropsychological testing. School information from interviews, rating scales, and records can be helpful in accurately interpreting results from the ability and achievement testing. Schools will often be able to do this testing themselves. This information is helpful not only for diagnostic purposes, but also for understanding other symptoms (e.g., a processing deficit that interferes with understanding directions may affect compliance with directions) and for intervention planning.

When there is evidence of depression, anxiety, trauma, or acute stress, further assessment may be needed to better define the problem and recommend interventions. Parent and teacher rating scales and interviews are useful for identifying symptoms such as social withdrawal, changes in eating and sleeping patterns, and increased inattentiveness. Such information needs to be supplemented with the child's own report of subjective experiences. Broad and narrow rating scales, interviews, and possibly projective methods can be used. Useful rating scales include the Revised Children's Manifest Anxiety Scale (Reynolds & Richmond, 1985), the Children's Depression Inventory (Kovacs, 1992), and the Reynolds Child Depression Scale (Reynolds, 1989).

In addition to comorbid disorders, biological and historical variables also function as child risk factors. Obtaining information related to these variables assists in identifying biological factors influencing behavior, generating hypotheses concerning comorbidity, supporting diagnoses, and providing the historical context for the current problem. Information should be obtained on the pregnancy and birth, especially information about prenatal exposure to alcohol and drugs, premature birth, and birth complications; early temperament; developmental milestones; medical history, including medications, history of elevated lead levels, hospitalizations, and significant illnesses and injuries; and family psychiatric history. This information is often obtained via questionnaires, unstructured or semistructured interviews with parents, and the review of medical records. Medical evaluations should be considered to further assess biological factors that may be affecting the ACP behaviors.

Defining Parent and Family Risk/Protective Factors

Multiple factors related to parent and family functioning affect the onset, maintenance, and expression of ACP behaviors. Parent factors related to ACP behaviors include depression, low levels of social support, antisocial behavior, substance abuse, stress, and negative cognitions. Parent–child interactions that are of concern include inconsistent and harsh discipline, poor monitoring and supervision, low levels of warmth/nurturance, negative verbalizations toward the child, and physical abuse. Family risk factors include sibling relationship problems, marital conflicts and violence, divorce/separation, and family instability (e.g., multiple moves, changes in primary caretakers, and homelessness). Protective factors include a close relationship with a parent, supportive and authoritative parenting, and functional family relationships.

Information on parenting and family factors is obtained through parent and child interviews and narrow rating scales. There are a number of measures to assess parenting practices, including the Parenting Scale (Arnold, O'Leary, Wolff, & Acker, 1993) and the Alabama Parenting Questionnaire (Shelton, Frick, & Wootton, 1996). The Parenting Stress Index (Abidin, 1995) assesses both child and parent factors related to parenting stress. Issues involved in the selection and use of family-functioning rating scales were reviewed by Tutty (1995). Frequently utilized measures include the Family Environment Scale (Moos & Moos, 1983) and the Family Adaptability and Cohesion Evaluation Scale–III (Olson & Killorin, 1985). Marital conflict can be assessed with the O'Leary–Porter Scale (Porter & O'Leary, 1980). These measures can be used to identify both risk and protective factors. In addition to narrow rating scales, the practitioner's use of informal observation of parenting practices and parent–child interactions during the assessment process is helpful. If practical, more formal direct observation procedures can also be used.

Defining Social and Peer Risk/Protective Factors

Children with ACP commonly have difficulties with peer relations. Factors to assess include rejection by peers, affiliation with aggressive children, limited communication skills, poor emotional regulation, and social information distortions and deficiencies. Protective factors include association with prosocial peers and adaptive social interaction skills. Information on social functioning is obtained through parent, child, and teacher unstructured interviews; rating scales; sociometric ratings; and direct observation with peers. Demaray and colleagues (1995) reviewed and evaluated six published social skills rating scales. Recommended measures included the Social Skills Rating System (Gresham & Elliott, 1990), which includes forms for teachers, parents, and children; and the Walker–McConnell Scale of Social Competence and School Adjustment (Walker & McConnell, 1988), a rating scale completed by teachers.

Defining Contextual Risk/Protective Factors

Contextual factors include school, neighborhood, and societywide influences on ACP behavior. Relevant school variables include child–teacher relationships, parental attitude toward and degree of involvement with school, existence of effective school programming to address child problems, and overall school climate (e.g., an effective school program acts as a protective factor). Information on school factors can be obtained from teacher rating scales, interviews, and school records. The teacher interview focuses not only on school risk and protective factors, but also on the child's behavior, the child's social functioning, and parent's involvement. In Table 3.6 we provide a more detailed description of the information obtained from the teacher.

Relevant neighborhood factors include poverty, the amount of violence in the neighborhood, the child's and parent's sense of safety, the presence of positive adult and child role models, and the availability of appropriate recreational opportunities. Societywide influences include exposure to violence in the media and games, and exposure to guns and weapons. This information is commonly obtained from the parent and child in unstructured interviews.

Defining Level of Impairment

Obtaining information concerning the type and level of functional impairment is important for determining diagnoses and interventions. Functional impairment is difficult to define and measure (Bird, 1999), but in general refers to the degree to which a child's ability to perform as expected is compromised. Determining a child's level of functional impairment is compli-

TABLE 3.6. Information Obtained from a Teacher Interview

1. Clarification of the teacher's main concerns
2. Identification of problem behaviors and their contexts (setting, frequency, duration, antecedents, and consequences)
3. Attendance
4. Academic ability
5. Factors affecting academic performance
6. Social skills and social acceptance
7. Teacher's relationship with the child
8. School programming for the child and its effectiveness
9. Teacher's perception of the child's needs
10. Parents' involvement in school
11. Teacher's willingness to implement interventions

cated by the fact that it will commonly differ from one domain to another (e.g., psychological, interpersonal, school, and family).

A number of options exist for determining level of impairment in children. Using DSM–IV, practitioners rate the level of impairment for children on the Global Assessment of Functioning Scale (American Psychiatric Association, 1994). This scale requires practitioners to consider psychological, social, and occupational (school) functioning to rate a child's overall functioning on a scale from 0 to 100. A similar measure, the Children's Global Assessment Scale (CGAS; Shaffer et al., 1983), is designed specifically for children. The Nonclinician Children's Global Assessment Scale is a modification of the CGAS designed to be completed by nonpractitioners (Bird & Gould, 1995). Other measures for determining level of impairment for children are discussed by Bird (1999).

Combining Data from Multiple Sources and Multiple Methods

Having obtained information from multiple informants and multiple settings, and having used multiple methods, the practitioner must integrate this information into a clear and productive case conceptualization. This is a challenging task involving a somewhat subjective process that is dependent on the skill and knowledge of the practitioner. It is also a process that can be influenced by the orientation and biases of the practitioner.

Integrating inconsistent information is problematic when trying to use classification systems that require a tabulation of the number of symptoms present (e.g., diagnoses). Simple approaches to combining data (e.g., count a behavior as present if any informant reports it) are equal to or better than complex approaches (e.g., employ different weighting for information from different informants)(Piacentini, Cohen, & Cohen, 1992). Kamphaus and Frick (1996) support a simple approach to combining data, but add two considerations. First, decisions on whether to count a symptom as present should take into account the risks of false positives (e.g., potential negative effects for a client who is mislabeled) and false negatives (e.g., a child who needs services is ineligible to receive them) in making diagnostic decisions. A second factor to be considered is the credibility of the informant and whether the informant could be expected to have good knowledge of the specific behavior. For example, adults are generally considered to report overt behavior problems more accurately than children.

Kamphaus and Frick (1996) proposed a five-step strategy for integrating information from a comprehensive assessment. The first step is to document all clinically significant findings. The second step involves identifying convergent findings across sources and methods. They recommended including findings that may be important, yet do not exceed the cutoff point for clinical significance. For example, suppose a child reported a high level of anxiety, a parent reported three symptoms of anxiety, and a teacher's rating resulted in a T-score of 64 on an anxiety scale. Only one informant's report results in "clinical significance," yet there is some convergence among the three informants.

The third step is to attempt to explain discrepancies. This chapter has highlighted many potential sources of discrepancies such as the effects of different settings on behaviors and the many factors that affect ratings.

In the fourth step the practitioner develops a profile and a hierarchy of strengths and weaknesses. The strengths and weaknesses should be evident from the previous steps, but prioritizing the concerns is more difficult. To better focus interventions, the practitioner must try to determine which problem areas are primary and which are secondary. For example, if a child becomes depressed following school and home conflicts resulting from noncompliance, the noncompliance is primary and the depression is secondary. Targeting the noncompliance with an intervention may also reduce the depression. Kamphaus and Frick (1996) offered three factors to consider when prioritizing concerns: the degree of impairment associated with different problems, the temporal sequencing of problems, and family history (e.g., a family history of depression).

The fifth step consists of determining what information to place in the report. They recommended that information be included in the report only if it contributes to the understanding of the case formulation or the treatment recommendations.

Developing a Risk Profile

Much emphasis has been placed on the identification of risk factors and their use to inform intervention efforts. The process of compiling and using information on risk factors is generally guided by clinical judgment.

Attempts have been made recently to develop more systematic approaches to the organization and utilization of risk information. Frameworks have been developed for assessing risk for aggression (Augimeri, Webster, Koegl, & Levene, 1998) and dropping out of treatment (Kazdin, 1996b; Kazdin, Mazurick, & Bass, 1993).

The Early Assessment Risk List for Boys (EARL–20B; Augimeri et al., 1998) is used to organize the information obtained in an assessment to specify the aggression potential for boys under age 12. The EARL–20B consists of 20 factors associated with aggressive behavior that are rated 0, 1, or 2 depending on the degree to which they are present. The items are organized into three categories: family (e.g., stressors, parenting style), child (e.g., impulsivity, school functioning), and amenability to treatment (family responsibility and child "treatability"). Aggression and violence are broadly defined by the authors and include such behaviors as lying, stealing, and noncompliance. The practitioner completes the EARL–20B based on information obtained from an assessment.

Potentially, the EARL–20B can help to organize risk factors and guide providers in planning interventions. For example, if the majority of risk factors are in the family area, the intervention may focus on parent training. The EARL–20B may also be helpful in determining the intensity of the intervention needed. Higher summary scores will likely indicate the need for more intensive interventions. While theoretically appealing, the treatment utility of the EARL–20B will require empirical verification. In addition, the EARL–20B is still in the development stage, with limited normative data available.

A similar approach to assessing risk was utilized by Kazdin and colleagues (1993). They developed scales for each of 10 variables associated with conduct problems and poor prognoses (e.g., family economic disadvantage, parent psychopathology, and child contact with antisocial peers). Scores on each scale were determined by multiple measures. For example, the score on the child antisocial scale was calculated from the number of conduct disorder symptoms reported in a structured parent interview, the range and severity of symptoms reported by parents on the Interview for Antisocial Behavior (Kazdin & Esveldt-Dawson, 1986), the history of antisocial behavior reported by the parents on the Risk Factor Interview, and the severity of self-reported antisocial behavior determined by the Self-Report Delinquency Checklist (Elliott, Dunford, & Huizinga, 1987).

Rather than using complex algorithms to summarize risk factors, Kazdin (1996) recommended use of a checklist that rates each risk factor as present or absent. Children and families with multiple risk factors are likely to drop out of interventions (Kazdin, 1996). Early identification of those children and their families allows the practitioner to intervene to promote retention (see Chapter 12 for strategies to retain families in interventions). It also promotes an economical use of resources, as services to promote retention can be focused on those most likely to need assistance.

While currently not available, protection profiles could also prove to be useful for treatment planning. Protective factors identify resources that are available to families that can be used to promote positive change. The development of a systematic procedure for organizing protective factors and relating them to specific interventions would be helpful.

Selecting/Designing an Intervention

The utility of most assessments is to be found in their ability to recommend effective interventions. As with risk factors, the process of moving from assessment results to intervention planning is generally guided by clinical judgment. This complex process is influenced by such factors as the nature of the presenting concern, the level of impairment, the functions the problems serve for the child and family, the type and severity of skill deficits and risk factors, the presence of skills and protective factors, and the level of motivation for change. Often there is a need to prioritize interventions, differentiate short-term from long-term goals, and consider the availability of services.

A simple framework for determining interventions involves categorizing risk/protective factors and interventions. Categories of interventions are then matched to categories of risk and protective factors (see Table 2.4 in Chapter 2). Chapters 4 through 10 identify risk and protective factors targeted by the interventions described. While admittedly simplistic, this approach can serve as a starting point for selecting interventions. Information related to the problem behavior and its function can be used to further refine the selection process.

The four categories of risk and protective factors evaluated in the assessment are child, parent/family, social/peer, and contextual. If the assessment identifies risk factors in the parent/family domain, they can be targeted with parent and family skills training (see Chapter 5). Risk factors in the social/peer domain can be targeted with social competence training (see Chapter 4). Interventions can also attempt to enhance or create protective factors. If a child has prosocial friends, efforts can be made to provide greater opportunities for involvement with these friends. Positive bonds with prosocial school and community institutions can be promoted through involvement in mentoring or after-school programs (see Chapter 10).

Factors such as when, where, and with whom problem behaviors occur can provide helpful information for selecting/designing interventions. For example, if problem behaviors occur more frequently when a child is tired, interventions may focus on factors related to increasing the amount of sleep for the child. This may involve the establishment of a consistent bedtime routine and behavior management training for the parent (see Chapter 5). If problems are associated with unstructured times at school, interventions can focus on these times (see Chapter 8).

Various strategies for functional behavioral assessment offer another approach for matching interventions to assessment results (Dunlap et al., 1993; DuPaul & Ervin, 1996; Maag & Reid, 1994). These assessments identify factors associated with the problem behavior and determine the function or purpose the problem behavior serves for the child (see the section below on functional behavioral assessment). Some of the functions identified in school settings include obtaining adult attention, obtaining peer attention, and avoiding tasks. The same behavior can serve different functions. For example, a child may disturb other children during class to avoid work, to attract the teacher's attention, or to obtain peer attention. If the function is to avoid work, interventions could target factors related to academic engagement (see Chapter 7). If the behavior is intended to attract teacher attention, the teacher can be advised to ignore the inappropriate behavior and to give attention and praise to appropriate behavior, or the child could be taught more appropriate ways to obtain the teacher's attention. If the goal of the behavior is to elicit attention from peers, the classroom could be rewarded for ignoring the child's inappropriate behaviors, the child could earn peer contact with appropriate behavior, or the child could be taught more appropriate behaviors for gaining peer attention.

Procedures for tailoring treatment to assessment results are not well defined and are generally dependent on the skills of the practitioner (Abikoff, 2001). In discussing treatment for ADHD, Abikoff acknowledged the potential usefulness of empirically based algorithms for matching treatment to assessed needs, yet noted their value has not been empirically demonstrated. He pointed out that effective matching requires a model that accurately links needs (e.g., social skills deficits) with the outcome variables (e.g., aggression), valid assessment procedures for measuring needs, and interventions that have demonstrated efficacy in targeting the needs.

Summary

Table 3.7 summarizes information on assessment of behavior, functioning, and risk/protective factors. Assessments should go beyond mere descriptions of problems to include recommendations for effective interventions. To do this, information on behavioral concerns and risk/protective factors in the child, family, social, and contextual domains is collected and organized in a manner that directs the selection of interventions.

FUNCTIONAL BEHAVIORAL ASSESSMENTS IN SCHOOLS

Schools are increasingly using functional behavioral assessment (FBA) to evaluate children with ACP and to inform their interventions. This increase

TABLE 3.7. Assessing Behavior, Functioning, and Risk/Protective Factors

Collect data

- Define problem behaviors.
- Define child risk/protective factors.
- Define parent and family risk/protective factors.
- Define social and peer risk/protective factors.
- Define contextual risk/protective factors.

Combine data from multiple sources and methods

- Document all clinically significant findings.
- Look for convergent findings across sources and methods.
- Try to explain discrepancies.
- Develop a profile and a hierarchy of strengths and weaknesses.
- Determine critical information to place in the report.

Develop a risk profile

- Identify categories in which risks are present.
- Determine overall level of risk.
- Use this information to inform intervention planning.

Select/design the intervention

- Match categories of interventions to the categories of risks present.
- Utilize information on the behaviors and functions of the behaviors to select and focus the intervention.

has been spurred, in part, by the 1997 amendments to the Individuals with Disabilities Act that mandate FBAs in certain situations. FBA refers to a range of processes used to identify factors that control target behaviors. These assessments determine when, where, and why problem behaviors occur. They should not be equated with functional analysis, which is a specific form of FBA. Functional analysis involves the systematic manipulation of variables thought to effect a target behavior in order to establish a causal relationship between the variable and the target behavior.

Until recently, FBA was used and evaluated primarily with children with developmental disabilities (Heckaman, Conroy, Fox, & Chait, 2000). It is now commonly used in schools with children exhibiting ACP. Interventions based on FBA have been found effective in reducing problem behaviors and increasing desirable behaviors for students with or at risk for developing emotional and behavioral disorders (Dunlap, White, Vera, Wilson, & Panacek, 1996; Heckaman et al., 2000) and students with ADHD (DuPaul & Ervin, 1996; Ervin et al., 2000). What has not been demonstrated is the cost-effectiveness of FBA in school settings, that is, whether it is more effective than procedures that require less time and fewer resources (Fox, Conroy, & Heckaman, 1998; Nelson, Roberts, Mathur, & Rutherford, 1999). Fox and colleagues (1998) concluded that the reliability and validity of FBA instruments and techniques for students labeled emotional/ behavioral disordered (EBD) have not been established.

When to Use Functional Behavioral Assessments

Due to the time and expense involved in conducting FBAs, guidelines are needed for when they should be used. Interventions for simple behavior problems can be designed without the time and expense involved in conducting an FBA. Sugai, Horner, and Sprague (1999) recommended that when problem behaviors do not respond to interventions, or when the behaviors are severe, violent, or intense, that a functional assessment be utilized. O'Neill and colleagues (1997) recommended that the intensity of the assessment match the complexity of the problem behavior. For example, if an interview is sufficient to identify controlling factors and to design an effective intervention, then there is no need to conduct a more involved assessment. However, guidelines indicating when FBAs are productive and cost-effective have not been empirically established.

Procedures for Functional Behavioral Assessments

The main purpose of an FBA is to improve the effectiveness of behavioral interventions (Sugai et al., 1999). The practitioner, rather than implementing a generic intervention, uses functional assessment to design an intervention to match the qualities of the student and the environment in which the problem behavior occurs. O'Neill and colleagues (1997) described five primary outcomes of a functional assessment:

1. A clear description of the problem behavior.
2. Identification of the events, times, and situations that predict when the problem behavior will occur.
3. Identification of the consequences that maintain the problem behavior, that is, the function the behavior serves.
4. Development of summary statements or hypotheses that describe specific behaviors, specific situations, and specific outcomes that maintain the behavior in the situation.
5. Collection of direct observation data that support the summary statements.

Much variety exists among the procedures used to implement FBAs. There have been some efforts to standardize procedures, with that of O'Neill and colleagues (1997) being one of the better known (Fox et al., 1998). As a result, O'Neill and colleagues' procedures for conducting functional behavioral assessments will be described in some detail.

Three methods are used to collect information: informant methods (interviews, questionnaires, rating scales), direct observation, and functional analysis manipulations. The first step is to talk to the student and those who know the student and the problem behavior. To assist with this procedure, O'Neill and colleagues developed semistructured interviews for school staff and parents (the Functional Assessment Interview) and students (the Student-Directed Functional Assessment Interview). The Functional Assessment Interview format can be used to interview school staff or school staff can complete the form on their own. Table 3.8 lists the content areas covered in this interview.

After the information is gathered, the final step in the interview is to develop summary statements for each major predictor and consequence. Summary statements integrate the information obtained and help in the development of behavior support plans. They describe the situation, the behavior, and the function the behavior serves. An example of a summary statement is: "When Andrea begins to have difficulty with a reading or math assignment, she will put her head down, refuse to respond, and close her books to try to avoid having to complete the assignment. The likelihood of this pattern increases if Andrea has received teacher reprimands earlier in the day" (O'Neill et al., 1997, p. 17).

The Student-Directed Functional Assessment Interview is a shorter interview that has the student define the problem behaviors, identify contexts

---

TABLE 3.8. Content of the Functional Assessment Interview for School Staff

---

1. Describe the behavior (specific description, frequency, duration, intensity, sequence).

2. Define potential ecological/setting events (medications, medical or physical conditions, sleeping and eating patterns, daily routine).

3. Define the immediate antecedents for occurrence and nonoccurrence of the behavior (time of day, setting, people involved, activity).

4. Identify the consequences or outcomes of the behavior that may maintain it.

5. Define the efficiency of the behavior (i.e., amount of effort required to obtain desired outcome).

6. Identify functional alternative behaviors the student already performs.

7. Identify the primary ways the student communicates with others (receptive and expressive language skills).

8. Identify things staff should do and should not do in working with this student.

9. Identify what is reinforcing for the student.

10. Specify the history of the problem behavior and efforts to correct it.

11. Develop summary statements for each major predictor and consequence.

Note. From O'Neill et al. (1997). Copyright 1997 by Thomson Learning. Adapted by permission.

where the problem occurs, and identify antecedents and consequences. Summary statements are developed and changes that would promote the desired behavior are identified. A Student Daily Schedule (see Figure 3.1) is used to help students identify when they exhibit the problem behavior and rate the severity of the problem behaviors.

The functional assessment process can end after the interviews if the practitioner has a high level of confidence in his or her summary statements. For complex problem behaviors the preliminary summary statements should be validated and clarified with direct observation. The Functional Assessment Observation (FAO) form was designed for this purpose. It is used across multiple settings and times for low- to moderate-frequency behaviors (less than 20 times a day). A time sampling procedure is used for high-frequency behaviors. Data should be collected until clear patterns emerge (typically a minimum of 2–5 days and a minimum of 15–20 occurrences of the behavior). The FAO form is used to record observations (see Figure 3.2). The form is organized around "problem behavior events" which begin with a problem behavior and end after 3 minutes without a problem behavior. The observer records the problem behavior, its predictor or antecedents, perceived functions of the behavior (what the student is trying to obtain or avoid), and the actual consequences. The behaviors, predictors, and functions listed on the form are determined by the previous interviews and common factors identified in the literature.

If the interviews and direct observation do not reveal consistent patterns, functional analysis manipulations can be conducted. Functional analysis tests hypotheses concerning controlling factors by systematically varying environmental events and observing the effect on the targeted behavior. For example, if it is hypothesized that the problem behavior is brought on by frustration with assignments being too difficult, assignments can be modified and the resulting behavior observed.

Once the problem behavior, situation, and function are understood, this information is used to design interventions. This is accomplished by first identifying a desired behavior to replace the problem behavior. Then antecedents, consequences, and skills are identified that will promote the desired behavior. The consequences take into account the function of the problem behavior. For example, if the function of the problem behavior was to obtain peer attention, consequences for the appropriate behavior would involve peer attention.

Summary

Table 3.9 summarizes functional behavioral assessments, a form of assessment that is increasingly being used with children manifesting ACP in schools. While requiring much time, effort, and skill, these assessments can produce useful information for designing effective interventions.

Please place an "X" in each column to show the times and classes where you have difficulty with the behaviors we talked about. If you have a lot of difficulty during a period, place an "X" on or near the 6. If you have a little difficulty during the class or hall time, place the "X" on or near the 1. We can practice on a couple together before we start.

Subject, Teacher	Before School none	1st Period Reading Hall	Hall none	2nd Period Math Jones	Hall none	3rd Period Science Elliot	Hall none	4th Period P.E. Bendix	Lunch none	5th Period Social Studies Smith	Hall none	6th Period Music Best	Hall none	7th Period Study Hall Ogan	Hall none	8th Period Special Matthew	After School none
Most Difficult 6				X													
5		X								X						X	
4			X		X		X	X			X	X	X				
3									X					X	X		
2						X											
Least Difficult 1	X																X

FIGURE 3.1. Student Daily Schedule. From O'Neill et al. (1997). Copyright 1997 by Thomson Learning. Reprinted by permission.

Name: *Yolanda M.*

Starting Date: *1/30/96* Ending Date: *2/1/96*

Functional Assessment Observation form with the following structure (rotated on page):

Time	Behaviors					Predictors							Perceived Functions									Actual Conseq.	Comments (if nothing happened in period, write initials)
	Yelling	*Desks*	*Hit Teacher*	*Hit Peer*	*Demand/Request*	*Difficult Task*	*Transitions*	*Interruption*	*Alone (no attention)*	*Problem Peers*	*Math Group*	*Don't Know*	Attention	Desired Item/Activity	Self-Stimulation	Demand/Request	Activity ( )	Person	*Other/Don't Know*	*Verbal Redirect*	*Sent to Corner*	
8:15 Open	1 5		5					1 5				1 5	1 5							1 5	1 5	R.O.
8:45 Reading																						R.O.
9:45 Science			2	3								2							2		2	R.O.
10:45 Math	6 3 6 9	3	10					10		3 6 9						3 6 9			3 6 9	1 5		R.O.
11:45 Lunch								10				10	10						10	10		V.K.
12:30 Story Group			7					7				7	7						7	7		V.K.
1:30 Seat Work	4 8							4 8				4 8	4 8						8			#4 Ignored V.K.
2:30 Art	11							11				11	11						11	11		V.K.
Totals	6 3		2 3	3																		
Events:	1 2 3 4 5	6 7 8 9	10 11 12 13 14 15 16 17 18 19 20 21 22 23 24 25																			
Date:	1/30 1/31 2/1																				

FIGURE 3.2. Functional Assessment Observation form. From O'Neill et al. (1997). Copyright 1997 by Thomson Learning. Reprinted by permission.

110

SCREENING FOR AGGRESSION
AND CONDUCT PROBLEMS

Screening refers to a universally applied assessment procedure used to identify children who are at risk or experiencing difficulties. Screening methods are briefer and more economical than comprehensive assessments. They are used to identify children for early intervention services. It is commonly recommended that intervention begin early in the development of ACP (Mulvey, Arthur, & Reppucci, 1993; Yoshikawa, 1994; Zigler, Taussig, & Black, 1992). For this to happen there must be effective methods of screening for ACP. Universal interventions preclude the need for screening. However, given limited resources, there is a need to focus more intense interventions on those who are experiencing problems or who are likely to experience problems in the future.

Screening Procedures

Screening procedures for ACP identify the presence of the risk factors discussed in Chapter 2. The manifestation of early forms of ACP is a commonly used factor. Other risk factors used include problems in social functioning and ineffective parenting practices. Information is obtained from teachers, parents, children, and independent observers.

A common approach used for screening for children with ACP is the "multiple-gating" approach. This involves a less expensive and less time-

TABLE 3.9. Functional Behavioral Assessments in Schools

When to use functional behavioral assessments

- Problem behaviors have not responded to interventions.
- Behaviors are severe or violent.
- There is a complex relationship among problem behaviors and controlling factors.

Procedures for functional behavioral assessment

- Information is collected from child, teachers, and parents with interviews, questionnaires, and rating scales.
- Information is integrated by describing the problem behavior, the situation, and the likely function the behavior serves.
- If uncertainty remains, direct observation is used to better understand the relationship among factors.
- If the relationship among the controlling factors is still unclear, functional analysis manipulations are utilized to clarify how variables are affecting the problem behavior.
- Based on the obtained information, interventions are designed to promote the desired behavior using antecedents, consequences, and skill-building.

consuming assessment procedure being applied to all the children in a group (e.g., all children referred to a clinic or all kindergartners in a school). Only those children identified as being at risk in the first "gate" go on to the next level of assessment.

Multiple-gating approaches used in research, clinical, and school settings have been described (August, Realmuto, Crosby, & MacDonald, 1995; Charlebois, Leblanc, Gagnon, & Larivee, 1994; Feil, Walker, Severson, & Ball, 2000; Lochman & Conduct Problems Prevention Research Group, 1995; Walker, Colvin, & Ramsey, 1995). The screening procedures generally involve two or three levels or gates. A simple two-gate procedure described by Walker and colleagues (1995) involves teachers nominating up to five children who consistently display antisocial behavior (behavioral examples are provided to teachers). Children identified using this first gate are rated by teachers on the Aggression Scale of the Achenbach Teacher Report Form. If a child's score is two or more standard deviations above the mean, the child is referred for services for antisocial behavior.

Lochman and the Conduct Problems Prevention Research Group (1995) described a three-gate procedure. The first stage involved teachers completing the Teacher Observation of Classroom Adaptation—Revised (Werthamer-Larsson, Kellam, & Wheeler, 1991). The second stage consisted of parents responding to 24 items on externalizing behavior selected from various checklists. For the third gate parents completed the Parenting Practices Screen, a questionnaire assessing parenting practices. The first two gates were found to be effective, but the parenting practices screen was not helpful for increasing the effectiveness of prediction.

Accuracy of Screening Procedures for Aggression and Conduct Problems

Accurate screening is an important factor in the success of targeted interventions, yet the screening of young children for ACP has not achieved high levels of accuracy (Bennett et al., 1999; Bennett, Lipman, Racine, & Offord, 1998). For example, the Lochman and Conduct Problems Prevention Research Group (1995) screening procedure identified only 50% of the children who eventually met their criteria for problem outcomes at the end of first grade. Prediction of future ACP is made difficult by the high base rate for behavior problems in young boys and the fact that the factors that best predict behavior problems vary by age, the criteria predicted, and the characteristics of the sample (Kazdin, 1995).

The accuracy of screening procedures can be determined in different ways (Derzon, 2001). Positive-predictive value (PPV) refers to the proportion of children identified as being at risk that go on to develop ACP. By increasing the stringency of the requirements to be labeled at risk, the PPV is increased. This also increases the number of children who are labeled as not being at risk, yet go on to develop ACP (i.e., false-negative classification). A high false-negative rate results in many children who would have benefited from the intervention not receiving services.

A second type of accuracy is sensitivity, or the proportion of children who develop ACP who are correctly identified as being at risk. Relaxing the requirements to be considered at risk will increase a procedure's sensitivity. However, this will also increase the number of children inaccurately identified as being at risk (i.e., false-positive classification). This results in children being needlessly exposed to the potential negative effects of labeling and resources being used in an inefficient manner.

In selecting/designing screening procedures, practitioners balance the demands for a high level of sensitivity with those for a high PPV. They must identify which form of accuracy best meets their needs. If resources are limited, an effort may be made to increase the PPV of the procedure to increase the probability that those receiving services actually need them (i.e., reduce false positives). If there are sufficient resources and the goal is to intervene with all children at risk for a certain problem (e.g., violent behavior), efforts should be focused on increasing the sensitivity of the screening procedure (i.e., reducing false negatives).

Summary

Table 3.10 summarizes screening procedures used to identify children at risk for ACP behaviors. Current procedures are only moderately successful

---

TABLE 3.10. Screening for Aggression and Conduct Problems

Multiple-gating procedures

- A relatively brief and inexpensive procedure for identifing children at risk for ACP.
- An initial screening procedure, or "gate," is applied universally.
- Those who are identified by the first procedure go through a second, usually more involved, screening procedure.
- Generally two or three "gates" are used.

Accuracy of screening procedures

- Current procedures have not achieved a high level of accuracy in screening for ACP.
- Relaxing the criteria for inclusion results in reduced false-negative and increased false-positive identification (high sensitivity).
- Increasing criteria for inclusion results in reduced false-positive and increased false-negative identification (high positive-predictive value).
- Type of accuracy desired influenced by the goal of the screening and the availability of resources.

---

at identifying children who will exhibit ACP behavior in the future. However, they provide sufficient accuracy to assist in identifying children in need of preventive or early interventions.

CONCLUSION

The assessment of children with ACP is the first step in providing effective services. Through the use of multiple methods, multiple informants, and information from multiple settings, data is gathered that is needed to design/ select effective interventions. This includes clear definitions of the problem behaviors, descriptions of functioning in multiple areas, and delineation of risk and protective factors. The assessment identifies targets for interventions and protective factors that can be utilized in addressing concerns. Having identified targets for interventions, the next step is to provide effective interventions. In the following chapters we describe best practices for interventions, targeting the factors identified through the assessment process.

PART III

CHILD AND FAMILY INTERVENTIONS

CHAPTER 4

Social Competence Training

Social competence training (SCT) refers to child-focused skills training procedures that enhance children's social-emotional competence (Beelman, Pfingsten, & Losel, 1994). In this chapter, SCT refers to training procedures that attempt to enhance many areas of children's social and emotional adaptation. Therefore SCT includes behavioral social skills training, social-cognitive training, and emotional skills training, as well as environmentally based strategies that support children's social and emotional skills development. The SCT methods we discuss in this chapter are used primarily with children who exhibit ACP, as well as with children manifesting hyperactivity/impulsivity.

We hypothesize that SCT reduces risk factors and promotes protective factors primarily in the child and social/peer life domains (see Tables 2.3 and 2.4 in Chapter 2). In particular, SCT diminishes the behaviors associated with ACP and influences the development of social, emotional, and self-regulation skills, thereby potentially leading to more adaptive social interactions and affiliations.

This chapter is divided into three main sections. We begin by presenting an overview and research evaluation of the SCT literature. Next we discuss the common delivery methods that are used to teach children the skills involved in SCT. Finally, we present typical content of what children actually learn in SCT. We also provide examples of different procedures and content.

OVERVIEW AND RESEARCH EVALUATION
OF SOCIAL COMPETENCE TRAINING

SCT for children manifesting ACP targets several relevant areas (Beelman et al., 1994; Crick & Dodge, 1994; Dumas et al., 1994; Kazdin, 1996a;

Lochman & Lenhart, 1993; McFadyen-Ketchum & Dodge, 1998). One target is reducing children's aggressive/disruptive behavior such as yelling, pushing, arguing, and butting in line. Another target is increasing children's prosocial interaction behaviors such as entering a group, starting a conversation, participating in activities, sharing, cooperating, asking questions, and listening. Still another target is correcting the cognitive deficiencies and distortions exhibited by many children with ACP. A final target includes ameliorating emotion regulation and self-control problems to reduce emotional lability, impulsivity, and inaccurate self-evaluation in children with ACP. There is considerable overlap across the four target areas; in actual practice SCT usually focuses on all of them simultaneously. Once these target areas have been improved, the child's social development should progress in a more normative or resilient fashion.

A variety of SCT interventions have been developed to improve children's functioning in the four target areas (Beelman et al., 1994; Bierman, Greenberg, & Conduct Problems Prevention Research Group, 1996; Greenberg, Kusche, Cook, & Quamma, 1995; Guevremont, 1990; Guevremont & Foster, 1993; Kazdin, 1996a; Prinz, Blechman, & Dumas, 1994; Webster-Stratton, 1996b). One category of intervention, based on operant behavioral techniques, reduces interfering behaviors in children such as hitting, name calling, and "bugging" others. Another category of interventions teaches children social behavior skills such as participating, joining a group, conversing, playing fair, cooperating, sharing, and communicating better (e.g., asking questions, listening to others). Still another category of interventions teaches children to use adaptive thinking skills such as perspective taking, situation interpretation, self-monitoring, verbal self-instructions, and problem solving. A final category of interventions teaches children to better understand/express their feelings and to control strong emotions such as anger or stress. Most SCT intervention models incorporate most or all of these different interventions. SCT methods have also evolved in recent years to include parental and teacher involvement in the training process.

Research reveals that SCT brings about improvements in the functioning of children with ACP. Contingency management interventions that reinforce prosocial behaviors and punish aggressive behaviors do modify children's behaviors in the training setting, but have little generalizable effect on their behavior outside sessions (McFadyen-Ketchum & Dodge, 1998). Yet most practitioners agree that external behavioral management is essential in conducting SCT with aggressive and disruptive children (Kendall & Braswell, 1993). When children are taught adaptive social behavior skills, their aggressive behavior declines and their adaptive social behavior increases (Bierman & Furman, 1984; Bierman, Miller, & Stabb, 1987; Prinz et al., 1994; Webster-Stratton & Hammond, 1997). These social behavior interventions are more powerful if combined with cooperative peer activities and/or with behavior management of children's misbehavior in the training sessions (Bierman & Furman, 1984; Bierman et al., 1987). Interventions that attempt to modify the way impulsive children and children with ACP think reduces hostile attribution biases (Hudley et al., 1998; Hudley & Graham, 1993), improves perspective-taking skills (Chandler, 1973; Urbain & Kendall, 1980), enhances self-monitoring abilities (Hinshaw, Henker, & Whalen, 1984a, 1984b), and enables children to use self-statements to control their behavior (Kendall & Braswell, 1993; Kendall, Reber, McLeer, Epps, & Ronan, 1990). In particular, Kazdin and colleagues found that problem-solving training improves aggressive/antisocial children's behavior in both school and home settings, with improvements maintained for 1 year (see Kazdin, 1996a, for a review). Training of children in emotional awareness, self-control, and problem solving has resulted in greater feeling expression/fluency, improved frustration tolerance, and better social relationships in school (Greenberg et al., 1995). Finally, "anger coping" interventions that combine anger management and social problem solving improve children's social problem-solving skills and reduce their disruptive behavior in school settings, with behavioral improvements maintained at 7-month follow-up and low substance use rates at 3-year follow-up (Lochman & Lenart, 1993; Lochman & Wells, 1996).

The Section on Child Clinical Psychology (Division of Clinical Psychology) of the American Psychological Association evaluated various interventions used with children and designated them as either "well established" (similar to proven) or "probably efficacious" (similar to promising) (see Lonigan, Elbert, & Johnson, 1998, for a discussion of the criteria). As part of this effort, Brestan and Eyberg (1998) examined numerous studies evaluating treatments designed specifically for children with ODD and/or CD. Brestan and Eyberg determined that problem-solving skills (Kazdin, Esveldt-Dawson, French, & Unis, 1987a, 1987b; Kazdin, Siegel, & Bass, 1992) and anger-coping training interventions (Lochman, Burch, Curry, & Lampron, 1984; Lochman, Lampron, Gemmer, & Harris, 1989) are probably efficacious SCT interventions with school-age children. These intervention protocols have been subjected to rigorous evaluation to support their efficacy.

Although the literature reviewed above suggests that SCT has efficacy, this positive view needs to be tempered by the conclusions of Taylor, Eddy, and Biglan (1999) in their examination of the SCT literature specifically applied to children with ACP. Taylor and colleagues reviewed 19 studies that (1) reported intervention results on measures of aggression/antisocial behavior, (2) used a randomized/controlled design, and (3) were published in peer-reviewed journals. Using these criteria, Taylor and colleagues identified one study with preschool children, 15 studies with school-age children, and three studies with adolescents. They found SCT interventions were "moderately" effective, but of "limited" value in and of themselves. According to Taylor and colleagues, most studies obtained short-term statistical improvements, but provided little evidence of long-term clinically significant effects. Taylor and colleagues concluded that SCT should only be used as part of a more comprehensive approach that includes evidence-based parent, family, and classroom interventions.

Another limitation we have observed in current research is the lack of attention to ACP subtypes. There are few SCT interventions specified for subtypes of ACP (e.g., SCT for relational aggression). Studies examining the usefulness of SCT protocols with ACP subtypes (e.g., problem-solving training with relationally aggressive children) are also rare. Research evaluating SCT applied to different ACP subtypes is needed.

To summarize, there are differences in the conclusions reached by researchers as to the utility of SCT for children with ACP. Many researchers have found that SCT improves the functioning of children with ACP, but the magnitude of such changes is not always clear. Taylor and colleagues (1999) suggested that SCT by itself will have limited utility in reducing ACP-related behaviors and enhancing development. In view of the research findings, we agree with Taylor and colleagues that SCT should be used as one component of an overall comprehensive intervention with children that have ACP (see Chapter 11 for a discussion of multicomponent interventions).

BEST PRACTICE MODELS FOR
SOCIAL COMPETENCE TRAINING

We selected nine SCT models for preschool- and school-age children with ACP and ADHD to derive best practices. These SCT models have been extensively evaluated and have demonstrated utility in improving the developmental status of children with ACP (see citations below for details). We integrate common practices across these models and highlight specific procedures. The nine SCT model programs include (1) Bierman and colleagues' (Bierman & Furman, 1984; Bierman et al., 1987, 1996) social skills training; (2) Webster-Stratton and colleagues' (Webster-Stratton, 1996b; Webster-Stratton & Hammond, 1997) Dinosaur School program for young children; (3) Prinz and colleagues' (Prinz et al., 1994) Peer Coping training; (4) Greenberg and colleagues' (Greenberg et al., 1995) Promoting Alternative Thinking Strategies (PATHS); (5) Hudley and colleagues' (Hudley, 1994; Hudley et al., 1998; Hudley & Graham, 1993) BrainPower attributional retraining program; (6) Hinshaw and colleagues' (Hinshaw, 2000; Hinshaw et al., 1984a, 1984b) self-monitoring training; (7) Kendall and colleagues' (Kendall & Braswell, 1993; Kendall et al., 1990) verbal self-instruction training; (8) Kazdin and colleagues' (Kazdin, 1996a; Kazdin et al., 1987a, 1987b) problem-solving skills training; and (9) Lochman and colleagues' (Lochman, Lampron, Gemmer, & Harris, 1987; Lochman & Lenart, 1993; Lochman & Wells, 1996; Lochman, Whidby, & FitzGerald, 2000) Anger Coping program. The rest of this chapter describes the best practices for SCT from these models. Braswell and Bloomquist's practice model for SCT will also be occasionally reviewed to elaborate standard procedures (Bloomquist, 1996; Braswell & Bloomquist, 1991).

BEST PRACTICE DELIVERY PROCEDURES FOR SOCIAL COMPETENCE TRAINING

Our focus in this section is on how the practitioner delivers or conducts the SCT intervention. Discussion includes the methods used by the practitioner to convey information and teach skills to children. We discuss the content of the SCT interventions later in the chapter.

Practitioner Characteristics

Effective practitioners are able to form positive relationships with children and maintain a position of authority when conducting SCT. The practitioner should be enthusiastic, outgoing, and use humor to establish rapport with children. At the same time the practitioner will need to be firm and provide limits as needed. The balance between building rapport and establishing a sense of authority can be a challenge. In our experience, those practitioners who emphasize one over the other are less effective.

It is also necessary that practitioners have proficiency in the application of SCT with children manifesting ACP. It is very important that practitioners are extensively trained prior to delivering SCT, and that less experienced practitioners are supervised throughout its implementation. Practitioners should strive to conduct SCT according to best practices (discussed below).

Training Methods

Typically four to eight children meet with two practitioners in a small-group setting. Often one practitioner uses methods to "manage" the behavior of the children, while the other delivers the SCT content. Both practitioners need to be actively involved in interacting with all of the children in the group and to provide them with feedback about their behavior.

The composition of group membership should be carefully considered. Most SCT models recommend that children in a group be no more than 2 years apart in age. With younger preschool children, it is best to have same-gender groups if possible. As children grow older, mixed-gender groups are effective. In our experience, it is ill-advised to conduct an SCT group comprised of only severely aggressive children. Too many children with severe problems can make it too challenging to conduct the group. The practitioners might end up spending most of their group time managing the aggressive and oppositional behaviors of children rather than teaching SCT skills. We recommend that each group be composed of children with a range of problem severity (from mild to severe).

Many practitioners advocate enrolling "normal" peers in SCT groups. These normal peers can be involved in the skills training interventions and/or serve as "buddies" in supervised structured dyadic cooperative activities. Normal peers can function as role models of prosocial behavior. There is also the potential for new affiliations to develop between children with ACP and prosocial children. Involvement of normal peers has been found to be beneficial for aggressive children as well as for the normal peers (Prinz et al., 1994).

Practitioners use behavioral training methods in conducting SCT with children. Skills are taught using instruction, modeling, role playing, practice, feedback, and reinforcement methods. Practitioners promote and reinforce the application of skills throughout the sessions. Practice of skills is facilitated through games and activities. Coping with actual problems that emerge within the group can also be a useful training task. For example, if two children have a conflict or the group cannot agree on what to do, the SCT skills can be used to solve these "real-life" social problems. Homework assignments are given to children so that they can practice using their skills outside of the training situation.

Guevremont's (1990) summary of behavioral instructional techniques used in teaching SCT skills is similar to those espoused in the best practice models:

1. Introduce the skill.
2. Verbally instruct the children about the skill (e.g., listening with good eye contact).
3. Model the skill for the children to observe. Typically a "bad" model (e.g., listening with poor eye contact) is contrasted with a "good" model (e.g., listening with good eye contact).
4. Practitioner role-plays with a child to demonstrate the skill.
5. Children perform role plays with each other to demonstrate the skill. It can be helpful to videotape these role plays.
6. Practitioner continues to coach, model, discuss, and provide feedback to the children regarding skill acquisition.
7. Role-play videos are reviewed and discussed. Practitioner offers feedback and additional instruction to the children.
8. The skill is summarized.
9. A homework assignment is given so the child can utilize the skill outside the group-training situation.

These instructional techniques are repeated with each new skill (we review specific skill areas below). Practitioners evaluate children's performance of the skill in role plays and in practice situations to determine whether or not they have mastered the skill. Once mastery is achieved, a new social behavioral skill is introduced for training.

Most SCT programs require children to demonstrate mastery of skills in the training situation before moving on to additional skills. This means that the practitioner has judged a particular child as having incorporated a skill into his or her repertoire. Sometimes different children in the same group master the skills at a different pace. If that occurs, it may be necessary to move ahead with the group content, but pause to review particular skills with those children who are struggling with their mastery.

Behavior Management

Most SCT programs incorporate behavioral management techniques into the group training process. Behavior management serves several purposes. First, it makes the group training process more feasible. Conducting group training with very active and potentially disruptive children can be challenging. Behavior management brings some order into the training situation. Second, behavior management can assist an individual child. It is helpful for a child's aggressive, defiant, hyperactive/impulsive behaviors to be brought under control so that he or she can be more receptive to learning new skills. Behavior management brings some order to the child's behavior and allows the child to acquire new skills.

One method of behavior management is to employ group rules. The group rules are often created during the first session with input from the children. These rules might include no hitting, raise your hand before speaking, maintain confidentiality (e.g., "what's said in group stays in group"), and so on. The practitioner should write down these rules and refer to them as needed to remind the children.

A token or point system is also recommended for use in SCT groups. Usually tokens are used for younger children (under age 8) and points are used for older children. Children can earn tokens or points for exhibiting specified behaviors. For example, they receive tokens/points for following directions, sharing, or employing the new social skill that day (e.g., problem solving). Some SCT programs use a response–cost technique in which children lose tokens/points for incorrect performance of the skills being trained or for disruptive behavior. For example, they lose tokens/points for noncompliance with directions, aggressive behavior, or interrupting others. The practitioner shapes children's behavior by verbally informing them when they have earned or lost tokens/points. The earned tokens/points can be traded in at the end of the session for small tangible rewards/privileges or can be "banked" (saved) over sessions to save up for bigger rewards/

privileges. Often the token/point system is gradually faded out over the sessions so children rely on them less and less as they learn new skills. Practitioners need to use their own judgment as to how children are progressing to determine if and when the token/point system is faded out.

A "strike" system can be used to manage behavior that cannot be brought under control using rules and tokens/points. It involves children receiving up to three verbal warnings (i.e., strikes) about their noncompliant and aggressive behavior. If a child receives a third warning (strike), he or she has "struck out" and must leave the group for the remainder of that session. The child is readmitted to the next session and allowed to participate in group.

Figure 4.1 is an example of a group points chart that incorporates points and strikes. The practitioner keeps track of the children's behavior and administers points and strikes accordingly. This particular example tracks general "positive" and "negative" behaviors. This allows the practitioner to shape unique behaviors in each child attending the group. For example, one child could be shaped for sharing, while another could be shaped for raising hands before speaking. Another option is to alter the group points chart to indicate *specific* positive behaviors such as sharing, following directions, or asking questions and specific negative behaviors such as disobeying adults, hitting, or name calling. In a similar fashion, points would be gained or lost for the specific behaviors. This specific approach allows the practitioner to shape certain behaviors in all of the children.

Time-out is often effective with mild-to-moderate forms of aggressive/defiant/disruptive behavior. This procedure entails the practitioner giving the child a command (directive), followed by a warning if the child is noncompliant with the command, followed by putting the child in a time-out area or taking away a privilege if he or she does not comply after the warning. Time-out is described in more detail in Chapter 5.

The structure and content of the group sessions need to be delivered in an engaging and fun way to reduce the likelihood of disruptive behavior in children. The presentation of session content and materials should be well paced. Structure is essential so that group norms and procedures are established and repeated each session. For example, a routine for each session might include "checking in," introducing a new skill, practicing a new skill, cleaning up, having snacks, and doing a fun activity. Interesting games, activities, and videos keep children involved and out of mischief.

Number of Sessions

Approximately 18–22 weekly sessions lasting 40–120 minutes each are employed in many SCT programs. The exact number of training sessions and the length of the sessions vary across each of the best practice model pro-

Date: _____

Child's name	Points earned (1 point for positive behavior and for using problem solving when reminded, 2 points for using problem solving without being reminded)	Points lost (for mild disruptive behavior)	Strikes (circle)	Total points (summary of points earned minus points lost)
1. Latoya	|||||||||||	|||	① 2 3	9
2. Michael	|||||||||	||	1 2 3	7
3. Malcolm	|||||||||||||||	|||||	① ② 3	10
4. Alisha	||||||||||||	|	1 2 3	11
5. Jordan	|||||||||||		1 2 3	11
6. Maria	|||||||||||||||	||	① 2 3	13
7.				
8.				

FIGURE 4.1. Group points chart. From Braswell and Bloomquist (1991). Copyright 1991 by The Guilford Press. Adapted by permission.

grams. Our experience has taught us that fewer and shorter sessions may be indicated for younger children learning a few skills, whereas more and longer sessions may be needed for older children who are being exposed to more skills training areas. Practitioners need to use their own judgment to decide the number and length of sessions.

Three to six sessions are typically devoted to any one specific content area. For example, four sessions might be devoted to learning specific social behaviors such as starting conversations, sharing, and maintaining eye contact, while six more sessions might be used to teach an anger management module. Obviously the main goal is for children to master the new skills they are learning. The number of sessions necessary to achieve mastery will vary for different children. Practitioners need to use their judgment to specify how many sessions will be needed to teach specific skills to a given group of children.

Training Materials and Games

Effective use of training materials enhances the delivery of SCT. Certain training materials aid in skill presentation. Puppets can be used to present information to children, to instruct them, to model skill use, and so forth. Puppets are particularly engaging for younger children. A picture stimulus that depicts the skill being taught (e.g., a picture of children sharing) can be shown to children to illustrate a skill and elicit discussion. Similarly, video modeling, in which children view videos of other children engaged in problematic situations or using specific SCT skills, can be useful. These videos serve as a stimulus for discussion and also function as a model for the skills being taught. Webster-Stratton (1996b), for example, produced over 100 video vignettes depicting children in different social situations and using a variety of SCT skills.

Training materials also facilitate children's practice of skills they are learning. For example, when learning problem-solving, games such as "problem-solving recognition charades" (Braswell & Bloomquist, 1991) help children continue to learn how to recognize problems. A "TV talk show" game (Guevremont, 1990) helps children practice conversational skills by taking turns being a "host" and a "guest" on a pretend TV talk show. Other games, skits, and activities that match the skills being taught can be developed by the practitioner to further the training process.

Many practitioners use charts and related training materials to facilitate skill usage outside the training situation. For example, a "problem-solving steps" chart might be given to children to take home to share with their parents, who in turn use it to prompt them to use the skill at home. Practitioners can design their own charts to fit the unique training content of the group of children being served.

Other games can be used to facilitate cooperation and sharing. Cooperative board and physical games have been found to increase cooperation among preschool children (Bay-Hintz, Peterson, & Quilitch, 1994). Teamwork activities, such as constructing a group poster, are useful to help children learn to work together. Practitioners can facilitate training of other social skills by creating other games or activities.

Making Adjustments According
to Children's Developmental Level

All SCT models advocate adjusting procedures and content to match the developmental level of the children being served. A general rule of thumb is to make the interventions more concrete and to rely more on environmental support when using SCT with younger children. For example, younger children can be taught how to solve problems. To do this, however, the practitioner should rely less on verbal didactic training and incorporate more games and role playing. It is especially important for adults to encourage, prompt, and reinforce younger children in the use of newly learned skills outside of the training situation.

Promoting Generalization and Maintenance

One goal of SCT is for children to use the skills they are taught in "real-life" situations. Careful use of specific training procedures will promote generalization. Children should learn and then practice skills with a variety of training tasks. For example, in training problem-solving skills, hypothetical problems are used to introduce and practice problem-solving skill application. Later, children bring in real-life examples of social problems, which can become the basis of a role-play exercise. After a while, problem-solving skills might be used to solve the actual problems that emerge between children while participating in the group. Other skills can also be taught and practiced using a variety of training tasks and situations.

After SCT has been completed, it is useful to have children come back into a training situation periodically for booster or follow-up sessions. If this cannot be arranged, it may be helpful to have long-term follow-up with an individual child and family for booster training. The follow-up provides the practitioner with the opportunity to determine if the newly acquired skills have been maintained and to plan further interventions if indicated.

Social Competence Training with Parent and Teacher Involvement

Parents are typically involved in SCT in one of two ways. The first method entails simultaneously training children in SCT and parents in parent management interventions (like those discussed in Chapter 5). The second method involves training parents to guide their children in using the skills they are learning in SCT. In other words, parents can be involved in learning to manage their children's disruptive behaviors and also in assisting them to use new social skills at home.

Practitioners need to make sure that the home and school environments are prepared to support the newly acquired skills that children have learned through SCT. Providing charts, handouts, or manuals to parents and teachers, for example, on how to prompt, remind, and reinforce the application of skills in the home and school environments would achieve this goal. Bloomquist (1996), for example, wrote a parent-focused instruction guide that explains different procedures and provides numerous charts to aid implementation of various SCT-related skills in the home environment. Figure 4.2 is an example of a worksheet that could be used by parents to promote social skills use at home.

Summary

Table 4.1 summarizes the best practices for the delivery of SCT. This table provides a list of key procedures that need to be incorporated in SCT. We recommend that practitioners use all of the delivery procedures to ensure that an effective SCT program is delivered to children with ACP.

BEST PRACTICE TRAINING CONTENT AREAS FOR SOCIAL COMPETENCE TRAINING

In this section we focus on what children learn during SCT. We break the training content down into specific skill areas. Children are trained in these specific skills using the training methods just reviewed.

Social Behavior and Communication Skills Training

All SCT programs provide for direct instruction and coaching of children to promote development of overt social behaviors. These social behaviors include helping, sharing, taking turns, starting conversations, expressing feelings, asking questions, listening to others, ignoring, complementing, talking briefly, working as a member of a team, being assertive, apologizing, accepting apologies, and so on. Usually an attempt is made to individualize the exact skills taught to match the skills deficits of the children receiving social behavioral skills training. In other words, the practitioner chooses the social behavior skills that are most important to work on for a particular child or group of children. The practitioner uses instructing, modeling, role playing, and practicing to teach children each skill.

Children can also be taught social behavioral communication skills through the Prinz and colleagues (1994) Peer Coping skills intervention. In this program, children learn to effectively express their thoughts, feelings, and experiences to other children. They learn nonverbal communication skills, such as maintaining eye contact and how to display appropriate affect, that is, affect that matches the content of what they are saying. The children also learn to listen to others. They learn to summarize what the other person is saying, ask questions, use good eye contact, remain silent until the speaker is finished, and show appropriate affect while listening. The Prinz and colleagues protocol also incorporates teaching children behavioral self-regulation and problem-solving strategies.

In Peer Coping skills training, children are exposed to a series of "probe challenges" as training tasks to learn the social information ex-

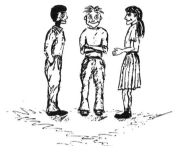

Name: _Tony_

Date: _Saturday_

Directions: The parent and/or child can complete the form, but all involved should discuss it. Complete Steps 1 and 2 before the social event and Steps 3, 4, and 5 after the social event.

Before Social Event

1. **I will work on these social behavior goals:**

   Speaking to other children and making eye contact.

2. **When and where I will work on the social behavior goals** (designate time and place):

   Saturday morning at baseball practice.

After Social Event

3. **How well did I accomplish my social behavior goal?** (circle one)

1	2	3	④	5
Not at all	A little	OK	Pretty good	Great
☹		☺		☺

4. **What did I do that tells me how to rate myself?** (Write down how you know you deserve the above rating.)

   I talked to Chris and Steve about the next game. I looked into their eyes when I talked to them. I asked Mr. Jackson to throw some balls to me. I looked into his eyes, too.

5. **If my parent agrees with my rating and it is a 3, 4, or 5, I get this reward:**

   Pizza for supper.

FIGURE 4.2. Practicing social behavior skills. From Bloomquist (1996). Copyright 1996 by The Guilford Press. Reprinted by permission.

TABLE 4.1. Summary of Best Practice Delivery Procedures for Social Competence Training

Delivery procedure	Best practices
Practitioner characteristics	Establish relationships, provide structure, display enthusiasm, follow standardized protocols.
Training methods	Carefully compose small groups and include "normal" peers; use instruction, modeling, role plays, practice, feedback, reinforcement, and homework.
Behavior management	Use group rules, token/point systems, time-out; provide structure and routines.
Number of sessions	Approximately 18–22 40- to 120-minute weekly sessions are needed to deliver an SCT intervention program; typically three to six sessions are needed to teach each content skill area.
Training materials and games	Use picture stimulus cards, videos, games, and charts to promote skill acquisition and practice.
Making adjustments according to children's developmental level	Incorporate more concrete training methods and environmental support for younger children.
Promoting generalization and maintenance	Vary training tasks, prepare natural environment to prompt and reinforce skills, and use "booster" sessions.
Social competence training with parent and teacher involvement	Train parents in behavior management; provide instruction to parents and teachers so they can prompt, guide, and reinforce skills usage at home and at school.

change skills. Table 4.2 displays these probe challenges. Dyads are formed and coached in conducting conversations. The dyads are given instructions to center their conversations around these probes. An example listening probe is "Find out about something that worries your partner this week." An example speaking probe is "Tell your partner about something that hurt you this week." Probes are calibrated so that some are easy and others are more difficult. The children must achieve mastery over easy probes before going on to more difficult probes.

Children are trained to reach the "cumulative goals" for listener and speaker probes outlined in Table 4.3 while responding to the previously described probe challenges. These cumulative goals are concrete behaviors they learn to emit while developing information exchange skills. The practitioner trains children to gradually master these behaviors. Prinz and colleagues hypothesized that the Peer Coping intervention not only helps children learn concrete communication skills, but also enables them to learn an adaptive coping style for dealing with adversities in life.

Affective Education

Affective education, commonly used in SCT, is a first step in helping children learn to control their emotions and behaviors. Children are taught to understand and express their feelings. This is accomplished by increasing their "feelings vocabulary," the words they use to identify and express feelings. Figure 4.3 displays an example of a feelings vocabulary chart. Children are instructed to practice using feeling words to describe their feelings about their experiences. Some practitioners employ a Feelings

TABLE 4.2. Probe Challenges Used in Peer Coping Skills Training

1	L	Find out something that makes your partner special.
1	S	Tell your partner about something that makes you special.
2	L	Find out something that made your partner laugh this week.
2	S	Tell your partner about something that made you feel happy this week.
3	L	Find out about your partner's family.
3	S	Tell your partner something that you like about school this week.
4	L	Find out about something that your partner did really well this week.
4	S	Tell your partner what you want to be when you grow up.
5	L	Find out about something that made your partner feel excited this week.
5	S	Tell your partner about one of your heroes.
6	L	Find out about something your partner thinks is beautiful.
6	S	Tell your partner about something that made you feel angry this week.
7	L	Find out about something that made your partner feel peaceful and quiet this week.
7	S	Tell your partner about someone you love.
8	L	Find out about something that is hard for your partner to do.
8	S	Tell your partner about something that scared you this week.
9	S	Tell your partner about something that embarrassed you this week.
9	L	Find out something that made your partner angry this week.
10	L	Find out about something that made your partner sad this week.
10	S	Tell your partner about something that made you jealous this week.
11	L	Find out about something that worries your partner this week.
11	S	Tell your partner about something that hurt you this week.
12	L	Find out about something that annoyed your partner this week.

Note. L, listener probes; S, speaker probes. From Prinz, Blechman, and Dumas (1994). Copyright 1994 by Lawrence Erlbaum Associates. Reprinted by permission.

Diary in which children write down experiences they have and how they feel about them. A child might write down, for example, that he or she was teased by some children and felt sad and lonely, or got a good grade on a school assignment and felt joyful and satisfied. Practitioners can model feelings expression and guide children to identify and express their own feelings.

Social Perspective-Taking Training

The goal of social perspective-taking interventions is to help children learn to understand how others think and feel. They typically begin with discus-

TABLE 4.3. Cumulative Goals for Listener and Speaker Probes Used in Peer Coping Skills Training

Listener probes

1. Follows instructions.
2. Remains silent during speaker's statement.
3. Maintains appropriate eye contact with speaker.
4. Uses nonverbal gestures to show understanding/interest in speaker's statement.
5. Shows affect appropriate to speaker's statement.
6. Asks one question about speaker's statement using speaker's words.
7. Asks several questions about speaker's statement using speaker's words.
8. Summarizes one of speaker's statements using speaker's words.
9. Summarizes several of speaker's statements using speaker's words.
10. Asks whether his or her summary of speaker's statement is accurate.
11. Asks a question to clarify an aspect of speaker's statement that was not understood.
12. Asks a question that requires speaker to expand statement.

Speaker probes

1. Follows instructions.
2. Readily heard and understood.
3. Begins speaking within 5 seconds.
4. Shows affect appropriate to statement.
5. Uses eye contact and other nonverbal gestures to capture the interest of listener.
6. Makes a unique statement and does not duplicate what others have said.
7. Makes coherent, meaningful statements that are readily understood and make sense.
8. Conveys details sufficient to tell story with beginning, middle, and end.
9. Makes personal statements when telling his or her story.
10. Tells how he or she felt or feels about his or her story using appropriate words to describe the feelings.
11. Makes only genuine statements evidencing an ability to distinguish fact from fiction such that his or her total narrative seems credible.

Note. From Prinz, Blechman, and Dumas (1994). Copyright 1994 by Lawrence Erlbaum Associates. Reprinted by permission.

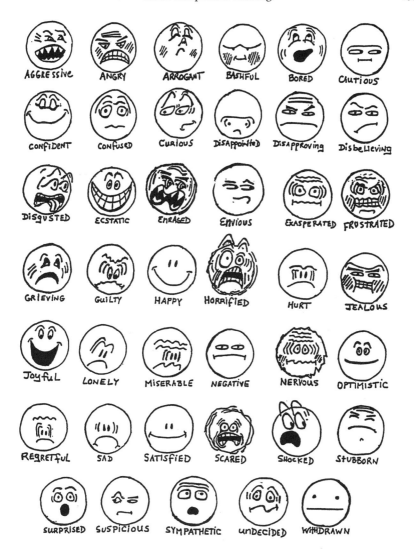

FIGURE 4.3. Feelings Vocabulary Chart. From Bloomquist (1996). Copyright 1996 by The Guilford Press. Reprinted by permission.

sions of others' thoughts and feelings in interpersonal situations. Practitioners present scenarios of social situations involving peers, teachers, and parents. These scenarios are often presented through picture stimulus cards or videos. For example, a picture stimulus might depict two children who want to use the same red crayon while they are coloring pictures, with one child using the crayon and the other looking at it. The group discusses the facial cues, body postures, and possible thoughts of the children depicted to determine the feelings of each child in the picture. Group members infer the thoughts and intentions of each child depicted in the scenario. Children are essentially taught to put themselves "in the other person's shoes."

Role-play exercises where children take turns acting out scenarios can be useful in training social perspective-taking skills. For example, children can act out the scenario involving the red crayon as described in the previous paragraph. During the middle of the role play the children stop to discuss their thoughts and feelings and what they perceive to be the thoughts and feelings of the other child. They switch roles halfway through the role-play exercise, act out the same scene again, stop again, and discuss their new role. Another technique involves videotaping the role-play scenarios and reviewing the videos later. While watching the videos, group members can talk about what they think others thought and felt.

Children can also be taught observable social behavior skills related to displaying empathy. To accomplish this, children are instructed to listen to others, express care and concern when others have hurt feelings, and engage in prosocial behavior such as sharing and helping. This intervention is similar to the communication skills training discussed earlier (Prinz et al., 1994). Children also discuss how good they feel inside by empathizing with and helping others.

Attribution Retraining

Attribution retraining focuses on remediating the hostile intent bias observed in many children with ACP. In the BrainPower program developed by Hudley (1994), aggressive school-age boys are engaged in a number of didactic, experiential, role-play, and homework experiences to learn to make accurate attributions for others' behavior. Children first learn a definition of intent such as "what someone meant to do." They discuss the consequences of making mistakes in determining others' intent and how such mistakes relate to the development of conflict between people. They learn to identify the intent of another person by examining the other person's facial expressions and their own feeling responses. Through discussion and role play, children learn to determine if someone did something to them on purpose, accidentally, or for some other possible reason. For example, social dilemmas are presented to children such as "A friend does not return a borrowed videogame." Children write down different explanations depicting hostile (e.g., "He's trying to steal it") or nonhostile (e.g., "He forgot") reasons for the other child's behavior. They discuss which one of the explanations might be the most likely one. They engage in discussion and role-play exercises about a variety of ambiguous situations and practice determining causes for them.

Other practitioners have incorporated similar procedures for attributional retraining. Braswell and Bloomquist (1991), for example, described "situation interpretation" training for school-age children. This involves determining the intent of other individuals in potential conflict situations. Children are educated about the tendency to "jump to conclusions" regarding others' behavior. They discuss the fact that sometimes people jump to conclusions without having satisfactory evidence to support those conclusions. They are trained to try to "find the evidence" to help them justify the conclusions that they reach. For example, children might discuss and then role-play getting bumped in the hallway by another child. They generate potential explanations for this behavior such as "he did it on purpose," "he slipped," or "he was pushed by someone else." Children learn to find the evidence, or "signals," that would justify any of these possible conclusions. This includes discussion of the facial expressions and the body postures of the individuals involved. They note the other person's reaction after the incident occurs. Eventually, the evidence is accumulated and examined so that an accurate attribution about the child who bumped into the other child can be made.

Braswell and Bloomquist also discussed a "Kids' Court" training exercise as an example of situation interpretation. This involves role-playing ambiguous conflictual situations and conducting a "trial." The child who receives the ambiguous provocation acts as both the "prosecuting and defense attorneys." The practitioner acts as "judge," and other group members act as the "jury." The child takes turns presenting the evidence to support the view of "he did it on purpose" or "he did it by accident." The judge and jury weigh the evidence, and finally make a decision regarding the "verdict." Through this process, children learn to examine evidence to justify the conclusions that they make regarding other peoples' behaviors and intentions. For example, the role play could center around one child spilling the milk of another child in the lunchroom at school. The trial could be used to determine if the child spilled the milk on purpose or for some other reason.

Self-Monitoring and Self-Evaluation Training

Enabling children to increase their self-awareness and to better observe themselves is the goal of self-monitoring and self-evaluation training. Hinshaw (2000) described a small-group training exercise to improve this skill in elementary school-age children. First, a social behavioral skill is introduced to the group—for example, paying attention, cooperating, or helping others. The children discuss the behavior extensively. They role-play positive and negative examples of the behavior until all the children know how to perform the behavior. Then they engage in tasks/activities that elicit the behavior (e.g., group members draw pictures with one box of crayons while working on sharing). Occasionally, practitioners will prompt children about the social behavior that they are working on for that session.

At different intervals during the meetings, children will stop and play the "Match Game." Figure 4.4 offers a Match Game chart. Two practitioners initially model the use of the Match Game. Later, each child "plays" the "game." It involves the child rating how he or she thinks the practitioner will evaluate him or her for working on a specified behavior (e.g., sharing) according to a scale of 1 (not at all good) to 5 (great). It is helpful for the child to explain why he or she thinks the practitioner will provide the anticipated rating. The practitioner then rates the child and explains his or her observations of the child's behavior to justify the practitioner's rating. Sometimes it is helpful to videotape and play back examples of behavior to the child so that he or she can learn to more accurately observe his or her own behavior. Points are awarded according to the practitioner rating. For example, 3 points are given to the child if the practitioner rates the child at a "3." To promote realistic self-appraisal, points are doubled if a match occurs. Accordingly, if the child and the practitioner both rate the child as a "3," he or she would earn 6 points.

Once the self-monitoring/self-evaluation skills have been learned, then procedures to promote generalization and maintenance are utilized. Initially, the Match Game is played several times a session, but eventually, as sessions progress, children play it only once per session. Eventually, they learn to utilize the Match Game procedure in home/school environments. Hinshaw argued that employing the Match Game with a variety of different behaviors, using it in multiple settings, and involving parents and teachers will enhance maintenance and generalization of this intervention.

Verbal Self-Instruction Training

Verbal self-instruction training helps children reflect on their behavior and use self-statements to guide and regulate it. Kendall and Braswell (1993) described verbal self-instruction training methods and procedures to train school-age children in using self-statements to guide their problem-solving efforts. The content of these self-statements is summarized in Table 4.4. Tasks are presented to children that allow them to apply and practice verbal self-instruction methods. For example, initially the tasks are impersonal, such as puzzles, matching tasks, games, mazes, mathematics problems, and so on. Eventually the tasks become more like "real life" and involve interpersonal problems and conflicts such as how to handle someone butting in line in front of you. Children role-play typical interpersonal problems that are initially supplied by the practitioner, but eventually use their own real-life problems. The children apply and practice the verbal self-instructions presented in Table 4.4 while performing these tasks.

The ultimate goal of verbal self-instruction training is for children to

The Match Game

name: ______________________________

date: ______________________________

working on:

____

1	2	3	4	5
NOT AT ALL GOOD	A LITTLE GOOD	OK	PRETTY GOOD	GREAT
______	______	______	______	______

FIGURE 4.4. Match Game used in self-monitoring/self-evaluation training. From Hinshaw (2000). Copyright 2000 by The Guilford Press. Reprinted by permission.

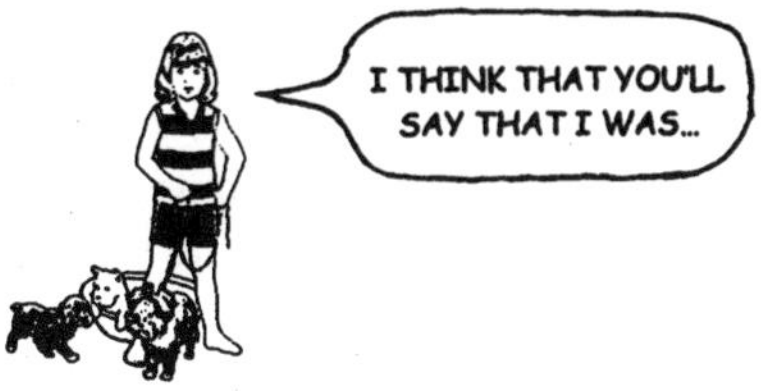

internalize the methodical self-statement sequence. This is accomplished by employing training experiences that allow them to gradually move from using the self-statements overtly to using them covertly. Table 4.5 summarizes the training steps involved in fading the self-instructions. The children continue to work on various tasks while using the self-statements in Table 4.4. The steps outlined in Table 4.5 are utilized to help children internalize the strategy.

Problem-Solving Skills Training

Problem-solving skills training targets the distorted/deficient cognitive processes characteristic of many children with ACP by teaching them interpersonal cognitive problem-solving and prosocial behavioral skills (Kazdin, 1996a). The intervention's main goal is to teach children how to think of the components of problems and learn how to solve them effectively. Children are trained to think and state a sequential set of problem-solving statements. Typically, the statements are presented so that the children are actually asking themselves questions and answering them so as to direct their own problem-solving efforts.

Figure 4.5 depicts an example of a problem-solving chart. It guides children to utilize seven steps to solve interpersonal problems. By going through these steps the child will recognize the problem (Step 1), interpret the situation (Step 2), determine another's perspective (Step 3), generate solutions (Step 4), think of consequences (Step 5), execute behavior (Step 6), and evaluate whether or not the "plan" worked (Step 7).

Children are taught to use problem-solving strategies with a variety of training tasks. Initially, they learn to utilize them with games and activities. Later they graduate to using problem-solving strategies for interpersonal problems involving peers, parents, siblings, and teachers. Initially, the problems are practitioner-derived. Eventually, the focus shifts to real-life problems that children bring to the training situation. This can be accomplished

TABLE 4.4. Content of Self-Instruction Procedures

Problem definition:	"Let's see, what am I supposed to do?"
Problem approach:	"I have to look at all the possibilities."
Focusing of attention:	"I better concentrate and focus in, and think only of what I'm doing right now."
Choosing an answer:	"I think it's this one . . . "
Self-reinforcement: or	"Hey, not bad. I really did a good job."
Coping statement:	"Oh, I made a mistake. Next time I'll try to go slower and concentrate more and maybe I'll get the right answer."

Note. From Kendall and Braswell (1993). Copyright 1993 by The Guilford Press, Philip C. Kendall, and Lauren Braswell. Reprinted by permission.

TABLE 4.5. Sequence of Fading Self-Instructions

1. The practitioner models task performance and talks out loud while the child observes.
2. The child performs the task, instructing him- or herself out loud (after sufficient practice).
3. The practitioner models task performance while whispering the self-instructions.
4. The practitioner performs the task using covert self-instructions with pauses and behavioral signs of thinking (e.g., stroking beard or chin).
5. The child performs the task using the self-instructional steps privately.

Note. From Kendall and Braswell (1993). Copyright 1993 by The Guilford Press, Philip C. Kendall, and Lauren Braswell. Reprinted by permission.

by solving actual problems that emerge as a result of children interacting together in the group. For example, two children may want to sit in the same chair. The practitioner could prompt the children to use the problem-solving steps to reach a satisfactory solution.

The sixth problem-solving step depicted in Figure 4.5 requires execution of specific behavior. Most problem-solving interventions therefore also involve the use of social behavioral skills training. Since many of these children have social behavioral skills deficits, they need to be trained how to implement the actual behaviors they think of in the process of solving problems.

Many problem-solving skills training protocols involve training within each of the component skill domains (e.g., problem recognition). For example, Braswell and Bloomquist (1991) described specific interventions to teach problem recognition, solution generation/consequential thinking, anticipating obstacles, and evaluating whether or not a solution works. To train problem recognition, they advise using games such as "problem recognition charades." During this game, children learn to recognize the signals or cues that tell them that a problem exists and then learn to interpret and define the problem. To learn solution generation/consequential thinking, children participate in brainstorming exercises in which they work to generate as many solutions to problems as possible, and then think about what would happen if the solutions were employed. To learn to anticipate obstacles, children participate in role-play exercises where their initial plans to solve a problem do not work and they need to "think on their feet" to deal with the obstacles. Evaluation of the effects of problem solving is also done through specific role-play exercises where children solve problems and think about whether or not they were effective in meeting their goals.

Anger Management Training

Children with ACP learn how to regulate emotions and behaviors through anger management training. Lochman and colleagues (1987, 2000) and Lochman and Wells (1996) articulated anger management procedures to

1. **Stop! What is the problem?**

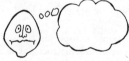

2. **Who or what caused the problem?**

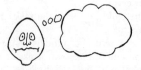

3. **What does each person think and feel?**

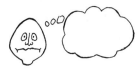

4. **What are some plans?**

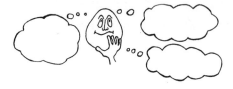

5. **What is the best plan?**

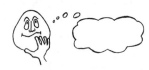

6. **Do the plan.**

7. **Did the plan work?**

FIGURE 4.5. Problem-Solving chart. From Bloomquist (1996). Copyright 1996 by The Guilford Press. Reprinted by permission.

help children reduce arousal, modify thoughts, and cope with stress. These procedures are based, in part, on adaptations of Novaco's (1978) stress-inoculation paradigm. Children learn anger management skills through the process of education, skills acquisition training, and practice. Groups of children participate in discussions, role-play exercises, and other activities to learn these skills.

The first step in anger management consists of children learning to recognize when they are angry. Children describe anger in their own words. They discuss situations that elicit anger responses ("triggers"). They learn to identify the cues ("signals") that indicate physiological arousal (accelerated heart rate, muscle tense, etc.), angry thoughts ("I hate you"; "They are so unfair"; etc.), and angry actions (throwing, hitting, yelling, making facial expressions, etc.). Children learn to recognize these signals in others and then in themselves. They do this by watching videos and participating in role-play exercises. They learn to recognize the levels of anger, which can range from frustration to irritation to anger to rage. Sometimes an Anger Thermometer (a picture of a thermometer calibrated with varying "anger degrees") is utilized to help children understand how anger can range in severity.

The second step involves teaching children to cope with anger by using coping self-talk, relaxation, and effective action strategies. They learn to say self-statements such as "Stay cool," "Chill out," "It's okay, I'm not going to let this bother me," and "Take some deep breaths" as a way of reducing their arousal. Younger children learn to take deep breaths, count to 10, or imagine themselves in a relaxing situation. Older children use these techniques plus muscle tension reduction procedures such as systematically tensing and releasing muscles.

Once the children have calmed down, they need to solve the problems that made them upset to begin with. It may also be useful for these anger-prone children to learn betters ways of interacting with others to avoid future anger episodes. Therefore anger management interventions frequently incorporate many of the other SCT strategies previously mentioned into the training experience. In particular, children who are prone to anger benefit from instruction in social behavior skills, affective education, attribution retraining, and problem-skills procedures.

Combining Social Competence Training Content

Most SCT models emphasize training children in a variety of skills training domains. For example, Webster-Stratton (1996b) described a comprehensive SCT intervention (the "Dinosaur School" curriculum) applicable for 3- to 8-year-old children with conduct problems. This program utilizes a video-modeling and discussion format. It is conducted over 22 sessions each lasting 2 hours. Training content is presented to improve empathy, problem-solving skills, anger control, friendship skills, communication skills, and school behaviors. The intervention is delivered through age-appropriate methods, including child activities, puppets, and video depictions of children of similar age. Webster-Stratton and Hammond (1997) found that this child training intervention was associated with improved social behavior, problem-solving, and conflict resolution skills in young children with ACP.

Deciding Which Skills to Emphasize in Training

We recognize that it may not be feasible to deliver interventions that focus on all content areas with a particular group of children. We therefore recommend that practitioners pick and choose content skills for a specific population of children. In our opinion, younger preschool- and early elementary-age children with ACP will derive benefit from all of the content interventions, but will profit most from an emphasis on social behavior and affective skills training. Older children with ACP will benefit from those same skills and can improve their functioning through training that emphasizes the more cognitively sophisticated skills such as attribution retraining, problem-solving training, and so on. As we noted earlier, it takes at least three to six sessions to initially train children in any one content area, so practical considerations will also dictate which content areas are emphasized. Practitioners are advised to consider the developmental capabilities

TABLE 4.6. Summary of Best Practice Training Content Areas for Social Competence Training

Training content areas	Best practices
Social behavior and communication skills training	Teach children observable prosocial behaviors and verbal and nonverbal communication skills.
Affective education	Teach children to identify and label feeling states in self and others.
Social perspective-taking training	Teach children to infer others' thoughts/feelings.
Attribution retraining	Teach children to accurately determine others' intentions and to interpret situations.
Self-monitoring and self-evaluation training	Teach children to accurately observe and evaluate own behavior.
Verbal self-instruction training	Teach children to use internal private speech to regulate behavior.
Problem-solving skills training	Teach children to use methodical steps to solve interpersonal problems.
Anger management training	Teach children to recognize and cope with angry feelings and reactions.
Combining social competence training content	Combine multiple social competence training content areas into one intervention.
Deciding which skills to emphasize in training	Consider the developmental status of children and practical matters in determining which skill areas to emphasize in training.

of the children they are working with and the goals of the intervention to figure out what skills should be emphasized.

Summary

Table 4.6 provides a summary of best practices for SCT training content that can be used for children with ACP. This table reveals that there are multiple potential content areas, with considerable overlap among them. Practitioners should match the specific needs and the capabilities of the children being served and deliver content areas accordingly.

CONCLUSION

SCT is a useful intervention program for children exhibiting ACP, especially when combined with other efficacious interventions (we discuss combining SCT with other interventions in Chapter 11). We have reviewed the most common delivery procedures and content areas employed in SCT interventions applicable to children with ACP. We believe that SCT can be incorporated into clinic, school, and community settings.

CHAPTER 5

Parent and Family Skills Training

*P*arent and family skills training (PFST) teaches parents and families skills that enhance child, parent, and family functioning (Miller & Prinz, 1990; Taylor & Biglan, 1998). PFST addresses the behavioral characteristics of children with ACP, and the parent and family factors that can exacerbate and escalate their problems. For purposes of discussion, we define a parent as any adult who assumes a primary caretaking role with a child (e.g., biological parents, foster parents, grandparents, other guardians) and a family as the group of individuals who reside with and take care of the child.

We hypothesize that PFST reduces risk factors and promotes protective factors in the child, parent/family, and social/peer life domains (see Tables 2.3 and 2.4 in Chapter 2). In particular, PFST reduces the aggressive/noncompliant/disruptive behavior of children with ACP, enhances the parent–child relationship, improves parents' personal functioning and parenting skills, and facilitates broader family relationships. Indirectly, PFST also improves children's social skills and minimizes the impact of antisocial peers.

We present PFST in three main sections in this chapter. The first section offers an overview and research evaluation of PFST. In the second section we discuss the common delivery methods used in working with parents and families. In the third section we address the content or skill areas taught to parents and family members. Our focus is on PFST interventions geared toward preschool- and school-age children.

OVERVIEW AND RESEARCH EVALUATION
OF PARENT AND FAMILY SKILLS TRAINING

PFST focuses on important child, parent, parent–child interaction and family target areas (Foote, Eyberg, & Schuhmann, 1996; Kazdin, 1997a; McMahon, Slough, & Conduct Problems Prevention Research Group, 1996; Taylor & Biglan, 1998). The first target is reducing children's overt aggression, conduct problems, and noncompliance. The second target is changing problematic parent behaviors such as inadvertent reinforcement of negative child behavior, frequent and ineffective commands, harsh and inconsistent discipline, poor monitoring, and inattentiveness to positive child behavior. The third target is improving the emotional bond between child and parent. The fourth target is dealing with the parent's personal problems (e.g., mental health, relational, financial, social, community difficulties) that cause stress for the parent and interfere with optimal parenting. The final target is improving the way family members communicate with one another and solve family problems. PFST protocols attempt to improve some or all of these target areas simultaneously. Once they are improved, the child will likely exhibit enhanced development in multiple domains of functioning.

Many specific interventions have been developed to effect change in the target areas just reviewed (Barkley, 1997; Foote et al., 1996; Forehand & McMahon, 1981; Kazdin, 1996a; McMahon et al., 1996; Patterson, Reid, Jones, & Conger, 1975; Webster-Stratton, 1996b). They can be grouped under two broad categories of PFST intervention. The first intervention category is parent training in behavioral child management strategies designed to strengthen positive behaviors and reduce negative behaviors in children. In many parent training protocols a portion of the intervention is devoted to teaching the parent how to be more reinforcing to the child and improving the parent–child bond by encouraging the parent to play with the child and give the child more noncontingent attention. The second intervention category focuses on the parents' personal problems and other family issues. Parents are trained in stress management and marital (relationship) skills, and also assisted in obtaining practical help. Family interactions are also improved by teaching communication and problem-solving skills to family members. Most PFST interventions incorporate both of these broad intervention categories.

PFST is very effective in bringing about change in child, parent, and family functioning when applied to children with ACP. We assume the reader would find it cumbersome to wade through the hundreds of studies that have evaluated PFST. Therefore we rely here on the narrative reviews of the literature that were conducted by Kazdin (1997a) and Taylor and Biglan (1998). Most of the studies reviewed by these authors focused on parent training to change children's behavior. These reviews indicate that children whose parents participated in PFST do improve, as evidenced by parent and teacher ratings and by direct observation of their behavior. Often "clinical significance" is achieved because children's behavior is brought to within normative limits. Researchers have documented maintenance of intervention gains for 1–3 years, and, in some instances, for up to 10–14 years. Children below age 6 years obtained slightly better outcomes with PFST than children who were 6 to 12 years old. Researchers have also found that siblings and parents are better adjusted after PFST. Direct observations have demonstrated that parent–child interactions improved. Kazdin found that more treatment sessions related to better outcome. He reported that some PFST protocols involve up to 50–60 hours of intervention. Both reviews noted that PFST has faired well when compared to alternate treatment programs (e.g., client-centered therapy). The reviewers observed that the more severe the child's and the family's problems, the lower the treatment efficacy.

As part of the American Psychological Association's efforts to document effective treatments for children, Brestan and Eyberg (1998) reviewed the intervention literature for children with ODD and CD. They evaluated interventions according to certain criteria to determine which interventions were "well-established" (similar to proven) or "probably efficacious" (similar to promising) (see Lonigan et al., 1998, for a discussion of the criteria). Brestan and Eyberg found that parent training programs based on Patterson and Gullion's (1968) *Living with Children* manual and Webster-Stratton's (1984, 1990b, 1994) video-modeling series were well-established interventions. In addition, those parent training models based on Hanf's (1969, cited in Brestan & Eyberg, 1998) two-stage behavioral intervention (i.e., parent–child relationship enhancement and child management) were probably efficacious (e.g., Eyberg, Boggs, & Algina, 1995; Hamilton & MacQuiddy, 1984; McNeil, Eyberg, Eisenstadt, Newcomb, & Funderburk, 1991; Peed, Roberts, & Forehand, 1977; Wells & Egan, 1988; Zangwill, 1983). Practitioners can be confident when employing PFST methods and strategies that draw upon these intervention models.

Serketich and Dumas (1996) conducted a meta-analysis of PFST for preschool- and school-age children. They selected 26 controlled studies that included adequate description of the intervention, demonstrated sound measurement, and employed rigorous scientific methodology. Most of the studies reviewed were evaluations of parent training. Across the 26 studies, the average age of the child was 6 years, the average number of sessions was 9.5, and 33% of the subjects had single parents. Although the outcome measures used across the studies varied, the authors collapsed them into broad categories of child adjustment and parent adjustment. The meta-analysis revealed that both children and parents benefited from PFST. Children whose parents participated in PFST exhibited a better outcome (e.g., reduced aggression/conduct problems) than 81% of children who received alternative or no treatments. There was a slightly lower rate of improvement for child functioning at school than at home. The parents who completed PFST were also better adjusted themselves (e.g., they had reduced stress, a higher sense of parental efficacy) than 67% of the parents who received alternative or no treatments. Clinical significance, where the scores on outcome measure fell within the normal range after intervention, was achieved for a majority of children. Only a few studies evaluated the long-term benefits of the behavioral parent training, but those that did demonstrated durable intervention effects.

Two factors have prompted practitioners to expand PFST beyond the traditional emphasis on the child's behavior and parent–child interaction. The first factor is that less favorable outcomes and higher dropout rates occur with severe multiproblem families (Kazdin, 1996b; McMahon & Forehand, 1984; Miller & Prinz, 1990; Patterson & Fleischman, 1979; Webster-Stratton & Hammond, 1990). The second factor is that even when the parent training is successfully completed, up to 38% of the time involved in the intervention is spent dealing with parental personal problems, marital problems, family crises, and so on (Patterson & Chamberlain, 1988). PFST practitioners recognized the need to deal directly with additional parent/family problems and contextual difficulties (as documented in Chapter 2) to enhance the overall impact of the intervention.

Several recent studies have shown that broader focused PFST that provides parent training and intervenes with parent's personal and familywide problems are effective. Webster-Stratton (1996b) described the BASIC and ADVANCE parent training programs. The BASIC program is parent training to improve children's behavior and parent–child interactions. The ADVANCE program promotes parent's social support and self-care, personal self-control, and marital/family interaction skills, and also presents strategies to assist children in problem solving. Webster-Stratton (1994) compared families of children with ACP who received only BASIC to those who received combined BASIC and ADVANCE. She found that children in both groups were comparable in improvements, but families in the combined group showed additional benefits in the realms of marital communication, parents' problem solving, children's problem solving, consumer satisfaction, and lower dropout rates. Sanders and McFarland (2000) examined the effects of Behavioral Family Intervention versus Cognitive Behavioral Family Intervention in treating families of children with ACP. The Cognitive Behavioral Family Intervention included the Behavioral Family Intervention's focus on child management training, but also added parent cognitive therapy components, including monitoring and managing mood, scheduling pleasant events, relaxation, cognitive restructuring, and stress coping. Sanders and McFarland found that both interventions improved children's behavior and reduced mother's depression at immediate posttest. The Cognitive Behavioral Family Intervention, however, maintained child behavior and maternal mood improvements at a higher level than did the Behavioral Family Intervention at a 6-month follow-up assessment. Finally, Sanders, Markie-Dadds, Tully, and Bor (2000) compared self-help PFST, standard therapist-led PFST, and enhanced therapist-led PFST interventions for preschool children who exhibited early-onset ACP. All three conditions provided parent training to reduce child behavior problems based on the Triple P—Positive Parenting Program model. The enhanced condition, however, also incorporated partner support (e.g., communication skills, partner supportive statements, problem solving) and coping skills for personal problems (e.g., cognitive therapy for depression, anger, and stress). All three intervention conditions were compared to a wait-list control condition. Sanders et al. found that the enhanced PFST model produced the most reliable improvement on dimensions of child functioning and parenting competence at posttest and 1-year follow-up assessments. Taken together, these studies demonstrated the utility of broader models of PFST that intervene with family adversity factors.

Like with SCT, we observe a limitation in PFST as it relates to intervening with children manifesting different subtypes of ACP. Most of the PFST programs were designed for overtly aggressive and defiant children. There are few specific PFST interventions for children with other ACP subtypes. Moreover, existing interventions have rarely been evaluated for their effects on children who display different forms of ACP (e.g., relational aggression, reactive aggression). Therefore research is needed to evaluate the usefulness of PFST with different ACP subtypes.

In summary, PFST is an effective intervention for children with ACP and their families. PFST that incorporates parent training and addresses broader parent personal and familywide problems is the most effective. PFST brings about clinically significant changes that generalize to other settings/persons and that are maintained over time. In our opinion, PFST is mandatory when providing interventions to children with ACP because of the clear role parent and family factors have in the escalation of their problems and because of the effectiveness of PFST.

BEST PRACTICE MODELS FOR PARENT AND FAMILY SKILLS TRAINING

We reviewed six PFST program models that focus on preschool- and school-age children with ACP to derive best practices. Each of these PFST programs has been extensively studied and has been shown to be effective (see citations below for details). What follows is an integration of techniques and strategies used in these models. The six PFST models are (1) Patterson and colleagues' Parent Training program (Forgatch, 1991; Patterson, 1975a, 1975b; Patterson, Cobb, & Ray, 1973; Patterson et al.,

1975); (2) Forehand and McMahon's Helping the Non-Compliant Child program (Forehand & McMahon, 1981; McMahon & Forehand, 1984; McMahon et al., 1996); (3) Webster-Stratton's Video Modeling Parent Training program (also known as The Incredible Years program) (Webster-Stratton, 1992, 1996b); (4) Eyberg and colleagues' Parent–Child Interaction Therapy (Eyberg et al., 1995; Eyberg & Boggs, 1998); (5) Barkley's Defiant Child Training program (Anastopoulos, Shelton, DuPaul, & Guevremont, 1993; Anastopoulos, Smith, & Wien, 1998; Barkley, 1997; Barkley & Benton, 1998); and (6) Sanders and colleagues' Triple P—Positive Parenting Program (Sanders, 1999; Sanders et al., 2000). In the remainder of this chapter we present best practices of PFST from these models. We will also periodically review Braswell and Bloomquist's practice model for PFST to elaborate standard procedures (Bloomquist, 1996; Braswell & Bloomquist, 1991).

BEST PRACTICE DELIVERY PROCEDURES
FOR PARENT AND FAMILY SKILLS

Delivery of skills training pertains to how the practitioner presents the PFST intervention to the family. It has to do with the methods the practitioner employs during the intervention to teach parents and family members new skills. We discuss the content of the PFST intervention later in this chapter.

Practitioner Characteristics

Successful PFST practitioners possess certain characteristics that enable them to be effective. Alexander, Barton, Schiavo, and Parsons (1976) found that successful practitioners employing PFST with adolescents and their families were able to establish good relationships with families (e.g., through communication, humor, empathy, acceptance) and were structured (e.g., directive, focused, active) in teaching skills. Patterson and Fortgatch (1985) determined that effective practitioners avoid teaching or confronting "resistant" parents, and instead offer support, ask questions, and engage those parents in discussion. Effective practitioners engage the family in dialogue to lead them to discover what they should work on and to assist them in reaching their goals (Braswell & Bloomquist, 1991).

The model PFST programs incorporate extensive training of practitioners to conduct the interventions. They are trained in relationship building and in behavioral methods of skills training delivery (to be discussed later). Often practitioners follow a manual to assist them in standardized delivery of PFST. For example, practitioners using Webster-Stratton's (1996b) successful PFST program follow a manual that informs them about what to do during each session. Rigorous training of practitioners and the use of standardized manuals ensures that a quality PFST intervention will be administered to families.

Practitioners do not necessarily need to be highly credentialed individuals to be successful. Success follows when practitioners are experienced in working with people, show commitment to their work, are properly trained, and follow best practice procedures. Ongoing supervision of less experienced practitioners by more experienced ones is also important for successful interventions.

Training Methods

Specific PFST-related skills are taught to parents and family members through instruction, modeling, role-play rehearsal, and practice. The practitioner observes the parents performing the new skills and then gives them feedback regarding their progress. A skill is introduced in one session (e.g., attending to prosocial behavior), homework is assigned regarding that specific skill, and the parent practices it until mastery has been achieved. The rate at which parents achieve skill acquisition will vary. Practitioners should emphasize mastery of skills rather than a set number of sessions or hours.

PFST can be delivered through individual or group training formats. Individual and group training have been found to be equally effective, but the group format is more cost-effective (Webster-Stratton, 1984). Typically, a group of 8–10 parents meets with one or two practitioners. Webster-Stratton's (1996b) Video Modeling Parent Training program is a good example of group training. Webster-Stratton produced over 250 video vignettes and an accompanying manual for her BASIC parenting skills program. The vignettes show both positive and negative examples of parenting behavior. The practitioner shows the vignettes to the parents and then asks them specific questions regarding the vignettes. The vignettes serve as a springboard for group discussion and role play. These techniques allow parents to give each other ideas and support, and also provide practitioners with an opportunity to collaborate with parents. Video modeling/discussion formats of intervention have been found to be superior to alternative conditions in overall treatment effects, in maintenance of effects, and in achieving parent satisfaction with the intervention (Webster-Stratton, 1990b; Webster-Stratton, Kolpacoff, & Hollinsworth, 1988).

The individual format for parent training is similar in many respects, but the support that group members provide each other cannot be replicated. There are advantages, however, to individual training. The practitioner is allowed to pinpoint exactly what skills should be worked on with a particular parent or family member. A common procedure for individual training involves use of a one-way mirror and a "bug-in-the ear" device (Eyberg & Boggs, 1998; Forehand & McMahon, 1981). While the parent(s) and child interact together in a training room, the practitioner observes the interaction through a one-way mirror. The practitioner coaches the parent by providing feedback and instruction through the bug-in-the-ear device. Another procedure that can be used with individual families is in-home delivery of PFST. This has the obvious advantage of bringing the intervention directly to the family in their natural environment. This enables the practitioner to see the "real" context within which families operate and cuts down on missed appointments.

Number of Sessions

The number of training sessions employed is different across PFST protocols. They vary depending on the goals of the program and the characteristics of the families being served. Serketich and Dumas (1996) found PFST is delivered an average of 9.5 hours (across 26 studies). There is variation, however, across specific intervention protocols. Sanders and colleagues (2000), for example, delivered the Triple P—Positive Parenting Program over 10–14 1-hour sessions. Webster-Stratton (1996b) stated that it takes 13–14 2-hour sessions to go through the BASIC program, and an additional 14 2-hour sessions to complete the ADVANCE program. In Kazdin's (1997a) review, more sessions are related to better outcomes. He suggested it may take up to 50–60 hours of intervention with some families.

It is important to use as many sessions as necessary for parents and family members to achieve mastery of content. More sessions will be needed as the program content expands or as the level of adversity in participants increases. Vitaro and Tremblay (1994), for example, conducted a parent-training program that called for adjusting the number of PFST sessions each family received according to each family's needs and progress in achieving mastery. Families in the Vitaro and Tremblay study received up to 46 sessions, with an average of 17.4 sessions.

We find it somewhat confusing to sort through different suggestions regarding the number of sessions for PFST. As we review this information, and reflect on our own experience, it is our opinion that approximately 10–18 sessions are necessary to conduct PFST with most families. We agree with Vitaro and Tremblay; the exact number of sessions should be adjusted to fit the needs of each family. Therefore it is conceivable that the number of sessions could be more or less depending on the strengths and needs of a given family. In addition, follow-up sessions will be needed after initial training to monitor a family's progress and deliver booster or additional interventions as indicated.

The number of sessions to teach a specific skill will also vary for each family receiving PFST. Experience indicates that it takes three to six sessions to teach parents or family members a specific content skill. For example, in teaching how to deal with noncompliant behavior in children, the practitioner might use four sessions to teach parents the procedures for avoiding power struggles and using time-out. Several more sessions may be needed to monitor progress in the implementation of the new skills and to make adjustments in the procedures as needed. The goal is for the parent and/or family members to master the new skill. Practitioners need to use as many sessions as necessary to accomplish this goal.

Promoting Generalization and Maintenance

The ultimate goal is for parents and family members to use the new skills they are learning at home and over time. PFST calls for the use of procedures that increase the likelihood of generalization and maintenance of skills training. Graduated training tasks and homework can be used to enhance generalization. First, the parent learns a skill (e.g., using time-out) and demonstrates mastery of it in the intervention setting. Next, the parent is given homework assignments to utilize the new skill at home. PFST practitioners often give the parents charts, handouts, or even manuals/books to assist them with this transfer. For example, books written by Webster-Stratton (1992), Patterson (1975a, 1976), and Bloomquist (1996) provide parents with information and ideas on how to use PFST-related skills to deal with a variety of children's behavior problems at home. Finally, once the parent has gained proficiency in using a new skill at home, he or she is ready to start employing it in the community. The practitioner and parent strategize to set up procedures for employing new parenting skills in other settings (e.g., a store, the park, grandmother's home).

PFST practitioners employ review, follow-up assessment, and booster sessions to ensure that the intervention will have lasting effects. This is necessary because skill development is difficult and there is always a risk of relapse. Review consists of discussing/modeling/role-playing a skill after some time has elapsed. This affords the practitioner an opportunity to see if a parent still understands and can use the skill. Follow-up assessment usually entails observing parent–child interactions. This gives the practitioner evidence about whether or not previous intervention gains were maintained. Booster sessions can be scheduled periodically—for example, monthly or as needed. The previously learned skills are reviewed in booster sessions.

Summary

Table 5.1 summarizes the best practices for delivering PFST. We recommend that these delivery procedures be followed to ensure that the PFST program is effectively provided to families.

TABLE 5.1. Summary of Best Practice Delivery Procedures for Parent and Family Skills Training

Delivery procedures	Best practices
Practitioner characteristics	Establish relationships, provide structure, lead parents to discover new skills, follow standardized protocols.
Training methods	Use instruction, modeling (including video modeling), role plays, practice, feedback, reinforcement, discussion, and homework; interventions can be delivered in small groups or with individual families.
Number of sessions	Approximately 10 to 18 sessions are utilized, although the number of sessions should be adjusted to allow for mastery of content; typically three to six sessions are needed to teach families one of the content skills.
Promoting generalization and maintenance	Use graduated training tasks, books that describe procedures, and charts to assist in homework exercises; use follow-up booster sessions.

BEST PRACTICE TRAINING CONTENT AREAS FOR PARENT AND FAMILY SKILLS TRAINING

In this section we review the content of PFST interventions from the various best practice models. Training content is what families learn as a result of participating in PFST. The practitioner picks and chooses which skills are most relevant to a particular family or group of families.

Understanding Social Learning Principles

Many child management-focused PFST protocols begin by educating parents about the social learning theoretical principles on which child management strategies are based (Forehand & McMahon, 1981; Patterson et al., 1993). Miller and Prinz (1990) summarized the social learning principles that parents are taught as follows:

1. The need to pinpoint and accurately label child behavior.
2. The necessity of refocusing parental attention away from the child's behavior problems to the child's positive and prosocial behavior.
3. The importance of tracking specific child behaviors on a daily basis.
4. How prosocial child behavior is increased by tangible and social reinforcements.
5. How aggressive/defiant behavior is reduced by effective discipline techniques.
6. The importance of effective commands and communication.

7. The utility of anticipating and solving ongoing parenting problems that emerge.

An example of this procedure is Patterson's two parent books, which are often utilized to convey social learning theory information and child management strategies to parents. Parents are often given copies of either *Living with Children* (Patterson, 1976) or *Families* (Patterson, 1975a) to convey this information prior to or during intervention. Parents must read the book and then demonstrate to the practitioner that they understand and have mastered the principles of social learning theory.

Observing and Tracking Child Behavior

The parent is taught to pinpoint and track specific child behaviors. Each behavior is carefully defined, observed, and recorded over time. For example, compliance with parental commands is defined as the child "listening and obeying the parent when told to do something." Initially, a baseline is established by counting the frequency of the specified behavior (e.g., the number of times the child complies with parental commands) during a specified time interval (e.g., evenings for 1 week). An intervention is then conducted (specific interventions are described below), and its effects are observed through ongoing tracking of child behavior. Different types of compliant and prosocial behavior can be observed and tracked. The targeted positive behavior should increase as a function of the intervention.

Figure 5.1 provides an example of a tracking chart. In this example the child's compliance with parental commands is tallied during the evening

Name: _Tony_

Dates: _Monday March 5th through Sunday March 11th_

Time of observation: _After supper to bedtime_

Behavior being tracked: _Compliance with parental commands_

	Monday	Tuesday	Wednesday	Thursday	Friday	Saturday	Sunday
YES	///	/	//	//	///	//	///
NO	//	////	///	//	////	///	///

FIGURE 5.1. Child behavior tracking.

hours. A similar procedure could be used to track different behaviors at different times.

Encouraging Child-Directed Interaction and Play

Child-directed interaction and play enhances parent–child relationships, makes the parent more reinforcing to the child, and shapes the child's prosocial behaviors. To accomplish this, parents and children are instructed to engage in play or "special time" activities. These activities include those that allow for back-and-forth interaction such as playing with cars or dolls, building something, baking or cooking, or playing catch. Watching television or playing a board game would not be conducive to reciprocal interaction. Parents are instructed to allow the child to choose the activity and set the pace for play. The parent is to give attention to positive, neutral, and prosocial child behavior, while deemphasizing attention to negative child behavior, during the child-directed activities.

Parents are instructed to *increase play-facilitating behaviors* such as the following:

1. Praising—verbally reinforcing the child during the activity.
   - "That looks good."
   - "You're doing a good job."
   - "Good boy [girl]!"
   - "It looks great!"
2. Describing—commenting on what the child is doing and how the child might be feeling.
   - "You put the car in the garage."
   - "You caught the ball!"
   - "You look happy [sad, angry, scared]."
   - "It looks like you're thinking."
3. Touching—appropriately touching the child during the activity.
   - Hugs
   - Kisses
   - Pats on the shoulder

Parents are also instructed to *decrease play-detracting behaviors* such as the following:

1. Questions—asking the child unnecessary questions during the activity.
   - "Why did you put the car in the garage?"
   - "Do you want to play this game?"
   - "Why are you so mad?"
2. Commands—telling the child what to do during the activity.

- "Put all the cars in the garage."
- "Throw me the ball."
- "You be the cowboy and I'll be the horse."
3. Criticism—negatively evaluating the child's behavior during the activity.
   - "That doesn't look right."
   - "Try harder."
   - "It doesn't go that way."

The frequency of the parent's behavior is sometimes counted in session by the practitioner or by another observer. A criterion is established for the amount of behaviors that are to be emitted by the parent during a certain interval. For example, in Parent–Child Interaction Therapy (Eyberg & Boggs, 1998), the parent is observed for 5 minutes while interacting with the child during child-directed activities. The parent is coached to emit up to 35 positive behaviors. The parent is also asked to emit three or fewer negative behaviors. Once the two criteria are met, the parent can move on to other training content.

Webster-Stratton's (1996b) program helps parents to understand the importance of play in children's development. They are educated about the benefits of play for enhancing cognitive and language development, imagination, and self-esteem in children. Parents are encouraged to play with their children and follow their lead during play activities.

Some debate exists about the timing of child-directed interactions and play in the intervention process. Forehand and McMahon (1981) argued that parents need to master child-directed activities before moving on to other parent training content. This argument is based on the assumption that parents need to establish a more positive tone in the parent–child relationship before applying discipline strategies. One study, however, found that training parents in child behavior management skills before training them in child-directed activities was associated with more improved child behavior and greater parental satisfaction than training in child-directed activities before discipline techniques (Eisenstadt, Eyberg, McNeil, Newcomb, & Funderburk, 1993). In practice it may be helpful to collaborate with parents and ask them what they would like to learn first.

Shaping Positive Behavior with Positive Attention and Reinforcement

PFST emphasizes "catching them being good" to help children increase compliant and prosocial behaviors. Parents are trained to pay attention to their children and praise them for these positive behaviors. First, the parent has to learn how to track the behavior and "see" it better (see "Observing and Tracking Child Behavior," above). When the child manifests the behavior, the parent is taught to give labeled praise that specifies what the child did and communicates the parent's satisfaction (e.g., "I like it when you share crayons with your sister").

Parents are also taught to administer tangible reinforcement to children for displaying specific behaviors. Sometimes this effort is orchestrated by using a behavior chart. Figure 5.2 displays an example of a daily child behavior chart. To use this chart, the desired child behavior is specified (e.g., Up and dressed by 7:00 A.M.), the behavior is tracked, and reinforcement is administered according to the child's behavior. Charts can be useful to "jump-start" behaviors, but they should be gradually faded out. Eventually, the desired behaviors should be maintained by using praise as described in the preceding paragraph.

Ignoring Mild Negative Behavior

Milder behavior problems such as whining, arguing, swearing, and protesting can be reduced with planned ignoring. Parents are trained to ignore these behaviors. When the child manifests these behaviors, the parent avoids verbal reinforcement (e.g., "Knock it off"), physical reinforcement (e.g., making annoyed eye contact), and physical proximity to the child. Instead, the parent remains quiet and physically removed from the child. Once the child's behavior has improved, the parent again attends to the child. The parent systematically selects certain behaviors that he or she would like to ignore in his or her child.

Defusing Power Struggles and Deescalating Parent–Child Conflict

Most PFST programs teach the parent how to defuse power struggles and deescalate conflicts that can emerge when trying to discipline or gain the compliance of a child with ACP. Parents need to be educated so they understand that their response to the child's problematic behavior can make the child increasingly angry and aggressive. In a worst-case scenario this could escalate to a physical confrontation between parent and child. To be successful, parents must learn to provide discipline in a firm and calm manner in order to defuse potentially volatile situations with their child.

One strategy is to train parents in stress management skills so they can "stay cool" (i.e., manage their own stress, frustration, and anger) when their child exhibits noncompliant and/or problematic behaviors. Stress management procedures are especially important to review with parents who have a history of overreacting and thereby escalating their child's behavior. Parents are taught stress management techniques through education, modeling, role playing, and fulfilling assignments. Four procedures are commonly used to teach stress management skills to parents:

Name: *Latoya*

Week of: *November 6–12*

Directions: Identify four (or fewer) target behaviors for your child to work on each day. Put a smiling face in the box if the behavior was completed. Put a frowning face in the box if the behavior was not completed. Always praise your child each time he/she gets a smiling face. At the end of the day, tally up smiling and frowning faces. Administer the reward or mild punishment sometime within 24 hours. There are two levels of rewards and one level of mild punishment.

Behavior	Mon.	Tues.	Wed.	Thurs.	Fri.	Sat.	Sun.
Up and dressed by 7:00 A.M.	☹	☺	☹	☺	☺		
Homework done before supper	☹	☺	☹	☺	☺		
Take dog out for walk	☹	☹	☺	☺	☺		
In bed by 7:30 P.M. with lights out	☹	☺	☺	☺	☺		
Total smiling faces	0	3	2	4	4		
Total frowning faces	4	1	2	0	0		

Daily reward: **Mild punishment:**
1–2 Smiling faces = *Special bedtime snack*   4 Frowning faces = *No TV for a day*
3–4 Smiling faces = *Special activity with parent*

FIGURE 5.2. Daily Child Behavior Chart. From Bloomquist (1996). Copyright 1996 by The Guilford Press. Reprinted by permission.

1. Teach parents to recognize stress and to be aware of stress "signals"—parents are instructed to recognize the "body signals" (e.g., accelerated breathing/heart rate, tense muscles, feeling hot), the "thought signals" (e.g., "That brat!"; "I can't handle this!"; "I give up") and the "action signals" (e.g., yelling, hitting, crying, withdrawing) associated with stress.

2. Teach parents to use relaxation strategies—parents are instructed to take slow deep breaths, to tense and release their muscles, and to count to 10.
3. Teach parents to use "coping self-talk"—parents are instructed to think self-statements such as "Take it easy," "I can handle this," "Stay cool," and "I'll try my best."
4. Teach parents to take effective action—parents are instructed to walk away, ignore it, express feelings, and solve the problem.

Once parents have learned to remain calm, they can then employ other strategies to gain their children's compliance and/or reduce other behavior problems.

The parent can also be trained to recognize different stages in the escalation process and employ commonsense strategies to deescalate the situation. Through discussion with the practitioner, the parent can learn to pinpoint the "triggers" or situations that commonly "set off" their child. The practitioner and parent can then strategize about different ways to proactively manage those situations instead of merely reacting to them. For example, if being told to do homework routinely sparks an angry response from the child, the parent could warn him or her every 5 minutes for 15 minutes prior to giving the command to do homework. The parent can also learn to reassure the child that they can work out their problems and firmly insist that the child calm down. It may be useful to discuss safety concerns that need to be considered when the child does spiral out of control. This may entail the parent physically removing others from the child or restraining him or her. The parent will also need to supervise the child once he or she has begun to calm down to avoid a recycling of the angry and explosive behaviors. See Table 9.3 in Chapter 9 for an elaboration of similar procedures that teachers can use to reduce escalating child behavior in schools.

Using Time-Out/Removal of Privileges for Noncompliance

All the PFST models incorporate time-out and removal of privileges as a way of enabling parents to improve the way they respond to their child's noncompliant behaviors. Eyberg and Boggs (1998) characterized this part of the training as "parent-directed interaction" in that the parent takes the lead to decrease noncompliant and angry behavior. All PFST models work with the parent to achieve control of the child first in the training situation and then in home and community settings.

The first step is educating parents to accurately define noncompliant behavior. Most PFST programs suggest that noncompliance occurs when a child resists or refuses to follow a parental command. The three most typical forms of noncompliance are the following:

1. Overt noncompliance—the child refuses to physically perform the task.
2. Bargaining—the child verbally tries to rationalize and/or strike up a "deal" with the parent and does not physically perform the task.
3. Resistance—the child complains and half-heartedly performs the task.

Parents learn that they need to take effective action (described below) when their child displays these forms of noncompliance.

In the second step parents are taught to improve how they give commands to their children. Parents are educated about a variety of *ineffective commands* including the following:

1. Vague command—telling the child about what is expected in a nonspecific manner (e.g., "Shape up"; "Knock it off").
2. Question command—giving a command in the form of a question (e.g., "Would you please brush your teeth?").
3. Rationale command—explaining the parent's reasons for why the child needs to follow the command (e.g., "You need to brush your teeth now because if you don't you'll have bad breath when you go to school and someday you'll get cavities.").
4. Multiple or chain commands—instructing the child to follow many commands simultaneously (e.g., "Turn off the TV, pick up the toys in this room, wash your hands, and then come to dinner.").
5. Frequent commands—repeating the same command (e.g., "Pick up the toys."; Come on, pick up the toys."; "I told you to pick up the toys!"; "PICK UP THOSE TOYS!").

To promote awareness, parents are instructed to self-evaluate. They also receive feedback from the practitioner about commands that are typical for them. Parents are told that these commands do not work in situations where the child's compliance is needed.

The parents are taught to use *effective commands* including the following:

1. Specific, one-step command—explicitly stating a directive in approximately 10 words (e.g., "Go to your room now."; "Take the dishes off the table and put them on the counter."; "Turn off the light.").
2. When–then command—telling the child that he or she can engage in a desired activity when a task is completed (e.g., "When your homework is completed, then you can go outside.").

If the child complies with the effective command, the parent provides labeled praise and attention to reinforce this behavior.

During the third step parents are taught to use warnings if the child remains noncompliant with an effective command. Parents are instructed to stay calm and give a warning in the form of an "if–then" statement. For example, with a child who refuses to pick up toys, the parent states: "*If* you don't pick up the toys and put them on the shelf, *then* you will have to go to the time-out chair." The parent states the warning only once. If the child complies with the warning, the parent administers labeled praise and attention for compliance. If the child does not comply with the warning, he or she is put in the time-out chair.

The fourth step involves the parent learning to put the child in a time-out chair for noncompliance with the warning. In a calm manner, the parent escorts the child to a time-out chair. The chair should be somewhere in the house that is free from distractions and also allows the parent to monitor the child from a distance. If the child refuses to cooperate with sitting in a chair, a warning is given that a backup procedure will be used if the child does not sit on the chair (e.g., spanking, holding the child in the chair, removing other privileges). For example, if a child refuses to comply with going to time-out, the parent states: "You will not be allowed to watch TV again until you go to time-out." If the child does not go to time-out, the backup procedure is administered until he or she goes to time-out. The command–warning–time-out (with backup procedure) sequence is repeated until the child eventually complies with the original command.

The backup procedure used for refusing to sit in a chair can become complicated and for that reason is sometimes resisted by parents. Eyberg and Boggs (1998) advised that parents should be given choices to use backup procedures that fit their unique beliefs or needs. Nonviolent and nonangry spanking (e.g., two swats on the buttocks) is recommended for some parents. Other parents are instructed to hold the child in the chair for 1 minute until the child sits quietly in the chair for at least 5 seconds. The practitioner should discuss with parents what they believe will be the most effective backup procedure.

The amount of time the child is required to sit in the time-out chair varies according to different PFST protocols. Eyberg and Boggs (1998) recommended that preschool children spend at least 3 minutes in the time-out chair, and that they be required to sit quiet for the last 5 seconds before being released. Barkley (1997) recommended that a child be given 1 or 2 minutes of time-out for each year of the child's age, with 2 minutes per year of age being reserved for more serious behavioral infractions.

The fifth step has to do with teaching the parent to use time-out in public settings. Initially, the parent is instructed to use time-out only at home. Once the parent is convinced that the procedure is going well at home, then the parent is encouraged to employ it in community settings. This involves the parent thinking very quickly when noncompliance occurs in public settings, and then determining the likely spot where time-out could be administered. The place should be free from distractions and potential reinforcement (e.g., a corner in a store).

The time-out procedure can be *modified somewhat for older elementary school-age children.* The sequence of events as described above would be similar for older children, although taking an older child to a time-out chair might not be age-appropriate. In this case, removal of privileges would be utilized (e.g., taking away a bike, computer time, or outside privileges). For example, if a parent wanted a 12-year-old child to turn off the TV, the parent would give an effective command, followed by a warning (if necessary), and then take away a privilege, such as a video game, for 24 hours (if necessary).

Practitioners need to work with parents so they understand that the privileges taken from the child do not need to be severe or extensive (e.g., "You're grounded for a month!"). In most instances, the older elementary-age child will learn to obey if a simple privilege is removed until the child complies or for 24 hours. A good frame of reference is to tell parents that the purpose of discipline is to "teach the child a lesson," not to "punish the child." Therefore the parent need not administer a harsh consequence.

Using Standing or House Rules for Behavior

"Standing rules" or "house rules" is used to describe what the parent expects the child to do on an ongoing basis without having to be told or reminded. These rules are designed to reduce aggressive and/or covert antisocial behaviors such as hitting, destroying property, teasing, or stealing, and to increase positive behaviors such as homework, chores, and brushing teeth. Parents are instructed to inform their child of the rules (e.g., "no hitting" or "homework before TV"). It is helpful to write down the rules and post them for all to see.

The child is informed that if he or she violates a rule, he or she will be taken directly to time-out or will lose a privilege. In essence, the rule serves as the warning for the child. Therefore, no additional verbal warning is needed. When the child violates the rule (e.g., hits a sibling or watches TV before completing homework), the consequence for the rule violation is automatically given.

Using a Token System for Behavior Management

A token system is an intensive intervention designed to modify behaviors of a child. The parent is instructed to define which behaviors he or she would like the child to increase. The parent is then asked to "weight" these behaviors for their importance. After this, the parent assigns values to the behaviors that correspond to the weight of that behavior. These assigned values can be transformed into chips or points that the child can earn for manifesting the behaviors. For example, the child might earn two chips/points for clearing the dishes off the table after dinner, three chips/points for picking up toys in the bedroom, eight chips/points for getting dressed in the morning, or 10 chips/points for doing 15 minutes of homework in the afternoon. It is recommended that chips be used for children ages 4–8 and that points be used for children ages 9–12. The parent should allow opportunity for the child to earn up to 50 chips/points per day with the token system.

Next, the parent has to define specific privileges/rewards that the child can earn for amassing different amounts of chips/points. The parent explains to the child that the chips/points are like money, which can be traded in for special privileges or rewards. For example, a social reward of playing a one-on-one basketball game with a parent might be worth 10 chips/points. A special reward of going to a movie with a parent might be worth 50 chips/points. The rewards do not necessarily have to be "extras." They could be everyday privileges that the child takes for granted. For example, the child is used to riding his bike after school or watching TV on Saturday mornings. These activities are privileges and not rights. The parent could require the child to earn these privileges by accumulating chips/points. It is also useful to obtain the child's input to be sure that rewards are actually reinforcing to the child.

Figure 5.3 from Barkley (2000) summarizes a home chip program for a 6- to 8-year-old child. This example lists specific "jobs" (behaviors) that the child could complete, with corresponding "payment" (chips), "rewards" (privileges), and costs for these rewards.

The parent is instructed to track the specific behaviors targeted and to administer chips/points accordingly. A "bank" (e.g., a box or a can) is utilized for collecting chips earned. A chart is utilized for keeping track of points earned. When the child manifests a specific behavior, the parent verbally acknowledges the behavior and informs the child of the chips/points earned. The parent and child keep track of the amount of chips/points earned and spent.

Barkley (2000) recommended that children be allowed to earn chips/points without losing them during the first week. This provides the child an opportunity to become familiar with the system and enjoy the rewards for good behavior. After about a week, however, the chips/points can also be utilized in a response-cost fashion. That is, in addition to earning chips/points for positive behavior, the child can also lose chips/tokens for negative behavior. Accordingly, if the child manifests noncompliant or aggressive behavior, he or she could receive a warning to stop the behavior or a specified number of chips/points will be taken away. If the behavior persists, then the child would lose the aforementioned number of chips/points. It is recommended, however, that parents give out many more chips/points for positive behavior than take away chips/points for negative behavior.

Job	Payment	Reward	Cost
Get dressed	5	Watch television (30 minutes)	4
Wash hands/face	2	Play video games (30 minutes)	5
Brush teeth	2	Play outside in yard	2
Make bed	5	Ride my bike	2
Put dirty clothes away	2	Use a special toy	4
Pick up toys	3	Go out for fast food	200
Take dirty dishes to sink after eating	1	Rent a video game or movie	300
Homework (per 15 minutes)	5	Go bowling/miniature golf or	
Give dog fresh water	1	roller/ice skating	400
Take bath/shower	5	Stay up past bedtime (30 minutes)	50
Hang up coat	1	Have a friend play over	40
No fights with sibling		Have a friend sleep over	150
Breakfast to lunch	3	Go to a video arcade	300
Lunch to dinner	3	Get my allowance ($1.00/week)	100
Dinner to bedtime	3	Choose a special dessert	20
Uses nice voice with Mom/Dad		Go play at a friend's home	50
when asking for something	1		
Get pajamas on	3		
Come when called	2		
Tell the truth when asked about	3		
a problem			
Positive attitude	Bonus		

FIGURE 5.3. Sample of a home chip program job and privilege list for a 6- to 8-year-old. Barkley (2000) estimated that this child would earn about 50 chips each day for doing just the daily routine tasks on a typical school day. Barkley then made sure that about 30 of these chips would be needed to buy the daily privileges of television (1.5 hours), video games (1 hour), playing outside, riding a bike, and playing with a special toy that Mom and Dad control access to (such as a remote-control car, a racecar set and track, a train set, an army battle station with troops, a doll with clothes and accessories, a personal tape player or CD player, in-line skates, skateboard). The remaining privileges were priced by determining how often the child should have access to that reward—that is, how many days of waiting and saving. From Barkley (2000). Copyright 2000 by The Guilford Press. Reprinted by permission.

The child should always have a positive balance of chips/points each day or he or she will get discouraged and refuse to cooperate.

The token system should be periodically reviewed, at the very least on a weekly basis, to determine its continued effectiveness. Over time, it may be necessary to adjust the target behaviors, chip/point values, and rewards depending on what has transpired. Parents need to make adjustments so that the program will stay exciting and rewarding to the child. Eventually, however, the token program should be faded out and finally discontinued altogether. This occurs when the parent is convinced that the child has made sufficient progress in deportment.

Monitoring and Supervising Children

PFST interventions routinely focus on improving parents' monitoring/supervision skills. Patterson and Forgatch (1987) defined monitoring/supervision as the "4 Ws." These 4 Ws include the parent knowing *w*ho the child is with, *w*here the child is going, *w*hat the child is doing, and *w*hen the child will return home. It also involves knowing the child's friends and their parents, as well as keeping informed about the child's progress at school. Finally, monitoring/supervision has to do with structuring a child's time so that he or she is involved in prosocial activities and does not have too much unstructured free time. Although monitoring takes different forms at different ages in a child's life, there is evidence that this concept is relevant for children of all ages.

Several steps are utilized to train parents in improving monitoring/supervision (Dishion & McMahon, 1998; Patterson & Forgatch, 1987). First, it is essential to motivate the parent to make monitoring/supervision a priority. Typically, the practitioner presents didactic information about the potential impact of poor monitoring/supervision on child development. A discussion of values is also relevant so that the parent is able to see that monitoring/supervision of children is a valued activity in our society. The parent is encouraged to be in charge of his or her child. This is followed by a presentation of commonsense procedures to improve monitoring/supervision such as communication with other parents, talking to the child's friends, being involved at school, and being aware of the child's progress at school. The next step involves delineation of specific rules and expectations. This might include defining a curfew, discussing boundaries concerning where the child can and cannot go in the community, reviewing homework times, and so on. It is important to communicate these rules and expectations to the child and all other adults who are involved in coparenting. Sometimes rules are written down in the form of a "contract." Another technique that can be used by parents is a home–school communication note system (see Chapter 7). This improves the parents' ability to monitor the child's functioning at school.

Intervening with Stealing

Patterson and colleagues (1975) described procedures for intervening with children who steal. Patterson and colleagues utilize the standard parent training protocol that they devised (much of which has been discussed in preceding sections of this chapter) to deal with general child behavior problems and parenting difficulties. Once a family has completed the standardized parenting training protocol, then additional interventions can be put into place for children who frequently steal. Patterson and colleagues state that it is necessary to operationalize stealing. This means defining what it is that the child typically steals and allowing the parent to rely on his or her "gut feeling" to determine whether or not a child has stolen. The parent is not required to have "proof" of the child's stealing behavior (because many children lie when confronted about stealing). The second step involves the parent monitoring the child's stealing behavior. This could include checking the child's room or checking his or her possessions to determine whether specific items have been stolen. Finally, a mild consequence is utilized for every occurrence of the stealing behavior. This might entail grounding, temporary removal of toys from the child, and so on.

Tremblay and Drabman's (1997) protocol is similar to the Patterson and colleagues (1975) intervention, but also incorporates the concepts of apology, restitution, overcorrection, and praise for alternative behaviors. Again, Tremblay and Drabman do not require parents to obtain proof of a child's stealing. Tremblay and Drabman described a five-step procedure. All steps must be complied with by the child. If he or she does not comply with each step, then consequences are put into place until the steps are completed (e.g., losing privileges of watching TV, playing videos, or going outside). The five steps are as follows:

1. Identify instances of stealing—this includes searching the child, observing the child, and monitoring the child's whereabouts and activities to determine whether or not he or she has stolen.
2. Apology—if the child is caught stealing, he or she must confess and apologize to the victim. The parent is required to supervise the apology.
3. Return or replace stolen item—the child is required to return the stolen item at the apology session. If the stolen item is missing, the child must replace it.
4. Restitution plus 100%—in addition to returning or replacing the stolen item, the child must also pay the victim an amount of money equal to the value of the item that was stolen (i.e., its replacement cost). In essence, the child is required both to replace the stolen item and add on this additional payment. If the child is unable to come up with the money for payment, he or she is required to do chores to earn the money.
5. Role reversal—the child is made to relinquish an item identical or similar to the item that was originally stolen (e.g., if the child stole a toy car, he or she would relinquish a toy car). This requires the child to experience the role reversal of what it feels like to have something taken. It also serves the purpose of an additional consequence.

Intervening with Firesetting

Kolko (1996) advised that practitioners fully understand the conditions and risk factors that support firesetting in children so they can be addressed in the intervention. It could be that the child is being exposed to individuals who model firesetting behavior. Perhaps the child lacks knowledge about the consequences of setting fires. It might be that the child exhibits other self-control problems (e.g., anger, reactive aggression, defiance) and/or anti-social behavior. Perhaps parents are providing insufficient monitoring of the child's whereabouts and activities. All these risk factors, if present in a particular child, will need to be addressed in the intervention.

A primary intervention for firesetting is to improve parent monitoring of the child and parent use of standing or house rules. The procedures for monitoring and supervising children were discussed earlier. This is critical for the parents of children who set fires. They need to provide structure and know the whereabouts and activities of their child. In particular, the parent needs to be vigilant in spotting potential incidents of firesetting by the child. In addition, it is important to make sure the child has ample opportunity to be involved in prosocial activities with other children or in the community (see Chapter 10 for a review of community-based programs). The parent should employ a standing rule that the child cannot play with fire or he or she will lose a privilege.

Educational and skills training interventions are also used for children who set fires (Kolko, 1996). Many community fire departments offer educational programs that teach the child about the dangers and consequences of setting fires. Children who set fires also benefit from learning self-control strategies such as problem solving, verbal self-instruction, and social skills (see Chapter 4).

Addressing Parents' Personal and Other Family Problems

Expanded PFST interventions teach parents coping skills, deal with marital/relationship problems, strengthen home–school ties, and promote parents' problem-solving skills to enable them to respond to ongoing personnel and child behavioral challenges. Socioeconomic and community factors are also attended to in broader applications of PFST. For example, it may be necessary to assist the parent or the family in accessing community resources to deal with financial problems or to obtain affordable housing. Most PFST programs address broader parent/family/contextual problems with the families being served.

One strategy is to evaluate the family and make additional referrals as needed. Chapter 3 of this volume discusses assessment procedures. If certain problems are noted in the assessment, then referral to other services would be warranted. For example, it may be determined that the child or a family member has additional problems not addressed in PFST (e.g., mental health problems, marital difficulties, domestic abuse, inadequate child care, lack of after-school activities, housing needs). If problems are identified, then referrals are made to appropriate mental health, marital/family therapy, domestic abuse, and social services agencies.

A second strategy is to teach parents to cope with chronic stress. The idea is to teach parents commonsense strategies to deal with mild to moderate stress levels. This is accomplished through education and discussion. Parents learn to cope with chronic stress by using the following strategies:

1. Relaxation—teach various relaxation procedures.
2. Obtain occasional respite from the children and family—assist parents in scheduling time for themselves and arranging for babysitting.
3. Seek out social support—strategize with parents who feel isolated about different ways that they can seek support from family members and neighbors or attend community events.
4. Schedule pleasant events—encourage parents to schedule specific pleasant events in their daily or weekly schedule (e.g., go for a walk).
5. Develop good health habits—educate parents about the importance of increasing one's exercise level, eating a healthy diet, getting enough rest, and generally taking care of themselves.
6. Join a parents support group—refer parents to support groups for children with ADHD, for grief and loss, for dieting, and so on.

A third strategy is to train parents in cognitive restructuring of upsetting and/or distorted thoughts. Typically, cognitive restructuring is accomplished by identifying "unhelpful" thoughts, understanding the unhelpful nature of these thoughts, and countering these unhelpful thoughts with more "helpful" thoughts. Bloomquist (1996) offered a list of unhelpful parent thoughts and helpful counterthoughts to be utilized in cognitive restructuring exercises with parents. Figure 5.4 displays examples of several unhelpful and helpful thoughts for parents. These example thoughts pertain to attributions, beliefs, and expectations the parent may have about child, self, and who needs to change. Bloomquist has parents determine whether or not these thoughts are typical for them, whether or not these thoughts are helpful, how the unhelpful and helpful thoughts influence their behavior, and how this behavior ultimately affects their child. Most parents are able to identify unhelpful thoughts and learn effective helpful counterthoughts.

A fourth strategy is to teach couples and family members practical skills for dealing with broader family interactions. This is accomplished by teaching parents and family members communication and family problem-solving skills. For example, Bloomquist (1996) provided a list of family communication "Do's" and "Don'ts" (see Figure 5.5 on page 171). Couples and family members are asked to evaluate themselves for the Don'ts that they typically do. Couples or family members then practice the Do's in the session and gradually learn to use the new communication skills in real-

Unhelpful Parent Thoughts

Listed below are a variety of common thoughts that parents of children with behavior problems may have. Read each thought and indicate how frequently that thought (or a similar thought) typically occurs for you over an average week. There are no right or wrong answers to these questions. Use the 5-point rating scale to help you evaluate your thoughts:

1	2	3	4	5
Not at all	Sometimes	Moderately often	All the time	Often

1. _____ My child acts up on purpose.
2. _____ My child is the cause of most of our family problems.
3. _____ It is my fault that my child has problems.
4. _____ It is his/her fault (other parent) that my child is this way.
5. _____ I give up. There is nothing more I can do for my child.
6. _____ I have no control over my child, I have tried everything, and so forth.

For each thought you rated a 3, 4, or 5, ask yourself the following questions:

1. What is unhelpful about this thought?
2. How would this thought influence my behavior toward my child?
3. How would my behavior, which relates to my thought, affect my child?

Helpful "Counter" Thoughts for Parents

Listed below are "counter" thoughts that parents can think instead of unhelpful thoughts. Unhelpful Thought #1 corresponds to Helpful Thought #1 and so on. Compare the unhelpful thoughts to the helpful thoughts.

1. It doesn't matter whose fault it is. What matters are solutions to the problems.
2. It is not just my child; I also play a role in the problem.
3. It is not just my fault; my child also plays a role in the problems.
4. It doesn't help to blame him/her (other parent). We need to work together.
5. I have to parent my child. I have no choice. I need to think of new ways to parent my child.
6. My belief that I have no control over my child might be contributing to the problem. Many things are in my control. I need to figure out what I can do to solve the problem.

Ask yourself the following questions about these helpful thoughts:

1. What is helpful about this thought?
2. How would this thought influence my behavior toward my child?
3. How would my behavior, which relates to my thought, affect my child?

FIGURE 5.4. Example of Unhelpful and Helpful Parent Thoughts. Other thoughts that are specific to a particular parent can be targeted using this procedure. From Bloomquist (1996). Copyright 1996 by The Guilford Press. Adapted by permission.

life family interactions. In addition, through the process of education and practice, family members can learn to solve family problems by going through the following problem-solving steps:

1. "Stop, what is the problem we are having?"
2. "What are some plans we can use?"
3. "What is the best plan we can use?"
4. "Do the plan."
5. "Did the plan work?"

Gradually, couples and family members are trained to employ communication and problem-solving skills at home to deal with ongoing marital and/or family problems.

Integrating Parent and Family Skills Training

Increasingly practitioners are integrating many of the previously discussed procedures into a comprehensive PFST program. McMahon and colleagues (1996) provided an example of an integrated model of PFST for children with ACP. The parent/family training program is part of their Fast Track Prevention Program that targets young aggressive children who are at risk for developing later significant conduct problems (see Chapter 11 for a discussion of the Fast Track program). McMahon and colleagues' model is a good example of integrating basic PFST content with expanded content.

Parents meet in small groups with two leaders for parent group training. The content of the parent group addresses parenting and broader family issues. First, there is an emphasis on promoting academic competence among children. Parents are taught to monitor their child's academic progress, collaborate with teachers, engage the child in reading and other academic enrichment activities, and work with their child by encouraging homework and general learning development. Teachers are also invited to visit the parent groups occasionally to discuss learning and classroom issues. Next parents learn personal self-control strategies to manage their own anger/frustration/stress. Parents learn to recognize their anger (and other feelings) and then learn how to interrupt the anger process. They learn strategies for calming down, such as counting to 10, taking deep breaths, and taking a break. They reward themselves for staying calm while interacting with their children. The program also focuses on changing the thoughts and expectations of the parents. Group facilitators lead parents to better understand what is developmentally appropriate for their children.

Much of the program concentrates on parents learning effective child management skills. The Discipline Pyramid pictured in Figure 5.6 on page 172 organizes this part of the training and graphically emphasizes what parents should use to manage their children's behavior. The lower and big-

DON'Ts	DOs
• Long lectures or "sermons"	• Use brief statements of 10 words or less.
• Blaming (e.g., "You need to stop _____," "It's your fault," etc.)	• Use "I" statements (e.g., "I feel _____ when _____") or take responsibility for your own actions.
• Vague statements (e.g., "Shape up," "Knock it off," "I don't like that," etc.)	• Use direct and specific statements (e.g.,"Stop teasing your sister").
• Asking negative questions (e.g., "Why do you always do that?," "How many times must I tell you?")	• Use direct and specific statements (e.g., "Stop teasing your brother").
• Poor listening while looking away, silent treatment, crossing arms, and so forth	• Actively listen with good eye contact, leaning forward, nodding, and so forth.
• Interrupting others	• Let each person completely state his/her thoughts before stating yours.
• Not checking to see if you really understand others	• Give feedback/paraphrase (e.g., restate what another said to you).
• Put-downs (e.g., "You're worthless," "I'm sick of you," etc.), threats, and so forth	• Be constructive (e.g., "I'm concerned about your grades," "Something is bothering me; can we discuss it?," etc.).
• Yelling, screaming, and so forth	• Use a neutral/natural tone of voice.
• Sarcasm	• Say what you mean, be specific and straightforward.
• Going from topic to topic	• Stay on one topic.
• Bringing up old issues, past behavior	• Focus on here and now.
• Not matching verbal and nonverbal communications (e.g., saying "I love you" while pounding one's fist angrily on the table	• Match verbal and nonverbal communication (e.g., saying, "I love you" while smiling).
• Keeping feelings inside	• Express feelings to others appropriately.
• Scowling, directing antagonistic facial expressions toward others	• Use appropriate facial expressions toward others.
• "Mind reading" or assuming you know what other people think	• Really listen to others' point of view; ask questions to make sure you understand.

FIGURE 5.5. Couple and family communication skills. From Bloomquist (1996). Copyright 1996 by The Guilford Press. Reprinted by permission.

ger part of the pyramid is the positive approaches that parents can use to increase positive behavior in their children. Parents are trained to use these strategies most of the time. The upper and smaller portion of the pyramid contains negative approaches that parents can use to decrease negative behavior in children. Parents are trained to use these strategies least.

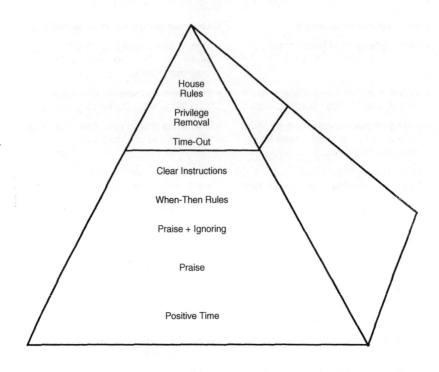

FIGURE 5.6. The Discipline Pyramid. From McMahon, Slough, and Conduct Problems Prevention Research Group (1996). Copyright 1996 by Sage Publications, Inc. Reprinted by permission.

Parents are taught all the skills in the pyramid and a problem-solving approach to solve specific child problems.

Deciding Which Skills to Emphasize in Training

We understand that practitioners cannot deliver all the previously discussed content interventions to families receiving PFST. Practitioners will need to select those skill areas that are most relevant for the family or group of families being served. In our opinion, the families of younger children will gain the most from interventions that focus on promoting parenting skills and parent–child cohesion. Of course, older children will benefit from these procedures too, but they also could be involved in learning family interaction skills. The PFST content that addresses broader needs of parents and families will certainly be relevant to most families. Obviously, the presenting problems of the families being served need to be considered in selecting

TABLE 5.2. Summary of Best Practice Training Content Areas for Parent and Family Skills Training

Training content areas	Best practices
Understanding social learning principles	Teach parents about the rationale and theoretical principles underlying specific interventions.
Observing and tracking child behavior	Teach parents to define and pinpoint specific child behaviors; plan when to observe the child; count the frequency of the behavior during child observation.
Encouraging child-directed interaction and play	Teach parents to increase relationship-enhancing behaviors and decrease relationship-detracting behaviors during child-directed play and activities.
Shaping positive behavior with positive attention and reinforcement	Teach parents to increase attention and reinforcement for prosocial child behavior.
Ignoring mild negative behavior	Teach parents to reduce attention for mild child problem behavior.
Defusing power struggles and deescalating parent–child conflict	Teach parents stress management skills to stay calm and commonsense strategies to avoid and defuse escalating child behavior.
Using time-out/removal of privileges for noncompliance	Teach parents to stay calm and use effective commands/warning/time-out or removing privileges procedures.
Using standing or house rules for behavior	Teach parents to explicitly state the rules and use time-out or removal of privileges when rules are violated.
Using a token system for behavior management	Teach parents to use tokens/points to shape child behavior.
Monitoring and supervising children	Teach parents to keep track of children; provide structure and expectations.
Intervening with stealing	Teach parents to define stealing, monitor stealing, and provide consequences for stealing incidents.
Intervening with firesetting	Teach parents to monitor child, provide contingent reinforcement for prosocial activity involvement, and provide contingent loss of privileges for firesetting. Teaching child self-control skills and educating him or her about fire safety may also help.
Addressing parents' personal and other family problems	Teach family members to use commonsense/practical strategies to deal with personal, parent/family, and contextual problems; teach them skills to cope with stress, restructure unhelpful thoughts, and improve marital/family interactions.
Integrating parent and family skills training	Combine multiple skills training content areas into one intervention.
Deciding which skills to emphasize in training	Consider the developmental status of children, their presenting problems, and practical matters in determining which skill training content areas to emphasize in training.

interventions. In addition, practical matters need to be taken into account. There is a limit to the amount of time that a practitioner can work with a family. Since it takes three to six sessions to initially train parents or family members in any one skill area, the practitioner needs to determine which are the most important skills to focus on. Practitioners are therefore advised to carefully consider the unique needs of the families they are working with and provide the most relevant PFST interventions. The practitioner will need to determine the amount of sessions he or she can deliver to a family and plan accordingly.

Summary

Table 5.2 provides a summary of best practices for training content in PFST. As the table demonstrates, there are multiple skills that can be taught and much overlap between them. Practitioners need to match the specific needs of the families receiving PFST and select those that are most in need of change.

CONCLUSION

PFST is an empirically supported intervention for children with ACP. We have presented the most common intervention ingredients for conducting effective PFST with the parents and families of children with ACP. PFST can be delivered in clinic, school, and community settings. We strongly advocate that practitioners include PFST in their work with most, if not all, children with ACP and their families.

CHAPTER 6

Mental Health Treatments

Children with ACP and related difficulties are frequently served in mental health treatment settings. In fact, children diagnosed with ODD, CD, and ADHD comprise the largest numbers of child cases receiving mental health services (Kazdin, 1995). In many instances it is necessary for children with ACP to receive mental health services as part of a comprehensive intervention plan.

In this chapter we describe mental health treatments for children with ACP who qualify for a psychiatric diagnosis and who exhibit functional impairment. This includes treatments for children with diagnoses of ODD, CD, and ADHD, as well as comorbid psychiatric conditions. The various mental health treatments fall somewhere on a continuum expressing the amount of restrictiveness experienced by the child. The level of restrictiveness corresponds to the level of symptoms and the amount of functional impairment the child exhibits. Less restrictive treatments include medications and clinic therapy (i.e., therapy provided by practitioners in mental health settings); more restrictive treatments include summer treatment programs, day treatment/partial hospitalization, residential treatment, and inpatient hospitalization. Typically, these interventions are conducted in a mental health setting by experienced mental health practitioners. We will discuss all these types of mental health services in this chapter.

We hypothesize that mental health treatments address risk factors and protective factors in the child, parent/family, and, to some extent, social/peer life domains (see Tables 2.3 and 2.4 in Chapter 2). Medications reduce risk in the child and parent/family life domains primarily through behavioral and emotional symptom reduction in the child. Clinic therapy and more restrictive treatments also reduce the same risks, but have the potential to enhance protective factors in the child and parent/family life domains (if they incorporate effective interventions such as social competence training, parent and family skills training, etc.). Although not typically a direct focus, mental health treatments can positively effect the social/peer life domain by reducing some of the negative child behaviors and characteristics that adversely impact social interactions and peer affiliations.

Our presentation of mental health treatments is divided into three main sections. First, we review common medications used to treat symptoms associated with behavior disorders. Second, we discuss procedures that can be used to improve the effectiveness of clinic therapy. Third, we provide information pertaining to increasingly restrictive treatments for children with severe levels of impairment. In each of these sections we review available research that evaluates treatment effects and present best practices for conducting them. We also give examples of different practices.

OVERVIEW AND RESEARCH EVALUATION OF MEDICATION TREATMENT

Medications are commonly administered to treat children with ADHD, ADHD with comorbid disorders, and aggression. These medications target ADHD symptoms, including hyperactivity, impulsivity, and inattentiveness. Aggressive behaviors, especially those associated with emotional lability and arousal, are also targeted by prescribing medications. Finally, various medications can treat comorbid conditions such as mood and anxiety disorders. Different medications, with different pharmacological effects, are used to reduce these target symptoms.

Childhood pharmacotherapy entails the use of six common classes of medications: stimulants, antidepressants, mood stabilizers, antihypertensives (adrenergic agonist), antipsychotics, and antianxiety medications (Wilens, 1999). Antipsychotic and antianxiety medications are not as commonly used for ACP and related problems as are the other classes of medications. Numerous studies exist evaluating the effects of these different medications on children; most of them focus on stimulants. We will attempt to summarize this research by discussing reviews of the literature conducted by the American Academy of Child and Adolescent Psychiatry (1997a, 1997b), Green (1996), Greenhill, Halperin, and Abikoff (1999), Schachar and Ickowicz (1999), Spencer and colleagues (1996), Waslick, Werry, and Greenhill (1999), and Wilens (1999). What follows is a research review of the most commonly used medications, the mechanisms by which they are hypothesized to impact children, and the observed effects on children's functioning.

Stimulants are by far the most widely prescribed medications in childhood pharmacotherapy. They are used primarily to treat children with behavior disorders. The six common types of stimulants include methylphenidate (Ritalin, Metadate, Concerta), dextroamphetamine (Dexedrine), magnesium pemoline (Cylert), amphetamine (Biphetamine), methamphetamine (Desoxyn), and amphetamine compounds (Adderall). Of all the stimulants, methylphenidate is the most commonly used. Stimulants improve neurotransmitter production of dopamine and norepinephrine in the central nervous system. The clinical effects of stimulants are short acting for the most part (approximately 3 to 6 hours), although there are longer acting variations of methylphenidate and dextroamphetamine (approximately 8 to 12 hours). Magnesium pemoline and amphetamine compounds are by their chemical nature longer acting medications (approximately 12 to 24 hours). Most studies have evaluated stimulant medications used with children with ADHD who may or may not have other commonly associated problems. This includes many randomized controlled research studies. The specific effects of stimulant medications are summarized in Table 6.1. These medications improve the core symptoms of ADHD, including hyperactivity, impulsivity, and inattentiveness, in a majority of children. Use of stimulants also results in a reduction of aggression, anger, noncompliance, and some covert behaviors. Importantly, stimulant medications also positively influence peer–child and parent–child interactions, as well as academic productivity. Higher doses are related to improved behavior and reduction of aggression.

Four types of antidepressant medications are prescribed for children exhibiting behavioral, mood, and anxiety disorders. One type is tricyclic antidepressants. The most common tricylics are imipramine (Tofranil), desipramine (Norpramin, Pertofrane), nortriptyline (Pamelor), and clomipramine (Anafranil). Generally, tricyclic antidepressants promote production of the serotonin and norepinephrine neurotransmitters. It can take weeks for an individual to achieve a therapeutic dose, but once such a dosage is achieved, these medications provide continuous coverage of symptoms. Research data is based on case reports, open trials, and several randomized controlled studies. Tricyclic antidepressants primarily reduce such behavioral dimensions of ADHD as disruptive behavior. They are less effective than stimulants, however, in improving behavior in children. They exert limited impact on children's academic productivity and cognitive performance. Although these medications reduce aggression in animals, this has not been studied in children.

The second type of antidepressants is the selective serotonin reuptake inhibitors (SSRIs). These SSRIs include fluoxetine (Prozac), sertraline (Zoloft), fluvoxamine (Luvox), paroxetine (Paxil), and citalopram (Celexa). These antidepressants enhance the production of the serotonin neurotransmitter. They also provide long-lasting coverage once a therapeutic dose has been achieved. There is limited research evaluating their effectiveness; what does exist is primarily case reports and open trials. Nonetheless, research

TABLE 6.1. Specific Effects Documented in Groups of ADHD Stimulant Responders

Motor effects

Reduce activity to the level of normal peers
Decrease excessive talking, noise, and disruption in the classroom
Improve handwriting
Improve fine motor control

Social effects

Reduce off-task behavior in classroom
Improve ability to play and work independently
Reduce anger
Decrease intensity of behavior
Improve participation when playing baseball
Reduce bossiness with peers
Reduce verbal and physical aggression with peers
Improve (but not normalize) peer social status
Reduce impulsive stealing and property destruction (in a laboratory setting)
Reduce noncompliance, defiance, and oppositional behavior with adults
Improve mother–child and family interactions
Parents and teachers become less controlling and more positive

Cognitive effects

Improve sustained attention, especially to boring tasks
Reduce distractibility
Improve short-term memory
Reduce impulsivity
Enhance use of cognitive strategies already in the repertoire
Increase amount of academic work completed
Increase accuracy of academic work

Note. From American Academy of Child and Adolescent Psychiatry (1997b). Copyright 1997 by Lippincott Williams & Wilkins. Reprinted by permission.

does suggest that SSRIs improve the behavioral dimensions of ADHD, but not attention. These medications have been found to reduce aggression in animals, but they have not been well studied for this effect in children.

Monamine oxidase inhibitors (MAOIs) are a third type of antidepressants. The MAOIs include phenelzine (Nardil) and tranylcypromine (Parnate). These medications stop the breakdown of norepinephrine and dopamine neurotransmitters. Their effects are also long-lasting once a therapeutic dose is reached. The research consists mostly of case studies and open trials, although some randomized controlled studies do exist. Tranylcypromine has been found to reduce behavioral symptoms of ADHD in children. The MAOIs impact on children's aggression has not been well studied.

The final type of antidepressants is the atypical antidepressants. The

Mental Health Treatments   179

atypicals include venlafaxine (Effexor), trazodone (Desyrel), nefazodone (Serzone), bupropion (Wellbutrin), and mirtazapine (Remeron). These medications enhance production of the serotonin and dopamine neurotransmitters. Among the atypical antidepressants, some are short acting, while others are long lasting. Bupropion is the most studied atypical antidepressant. The research consists of case studies, open trials, and a few randomized controlled designs. Bupropion has been found to reduce children's ADHD symptoms, but not as well as methylphenidate. Irritable moods in children have also improved with bupropion.

Mood stabilizers are designed to control and level out mood swings. These include lithium, carbamazepine (Tegretol), and valproic acid (Depakote). Mood stabilizers have nonspecific effects on hormones and neurotransmitters. They provide continuous coverage of symptoms after a therapeutic dose is reached. The research is sparse, but there are case studies, open trial studies, and some randomized controlled trials (especially with lithium). These medications have been mostly evaluated with children who have severe levels of aggression. They have been found to reduce volatile moods, aggressive behavior, and ADHD symptoms in children.

The antihypertensives (adrenergic agonists) were originally designed to treat high blood pressure in adults. They include clonidine (Catapres), guanfacine (Tenex), propranolol (Inderal), and nadolol (Corgard). The antihypertensives promote the release of the norepinephine neurotransmitter. They have a short half-life and are sometimes administered through a skin patch. The research evaluating these medications mostly consists of case studies and open trials. Most of the research has been on clonidine. These medications, especially clonidine, have been found to reduce aggression and anger outbursts in children, as well as some of their ADHD symptoms.

Antipsychotic and antianxiety medications are rarely applied specifically to ACP or the disruptive behavior disorders in children. Antipsychotic medications such as haloperidol and antianxiety medications (tranquilizers) such as benzodiazepines reduce severe aggression in children and adults. These powerful drugs are still rarely used with children because of the potential for significant side effects. These medications may be useful, however, when children exhibit comorbid psychotic or anxiety symptomatology. Readers interested in more information regarding antipsychotic and antianxiety medications should consult Wilens (1999).

Different classes of medication are frequently combined in clinical practice. This is done to address comorbid diagnoses/multiple symptoms and/or nonresponding children. For example, a stimulant might be combined with an antidepressant, a mood stabilizer, or an antihypertensive. Different combinations of medications produce different effects. Although combining medications is common in clinical practice, it has not been subjected to extensive research.

There are limitations regarding the effects of medications and the research that has been conducted to evaluate them. For example, information about the long-term benefits of medication to improve functional outcomes in children such as academic achievement, peer relationships, and antisocial behaviors is sparse. An exception to this is a recent retrospective study conducted by Biederman, Wilens, Mick, Spencer, and Faraone (1999), which determined that boys with ADHD who received medications (primarily stimulants) were less likely to abuse substances 4 years later than nonmedicated boys. Another problem with the research is that most of it evaluates elementary school-age Caucasian boys. Studies examining the effects of medications on children of different ages, genders, and races are rare. In particular, there is a pressing need to evaluate the impact of medications with preschoolers.

In summary, different medications can be used to treat the core symptoms of ADHD, ADHD with comorbid disorders, and aggression in children. In most cases, stimulants are the first-line medications because they have the most research support for treating these children. In general, the antidepressants are best suited for treating ADHD symptoms and comorbid depression and anxiety difficulties. Some preliminary evidence suggests that mood stabilizers and antihypertensives may assist children who are prone to labile moods and aggressive behavior. By reducing their disruptive and aggressive behaviors with medications, children with ACP and related problems may be more amenable to other interventions (see Chapter 11 for a discussion of medications combined with other interventions).

BEST PRACTICES FOR MEDICATION ADMINISTRATION AND MANAGEMENT

We utilized several sources to derive best practices for medication administration and management. These sources include (1) several textbooks/chapters that provide extensive information regarding the clinical practice of pharmacotherapy, including Barkley (1998), Green (1996), and Wilens (1999); (2) the American Academy of Child and Adolescent Psychiatry's (1997a, 1997b) practice parameters for assessment and treatment of children and adolescents with ADHD and CD; and (3) Greenhill and colleagues' (1996) review of medication treatment strategies used in the multimodal treatment of ADHD study (MTA) (see Chapter 11 for a review of the MTA study). These sources present detailed practical information and describe the roles of practitioners, parents, teachers, and children in the administration and management of medications. Typically, a physician is the lead practitioner who manages the medications, with other practitioners and parents assisting in the monitoring process.

Making a Careful Decision to Medicate

It is incumbent upon practitioners to collaborate with parents and children to make a careful decision regarding medication. There are many options and practical matters to consider in deciding whether or not medication should be tried. Barkley (1998) suggested that 14 questions be considered to determine the appropriateness of medications for a given child:

1. Has the child had adequate psychiatric and physical evaluations? Medications should only be given to healthy children with a psychiatric diagnosis.
2. How old is the child? Medications are rarely administered to preschool children.
3. Have other therapies been tried? Ideally other interventions have been attempted before a medication trial.
4. How severe are the child's current symptoms? In some instances, the level of symptoms are severe enough to warrant an immediate medication trial.
5. Can the family afford medications and associated costs? Medications and follow-up visits with physicians are expensive.
6. Are the parents sufficiently able to adequately supervise the use of medications and guard against their abuse? Parents must be able to monitor medication use and/or coordinate with school officials in this regard.
7. What is the parent's attitude toward pharmacotherapy? Ideally a parent would have an open mind regarding medications for his or her child.
8. Is there a substance-abusing sibling or parent in the household? To avoid possible illicit use or sale, alternative medications with little or no street value could be utilized.
9. Does the child have a history of tics, psychosis, or thought disorder? Stimulants may be counterindicated for these conditions.
10. Is the child highly anxious, fearful, or more likely to complain of psychosomatic disturbances? Such children should perhaps be tried on antidepressant medications.
11. Does the physician have the time to monitor medication effects properly? This includes initial assessment of drug efficacy, determining optimal dosage, and monitoring drug effects.
12. How does the child feel about medication and its alternatives? A particular child should be willing to take the medication.
13. Is the child or adolescent involved in competitive sports in which urine screens for illicit drug use is routine? Family members should be made aware of the possibility of disqualification from

competitive sports events while using medications (e.g., methyl-phenidate).

14. Is the older adolescent being considered for medication treatment planning on entering the military? There have been reported cases in the United States where adolescents were denied entrance into the military because of a history of ADHD and/or stimulant medication usage.

Practitioners should consider these 14 questions with family members. This will help determine the applicability and feasibility of medications with a particular child. Additionally, the parent should be fully informed as to the possible benefits and side effects of medications before they are prescribed.

Medications are not to be used as a "quick fix" or to satisfy a stressed parent or teacher. The practitioner should be aware of the influence of family adversity (e.g., chaotic living circumstances, evidence of child abuse, maternal depression, etc.), and not rush to prescribe medications when family adversity and other stressors might account for the presence or exacerbation of symptoms. In such cases, alternative interventions may be indicated or used with medications.

Selecting Medication Type

The selection of specific medications is based on current symptoms, past history of medication usage, and practical considerations. Different diagnoses and/or symptoms warrant different medications or combinations. Table 6.2 from Wilens (1999) can assist practitioners in deciding which medications to use with children that have ADHD and/or ODD/CD. Generally stimulants are the first-line drug. If there is a past history of limited clinical effectiveness and/or significant side effects with a particular stimulant, then consideration should be given to another stimulant or an alternative medication. Finally, certain medications may be impractical. For example, some children "forget" to take an afternoon dose of a shorter acting stimulant (e.g., methylphenidate), so it may be efficacious in some situations to consider using a long-acting medication (e.g., Dexedrine spansules, Wellbutrin, etc.) instead. The practitioner should weigh these issues and collaborate with the family to determine which medications will work best for their child.

Assessing Functional Domains

An assessment methodology needs to be established so that the effects of medications can be monitored during the initial dosage titration and over time. At least three domains of functioning should be assessed to determine the impact of medications. Parents and teachers can be asked to provide

TABLE 6.2. Pharmacotherapy of ADHD and the Disruptive Behavioral Disorders

Disorder	Pharmacotherapy

Attention-deficit/ hyperactivity disorder	Stimulants—Ritalin, Dexedrine, Adderall
	  First-line drugs of choice
	  Caution in patients with tics or marked height/weight
	    problems
	
	Cylert
	  Caution with liver problems
	
	Clonidine, Tenex (guanfacine)
	  Good for overactivity and impulsivity, preschoolers
	  First line for patients with ADHD and tics
	
	Tricyclic antidepressants—desipramine, nortriptyline, imipramine
	  Second line after stimulants
	  Good for co-occurring depression, anxiety, or tics
	  Caution if cardiac problems
	
	Wellbutrin (bupropion)
	  Second line after stimulants
	  Caution if tics or seizures
	
	Combined pharmacotherapy for resistant cases

Conduct disorder, oppositional defiant disorder	No specific pharmacotherapy available for core disorders
	
	Look for and treat other disorders (e.g., ADHD, depression)
	
	Consider stimulants, antidepressants
	
	For agitation, aggression, and self-abuse
	  Beta blockers (e.g., propranolol)
	  Clonidine, guanfacine
	  Benzodiazepines (e.g., Valium, Klonopin)
	  Lithium, anticonvulsants (e.g., Tegretol, Valproate, Neurontin)
	  Naltrexone
	  Antipsychotics (e.g., Thorazine, Mellaril, Zyprexa)

Note. From Wilens (1999). Copyright 1999 by Timothy E. Wilens. Reprinted by permission.

ratings or interview information to assess these three functional domains. The first domain is symptoms. Generally, ratings should reflect the symptoms being targeted with the medication such as impulsivity, hyperactivity, inattention, aggression, and defiance. The second domain is impairment. Ratings that assess the child's academic performance and social functioning at school and home are the most relevant and helpful in determining medication effects. Different examples of rating scales to assess symptoms and impairment were described in Chapter 3 (e.g., Connors Behavior Rating Scale, Home or School Situations Questionnaires, etc.). The third domain is side effects. All medications have the potential for side effects, so it is very important to carefully monitor them. Figure 6.1 reproduces Barkley's (1998) Stimulant Drug Side Effects Rating Scale. This scale can be adapted to monitor the side effects of other medications.

Determining Best Dosage and Schedule

It is essential to titrate medications to find the precise dosage that will achieve maximum positive benefits with minimal negative side effects. In fact, the positive findings associated with the medication intervention in the MTA study (discussed in Chapter 11) were largely attributed to the careful titration procedure used to define the optimum dosage for each child. Therefore careful and effective titration is imperative.

Most medications come with manufacturer-recommended dosages based on a fixed dose range (lower to upper limits) and/or according to body weight (milligrams of medications per kilograms of child's weight). It

---

Name _____ Date _____

Person completing this form _____

Instructions: Please rate each behavior from 0 (absent) to 9 (serious). Circle only one number beside each item. A zero means that you have not seen the behavior in this child during the past week, and a 9 means that you have noticed it and believe it to be either very serious or to occur very frequently.

Behavior	*Absent*									*Serious*
Insomnia or trouble sleeping	0	1	2	3	4	5	6	7	8	9
Nightmares	0	1	2	3	4	5	6	7	8	9
Stares a lot or daydreams	0	1	2	3	4	5	6	7	8	9
Talks less with others	0	1	2	3	4	5	6	7	8	9
Uninterested in others	0	1	2	3	4	5	6	7	8	9
Decreased appetite	0	1	2	3	4	5	6	7	8	9
Irritable	0	1	2	3	4	5	6	7	8	9
Stomachaches	0	1	2	3	4	5	6	7	8	9
Headaches	0	1	2	3	4	5	6	7	8	9
Drowsiness	0	1	2	3	4	5	6	7	8	9
Sad/unhappy	0	1	2	3	4	5	6	7	8	9
Prone to crying	0	1	2	3	4	5	6	7	8	9
Anxious	0	1	2	3	4	5	6	7	8	9
Bites fingernails	0	1	2	3	4	5	6	7	8	9
Euphoric/unusually happy	0	1	2	3	4	5	6	7	8	9
Dizziness	0	1	2	3	4	5	6	7	8	9
Tics or nervous movements	0	1	2	3	4	5	6	7	8	9

FIGURE 6.1. Stimulant Drug Side Effects Rating Scale. From Barkley (1998). Copyright 1998 by The Guilford Press. Reprinted by permission.

is beyond the scope of this chapter to provide suggested dosage levels for the many medications used to treat children with ADHD, ADHD with comorbid conditions, and aggression (interested readers should consult Wilens, 1999). Most practitioners advocate starting low and working up to achieve the best effects. Over time, parent and teacher ratings of symptoms, impairment, and side effects can be utilized to determine the precise dosage.

We use stimulants as an example to describe titration procedures because they are the most commonly utilized medications for children with ADHD and associated problems. Barkley (1998) advocated starting at the lower end of the recommended dosage and gradually raising the dosage in small increments on a weekly basis. Barkley obtains teacher's ratings at least once per week and parent ratings at least two times per week to evaluate medication effects. The procedure can be utilized to determine ideal dosage and the schedule of administration.

The titration procedure used in the MTA study, as described by Greenhill and colleagues (1996), can be used as a model for best practices. All children with a prior medication history first go through a "washout" period prior to initiation of medication. The child is taken off all medications (if he or she is already on medications) for a period long enough to make sure that all prior medications are inactive. Then there is a 4- to 11-day lead-in titration trial. The child receives a typical dosage depending on his or her weight and side effects are monitored. If no side effects occur, then the child is placed on a 28-day, double-blind, placebo-controlled titration trial. The child is given methylphenidate dosages that vary daily from 5 mg. (5 mg. three times a day), to 10 mg. (10 mg. twice a day and 5 mg. once a day), to 15 mg. (15 mg. twice a day and 5 mg. once a day), to 20 mg. (20 mg. twice a day and 10 mg. once a day). Parents and teachers ratings are completed on a daily basis regarding symptoms, impairment, and side effects. Parent and teacher data are combined and summarized on a daily basis. After the titration trial, the dosage code for each day is revealed to determine the dosage that yielded maximum benefits and lowest side effects. In this way, individualized dosages are determined for all children in the MTA study. Greenhill and colleagues recommend that a similar procedure be adopted in titrating medications in clinical practice.

It is also important at the titration stage to manage side effects. This can be accomplished by altering dosage, schedule, and/or type of medications. Finally, additional interventions (e.g., clinic therapy) could also be used with medications. These procedures may reduce side effects. Occasionally, it is necessary to stop medications altogether because of significant side effects.

Practitioners have discretion in determining the schedule of stimulant medication administration. The decision about when to administer stimulants should be made on a case-by-case basis. Preferences and circumstance for each child and family should be considered. With some children it is preferred to administer the stimulants only during school hours, but with other children it is preferred to administer medications while the child is inside and outside of school. Increasingly practitioners are recommending daily administration of stimulants, including weekends and summer vacations, so the child can derive the benefits across time and in many situations.

Monitoring Medication Effects over Time

Medications need to be monitored over time to make sure that the benefits are maintained in a safe manner. Most practitioners advocate monthly contact with the family. Barkley (1998) and Greenhill and colleagues (1996) suggested collecting monthly parent and teacher ratings to monitor medication effects. Practitioners should also directly interview parents, teachers, and children on a monthly basis. This information can be utilized to make adjustments in dosage or medication administration schedules. Medication dosages can be raised, lowered, or discontinued depending on this information.

Medications also require medical monitoring by a physician. Biological processes such as pulse, blood pressure, weight/height, and liver function are monitored to determine continued safety with various medications. Routine evaluation of serum levels and metabolites allows the physician to determine if certain drugs are being metabolized at a level of therapeutic dose and to guard against toxicity.

Discontinuing Medications

There are no strict guidelines or procedures for discontinuation of medications. The decision to discontinue is made on a case-by-case basis. The practitioner collaborates with the family and utilizes clinical judgment regarding the child's functioning. If the child is doing well in home, school, and community settings for an extended period of time, then discontinuation of medications can be considered. If medications are discontinued, the child should be monitored to assess whether or not he or she maintains adaptive functioning without them. Medications are also discontinued if side effects are judged to be significant.

Summary

Table 6.3 provides a summary of best practices for medication administration and management for children. We strongly recommend that practitioners use the best practices discussed in this section to determine if a trial of medications is indicated and to provide safe and effective medication treatment.

TABLE 6.3. Summary of Best Practices for Medication Administration and Management

Procedures	Best practices
Making a careful decision to medicate	Consider a variety of clinical and practical questions to determine the appropriateness of medications, and whether or not they can be used in an effective and safe manner.
Selecting medication type	Consider the child's diagnosis and prior medication history to select a medication type.
Assessing functional domains	Use assessment procedures (ratings, interviews, etc.) to monitor symptoms, impairment, and side effects of medications.
Determining best dosage and schedule	Try varying dosages and schedules of medication administration; assess the impact of medications on symptoms, impairment, and side effects; choose the dosage and schedule that achieves the best improvement in functioning with minimal side effects.
Monitoring medication effects over time	Continuous assessment of clinical and side effects while the child is on medication.
Discontinuing medications	Discontinue medications if the child maintains improved functioning over an extended period of time; continue to monitor the child's functioning.

OVERVIEW AND RESEARCH
EVALUATION OF CLINIC THERAPY

Clinic therapy (also known as "traditional therapy") is delivered in clinic settings by mental health practitioners and utilizes individual verbal therapy, individual play therapy, child and parent group therapy, family therapy, and marital therapy modalities (Tuma, 1989a; Weiss, Catron, Harris, & Phung, 1999; Weisz, Donenberg, Han, & Weiss, 1995). These therapies commonly incorporate client-centered, psychodynamic, and behavioral/cognitive therapeutic approaches and are delivered in an eclectic manner. The goals of clinic therapy are to develop a therapeutic relationship with the child, help the child get in contact with his or her feelings, promote the child's self-awareness and self-control, assist the child in school adjustment, assist parents in learning effective child-rearing strategies, and help family members to work out their problems.

Weisz and colleagues (1995) identified only nine studies (spanning 50 years) that examined clinic therapy up to 1995. The criteria used to identify these studies included subjects being referred for a variety of mental health problems, services being conducted in clinics, therapy being conducted by clinic-based practitioners, and the therapy being part of ongoing services for that clinic. Most of the studies employed quasi-experimental designs where clinic therapy was compared to a control with placebo conditions. Many of the children served in these studies had behavioral problems. Weisz and colleagues conducted a meta-analysis of these nine studies on various measures of adjustment. They found a very small overall (almost negligible) statistical effect size showing that clinic therapy had virtually no effect on children who received it.

Two recent studies have also examined clinic therapy. Weiss and colleagues (1999) randomly assigned elementary school-age children to two conditions: clinic therapy delivered in a school-based mental health clinic or an academic tutor control group. A majority of the children had problems related to aggression, attention/hyperactivity, and delinquency. The practitioners who worked with them had an average of 6 years of clinical experience. Children received an average of 2 years of clinic therapy delivered over 60 individual sessions; practitioners also provided 18 parent sessions and other consultation services. Children in the academic tutoring group received an average of 53 sessions. Numerous statistical comparisons were conducted on multiple measures. No significant between-group differences emerged. There were also no group differences at a 2-year follow-up assessment (Weiss, Cantron, & Harris, 2000). Children in both groups improved a similar amount. In another study, Andrade, Lambert, and Bickman (2000) reported on a quasi-experimental study where children who received clinic therapy (average of 22 sessions over 2 years) were compared to children who dropped out early and received negligible therapy (average of three sessions). At the end of the study, the children who received clinic therapy were no better off than the children who received negligible therapy.

The data evaluating clinic therapy stands in stark contrast to the data that has evaluated research therapy. This type of therapy is characterized by tightly controlled conditions and services delivered under ideal circumstances. Weisz, Weiss, Han, Granger, and Morton (1995) examined 150 studies evaluating the effects of research therapy for children with an average age of 10 years. Typically, a homogeneous group of children received a specific intervention for a specific problem. Interventions were most commonly conducted in laboratory or school settings. Practitioners were extensively trained to administer a prescribed intervention. For the most part, the interventions were based on behavioral approaches delivered in a standardized manner guided by a manual. Weiss et al. conducted a meta-analysis on various measures of adjustment. Children who received research therapy were compared to children in a variety of different control and comparison groups. A large overall effect size was obtained, suggesting that research therapy improved children's adjustment better than no intervention or alternative interventions. When long-term follow-up was conducted, the results were typically maintained up to nearly 1 year. The interventions used to treat children with externalizing and internalizing problems were equally effective.

We want to highlight Tynan, Schuman, and Lampert's (1999) example of a research therapy protocol being imported into a real-life clinic setting for children with behavior disorders. They employed empirically supported child social competence training and parent and family skills training interventions in an outpatient mental health clinic. The program evaluation they described did not involve use of control or comparison groups. School-age children who were diagnosed as ODD and ADHD and their parents received the interventions. It was an 8-week program of concurrent child and parent groups (see Figure 6.2 for an overview of session content). Tynan et al. found that the treatment was feasible and that treated children displayed improvements on parent ratings of conduct problems at a level that was comparable to improvements found in research therapy studies. Of course, the lack of control or comparison groups limits conclusions, but the study provides preliminary evidence that empirically supported interventions can be successfully used in a clinic setting with children exhibiting behavior disorders.

In summary, clinic therapy has not been demonstrated as effective. In fairness, though, this conclusion should be characterized as tentative due to the limited amount of research evaluating therapy in real-life clinic settings. In addition, many of the studies that do examine clinic therapy have methodological problems. On the other hand, research therapy has been found to improve the adjustment of children. This may be due in part to the rigorous methods employed in research. Of course, it is difficult to replicate the conditions under which research therapy is conducted in a clinic setting. It is hard to argue, however, with the premise that practitioners in clinic settings should strive to approximate research therapy as much as possible. The Tynan and colleagues (1999) program evaluation report revealed that it is possible to bring research-supported intervention protocols into clinic settings. In the next section we review ideas to bridge the gap between clinic therapy and research therapy.

Before presenting ideas to bridge that gap, however, we want to put clinic therapy into perspective. We are not saying that clinic therapy should be discarded. In our opinion, clinic therapy is useful for children with ACP as long as it is not the only modality of intervention. It can be helpful for the children and families to talk, obtain support, and achieve insight regarding life circumstances. It may be beneficial to discuss past events and current problems. Our message is simply that empirically supported interventions should be emphasized in the clinic setting when providing interventions for children with ACP and their families.

SUGGESTED BEST PRACTICES FOR CLINIC THERAPY

This section will be different from other best practice sections in the book because it is based on limited research. Presently, there are few studies where effective clinic therapy practices have been evaluated and supported. More research is needed to test the importation of empirically supported interventions into real-life clinic settings. In other words, research needs to move beyond efficacy trials (i.e., evaluating interventions under ideal and controlled circumstances) to effectiveness trials (i.e., evaluating empirically supported interventions under real-world conditions) (Hoagwood, Hibbs, Brent, & Jenson, 1995).

Given the current state of affairs, here we offer "suggested" best practices that are based on the premise of making clinic therapy more like research therapy. There are many distinctions between how practice is conducted in clinic therapy versus in research therapy. Some of these distinctions may serve as practice parameters to enhance the effectiveness of clinic therapy. Information in this section is derived from six primary sources: (1) Weisz and colleagues' (Weisz et al., 1995; Weisz, Huey, & Weersing, 1998) suggestions for "bridging the gap between the laboratory and the clinic" in the delivery of child therapy; (2) Kazdin's (1997b) recommendations about how to integrate theory, research, and practice in developing effective child treatments; (3) Brestan and Eyberg's (1998), Pelham, Wheeler, and Chronis's (1998), and Ollendick and King's (2000) descriptions of empirically supported interventions; (4) the American Academy of Child and Adolescent Psychiatry's (1997a, 1997b) best practice parameters for treatment of children with CD and ADHD; (5) Tynan and colleagues' (1999) effort to bring empirically supported interventions into the clinic when treating children with behavior disorders; and (6) Henggeler and colleagues' (Henggeler et al., 1998; Schoenwald, Brown, & Henggeler, 2000) review of training and supervision procedures for incorporating empirically supported interventions into multisystemic therapy. Several other sources will also be cited as they pertain to treating comorbid conditions in children who present in clinic settings.

Incorporating Research-Supported
Interventions into Clinic Settings

Here we offer suggestions on how to incorporate research-supported interventions into the clinic setting. Conducting research therapy in a clinical setting may be difficult because of the different circumstances in research and clinic therapy. Practitioners who work in clinic settings usually have high caseloads, little preparation time, and minimal ongoing training and supervision; moreover, they are under pressure to contain costs. These practitioners often employ eclectic treatment methods. The clients commonly present with heterogeneous symptoms and multiple problems. Typically, research therapy is not conducted under these circumstances. Therefore incorporating research therapy into clinical settings can only be accomplished with modifications of usual clinic procedures.

One of the hallmarks of research therapy is the utilization of empirically based decision rules regarding treatment. Clients with specific characteristics are matched to specific interventions. To approximate this procedure, practitioners in clinic settings need to be aware of research findings to guide their decisions about matching specific client problems with specific interventions. In the case of children with ACP, practitioners in clinical settings should utilize many of the empirically supported procedures described in this book with their clientele.

It is recommended that clinic-based interventions be "well established" (similar to proven) or "probably efficacious" (similar to promising) according to the American Psychological Association (Lonigan et al., 1998) and conform to best practices established by the American Academy of Child and Adolescent Psychiatry (1997a, 1997b). Brestan and Eyberg (1998) and Pelham and colleagues (1998) provided a description of well-established and probably efficacious interventions for children with ODD, CD, and ADHD. Their reviews showed that parent training and behavioral classroom management of disruptive/aggressive behaviors have been designated as well established. In addition, social competence training procedures emphasizing problem solving and anger management are probably efficacious for this group of children. The Academy has articulated best practices for the treatment of children with CD and ADHD, recommending utilizing similar empirically supported interventions in the clinic setting. Therefore these two respected professional organizations support the use of parent and child social competence skills training approaches in clinic therapy, and suggest that mental health practitioners should consult with schools regarding classroom behavior management. Best practices for these interventions should be utilized when conducting them (see Chapters 4, 5, and 9).

Modifications of typical clinical service delivery may be necessary to effectively incorporate empirically supported interventions in clinic practice. Practitioners need to have smaller caseloads, and should be afforded more time to plan and prepare for sessions. It is helpful to measure client outcomes (i.e., administer outcome measures before and after clinic therapy) so as to inform ongoing clinical practice. In addition, continuous training, supervision, and monitoring of staff aimed at clinical effectiveness would need to be a priority (this topic receives more attention below).

Tynan and colleagues (1999) provided a good example of incorporating research-supported interventions into a clinic setting. Their program utilized empirically based decision rules to match client characteristics to interventions. Children were carefully diagnosed as ODD and ADHD and were referred to a specialty program. The interventions that were subse-

Patient name _____

D.O.B. _____   SSN:_____

MR: _____   Group: _____

Diagnosis: 313.81   oppositional defiant disorder
                    314.01   attention-deficit/hyperactivity disorder

Both the American Psychological Association and the American Academy of Child and Adolescent Psychiatry have endorsed parent training, and child social skills training, as both effective and essential in the treatment of children with these diagnoses. I am requesting that this child and his parent be enrolled in our 8-week group therapy program that has concurrent child and parent groups.

REQUEST: 8 sessions of 90852 Medical Group Therapy for parent training
                  8 sessions of 90852 Medical Group Therapy for child social skills
                  2 sessions of 90844 Follow-up Individual Therapy

GROUP SESSION CONTENT:

1. Parents: How ADHD and impulsive behavior effects the family.
   Child: Initial rules and guidelines for social skills group.

2. Parents: Special, one-to-one positive time.
   Child: Introduction to role playing.

3. Parents: Charting behaviors.
   Child: Introduction to problem solving.

4. Parents: Establishing reward systems.
   Child: Practice role play and problem solving.

5. Parents: Review of behavior charts, modifying reward systems.
   Child: Learning relaxation.

6. Parents: Natural and logical consequences.
   Child: Review of relaxation.

7. Parents: The use of time-out.
   Child: Using stop-and-think game.

8. Parents: Working with your local schools.
   Child: Review of home practice.

All sessions will be conducted at our office under my direct care and supervision.

William Douglas Tynan, PhD, ABPP
Licensed Psychologist

FIGURE 6.2. Sample treatment plan for managed care organizations. From Tynan, Schuman, and Lampert (1999). Copyright 1999 by the Association for Advancement of Behavior Therapy. Reprinted by permission.

quently used for these children and their families fulfilled the American Psychological Association's criteria as well established and probably efficacious, and conformed to best practices as suggested by the American Academy of Child and Adolescent Psychiatry. Several practitioners worked together to offer child social competence and parent skills training programming in the evenings. Highly experienced practitioners conducted the intervention or supervised the provision of services. They were able to deliver 12 consecutive 8-session programs (see Figure 6.2) over a 15-month time period. They measured client outcomes using a brief parent rating scale. They also developed a standardized treatment plan for submission to managed care organizations to obtain reimbursement for professional services. The sample treatment plan is duplicated in Figure 6.2. Apparently, no requests for services were denied by the managed care organization. As discussed in the preceding section, children's behavior improved after the intervention. Therefore, Tynan and colleagues were able to successfully deliver an empirically supported intervention in a clinic setting that was cost-effective and that achieved a good outcome.

We are aware that children who come to clinic settings often present with comorbid conditions. Comorbid problems related to anxiety disorders, mood disorders, and other psychiatric conditions obviously need to be addressed in providing effective clinic therapy for children with ACP. It is beyond the scope of this book to review the procedures involved in therapy for other psychiatric disorders. We refer readers to other sources that describe effective child-focused therapy for anxiety disorders (e.g., Kendall, Chu, Pimental, & Choudhury, 2000; Ollendick & King, 1998), mood disorders (e.g., Kaslow & Thompson, 1998; Stark, Boswell Sander, Yancy, Bronik, & Hoke, 2000), and a variety of other childhood problems (e.g., Mash & Barkley, 1996).

Enhancing Client Engagement

To effectively incorporate empirically supported interventions into clinic practice, it is necessary for clients to receive the entire intervention. Unfortunately, high no-show rates and client dropout are common in clinic settings (Kazdin, 1996b). Employment of strategies to effectively engage families is necessary to ensure that they receive a full intervention. These strategies include preparing families for intervention, enhancing "bonding" with a program, identifying risk factors and barriers related to dropout, providing practical assistance, using interpersonal and cognitive strategies to enhance motivation in parents, collaborating with parents and community members, and conducting interventions in accessible locations. It is also important to make interventions culturally compatible for the families receiving them. Each of these strategies is reviewed in Chapter 12 of this volume (see Tables 12.1 and 12.2). They are relevant not only for engaging families in mental health interventions, but for all the interventions that are described in this book.

Providing Continuous Training, Supervision, and Monitoring of Intervention Staff

Adherence to empirically supported intervention protocols can be enhanced through effective training, supervision, and monitoring of intervention staff. Unfortunately, many practitioners in clinic settings receive minimal ongoing training and supervision. Yet to effectively utilize empirically supported interventions, it is necessary to adhere to a rigorous standardized protocol.

Extensive training prior to the implementation of an empirically supported intervention is required. It is unlikely that a workshop would provide a sufficient level of training. Rather, extensive training involves reading of treatment manuals and other clinical materials, didactic instruction, observation of experienced practitioners or modeling, and role-playing or "practice." Practitioners who complete such training are required to demonstrate mastery of content and delivery procedures.

Ongoing supervision and monitoring is also important. The multisystemic therapy supervisory model (Henggeler et al., 1998; Schoenwald et al., 2000) seems to us to be an excellent example of supervision that could potentially be incorporated into clinic settings. It calls for small-group supervision meetings that are conducted on a weekly basis. Individual supervision is utilized as necessary. It is the supervisor's job to ensure that interventions are carried out by supervisees according to protocol, thus maintaining intervention fidelity. Supervisors and supervisees are prepared to discuss cases and clinical issues. Typically, the group discusses 12–15 cases in a 1- or 2-hour supervisory meeting. To accomplish this task, the supervisor and supervisees must stay on task and focus on the most clinically relevant details of each case. The progress of clients is monitored on a weekly basis. Supervisors and supervisees strategize about ways to help clients achieve their (clients') goals using empirically supported procedures. It is both the supervisors and the supervisees' responsibility to assist clients in making sufficient progress toward meeting treatment goals. It seems to us that a similar level of supervision and monitoring of staff would be required to realistically achieve the goal of incorporating empirically supported therapy approaches into the clinic setting.

Summary

Table 6.4 summarizes suggested best practices for incorporating empirically supported interventions into the clinic setting. These best practices should result in more effective clinic therapy interventions for children with ACP

TABLE 6.4. Summary of Suggested Best Practices for Clinic Therapy

Procedures	Best practices
Incorporating research-supported interventions into clinic settings	Utilize empirically supported interventions; incorporate accepted best practices; modify clinic practice procedures to emphasize client outcome (e.g., small caseloads, ongoing training, etc.).
Enhancing client engagement	Utilize strategies that maximize the probability of clients successfully completing intervention (see Chapter 11).
Providing continuous training, supervision, and monitoring of intervention staff	Ensure continuous development of staff skills and active monitoring of clients' progress.

and related problems. More research is needed, however, to verify that this approach will ultimately work.

We recognize that it will be challenging to make the recommended changes in clinic therapy practice within the current mental health system. Indeed, substantial changes will likely need to be made at the systems and organizational levels to accommodate the suggested best practices for clinic therapy. Chapter 12 provides ideas for making organizational and system changes so as to increase the probability that these suggested best practices could be implemented.

OVERVIEW AND RESEARCH EVALUATION OF RESTRICTIVE TREATMENTS

If the level of ACP in a particular child is severe and/or unresponsive to medications or clinic therapy, or if the child presents a danger to self or others, then restrictive mental health services may be needed. It seems to us that restrictive services can be designated on a continuum of restrictiveness ranging from summer treatment to day treatment/partial hospitalization to residential treatment to inpatient hospitalization. These restrictive treatments target severe levels of ACP, ADHD, and other comorbid diagnostic conditions. Restrictive treatments offer a more intensive intervention than what can be otherwise achieved with less restrictive services. Typically, the child is the focus, but parents and family members are also involved to varying degrees. The various models of restrictive treatments offer similar components with varying degrees of intensity.

Pelham and Hoza (1996) described an 8-week summer treatment program for elementary-age children with ADHD. Many of the children treated in this program also have ACP. Children are placed in the summer treatment program to obtain more intensive services than what is possible with outpatient services. Children receive intensive behavioral, social skills, milieu, recreational, and education-focused interventions 5 days a week for 8 weeks. Some also qualify for medications. Pelham and Hoza (1996) summarized several years' worth of research utilizing a noncontrolled design. The children were mostly Caucasian, elementary-age boys. The results showed that children who attended the summer treatment program exhibited significant improvements on parents', program counselors', and teachers' ratings in the areas of behavior and social skill development. Standardized parent rating scales also showed positive effects. Self-report measures completed by the children indicated improved self-esteem. Parents were highly satisfied with the program. Pelham and Hoza noted that the summer treatment program is used in other university-based and private treatment programs. The summer treatment program was also one component of the MTA study (discussed in Chapter 11).

Day treatment and partial hospitalization services are provided during the daytime in hospital, school, or clinic settings. Most of these programs offer clinic therapy, child skills training, milieu interventions, and academic or school assistance. Many of these programs are time-limited. Partial hospitalization usually lasts about 8 weeks, while day treatment can last months. The goal is to stabilize the child and return him or her back to community providers as soon as possible. Very few randomized controlled research studies have been used to evaluate day treatment or partial hospitalization. Grizenko (1997) and Heston, Kiser, and Pruitt (1996) reviewed the available research in this area. They found that elementary-age children are most often admitted to day treatment or partial hospitalization programs because of significant behavioral problems. These programs are noted to improve child behavior and family functioning. Long-term effects are maintained, even up to 5 years, if the family cooperates with the treatment and follow-up services.

Residential treatment involves a child receiving mental health services while residing in an institution. He or she participates in ongoing mental health services, milieu interventions, behavior management, verbal individual and group therapies, recreational activities, medication management, and academic/vocational training. Residential treatment is utilized for children who exhibit severe and chronic difficulties. In years gone by, residential treatment was often very long term, but now, with the advent of managed care and mixed research results regarding the effectiveness of residential treatment, children are placed for shorter time periods. Children who are diagnosed with CD and comorbid problems are often among the clientele most often placed in residential treatment. Asarnow, Aoki, and Elson (1996), Mulvey, Arthur, and Reppucci (1993), and Lewis, Summerville, and Graffagnino (1996) discussed the research pertaining to residential treatment. They found that it was a good treatment to bring about

short-term gains, but that it was ineffective in altering the long-term trajectory for many of these children. Given how costly residential treatment is,
this research does not bode well as to its effectiveness. Intensive aftercare
needs to be utilized to maintain the benefits of a residential treatment placement.

A final type of restrictive treatment is inpatient hospitalization. This
involves a child being admitted to a hospital inpatient unit. Some children
with CD and comorbid difficulties receive this treatment because they are a
threat to harm themselves or others. Hospitalization is designed for short-
term stabilization of children who have severe and acute mental health
problems. Since the 1990s the average stay in an inpatient unit is several
weeks. Children are referred back to outpatient and other community services upon discharge. While admitted, these children are exposed to a variety of interventions similar to those found in residential treatment. Blanz
and Schmidt (2000) reviewed research evaluating the effectiveness of hospitalization. Most of the research consists of uncontrolled studies. The research demonstrated that children exhibit short-term stabilization and
some long-term maintenance of treatment gains. The results are better if effective interventions are employed on the inpatient unit and if families follow through with aftercare mental health services. Inpatient treatment is
least effective with children and families manifesting severe dysfunction.

BEST PRACTICES FOR RESTRICTIVE TREATMENTS

We integrated different practice sources to describe best practices for various types of restrictive treatment modalities. These sources include (l)
Grizenko's (1997) and Heston and colleagues' (1996) review of procedures
for day treatment and partial hospitalization; (2) Pelham and Hoza's
(1996) description of their innovative summer treatment program; (3)
Lewis and colleagues' (1996) discussion of residential treatment procedures; and (4) Blanz and Schmidt's (2000) and Woolston's (1996) presentation of effective inpatient hospitalization practices. We take the stance that
these modes of restrictive treatment are similar but offer different degrees
of intensity corresponding to the level of restrictiveness. In this section we
summarize best practices that are common across the different forms of restrictive treatments.

Making a Careful Decision to Place a
Child in a Restrictive Treatment Setting

As we noted above, placement of children in a restrictive treatment setting
is costly and not always effective. Moreover, the child placed in a restrictive
treatment setting may find that setting traumatizing and difficult. Therefore
good clinical judgment is needed to determine whether or not a child

should be placed in a restrictive treatment center. Typically, the criteria utilized to make this determination are that a child exhibits severe and refractory levels of problematic behavior and associated impairment in functioning. For example, the child has not benefited from outpatient therapy and specialized school services and/or the parents are unable to contain the child's behavior. Children are also admitted to inpatient hospital settings if they are a danger to self or others. The more severe the level of problems, the more restrictive the placement, ranging from summer treatment to day treatment/partial hospitalization to residential treatment to inpatient hospitalization.

Incorporating Effective Intervention Components into the Restrictive Treatment Setting

It is recommended that effective assessment and intervention components be utilized in restrictive treatment settings. We view restrictive treatments as more of a delivery methodology than as an intervention content area. The restrictive setting enables the child to experience interventions at varying levels of intensity. Many of the interventions that we have described previously, or that we will describe later in this volume, are the effective components of interventions delivered in a restrictive treatment setting.

Comprehensive assessment and diagnosis is required. Typically, children are placed in a residential treatment center with a diagnosis. The restrictive treatment setting, however, affords the opportunity to fine-tune diagnoses and treatment planning. It creates an opportunity for extensive observation of the child and for the child to receive a variety of assessment procedures. Comprehensive assessment and diagnostic activities should lead to more effective programming both while the child is in the restrictive treatment setting and after his or her discharge. Chapter 3 of this book reviews assessment procedures.

Medications are often employed in restrictive treatment settings. This enables practitioners to carefully monitor and manage medications. Pelham and Hoza (1996), for example, use double-blind, placebo-controlled evaluations to determine the effects of stimulant medication on children with ADHD enrolled in their summer treatment program. Since the child spends many hours in the intervention setting, the practitioner has an excellent opportunity to determine an optimal medication dose level and schedule. The child's behavior can be assessed in a variety of contexts (e.g., classroom, recreational activities, social interactions). The practitioner has access to various sources and types of assessment information to evaluate the effects of the medications with children. Restrictive treatments create an opportunity to develop an effective medication plan for the child that can be used when he or she leaves the restrictive setting.

Many restrictive treatment settings employ milieu interventions. One milieu intervention is behavior management. It provides an opportunity to shape the child's behavior. Effective behavior management reinforces positive behavior such as compliance, rule following, sharing, and playing fairly. It also reduces negative behaviors such as aggression, noncompliance, stealing, and interrupting. Behavior management provides immediate feedback and corrective experiences for children's behavior. Chapter 9 of this volume reviews procedures for behavior management in the classroom. Similar procedures are employed in restrictive treatment settings. Another milieu intervention involves the formation of positive relationships with adult staff and peers. The staff members provide attention for positive behavior, corrections and limits for negative behavior, and are available to talk to the children about their problems. Most restrictive settings also have opportunity for recreational activities that can be experienced with peers who are all being supervised by adult staff.

Social competence training is typically conducted in restrictive treatment placements. The level of social competence training varies across programs. The restrictive treatment setting creates an ideal situation for more intensive social competence training and provides numerous opportunities for staff to prompt and reinforce children for applying newly acquired skills in the milieu. Social competence training interventions are described in Chapter 4.

Most restrictive models of intervention employ academic engagement and skills building approaches. Children who are enrolled in such programs are often struggling with academics. Most of the programs offer regular classroom teaching and/or academic tutoring opportunities. This could present a good opportunity for children to make academic gains or possibly catch up to a level more consistent with their peers. Academic skills building interventions are reviewed in Chapter 7 of this book.

Another intervention utilized to varying degrees in restrictive treatment is parent and family skills training. Usually, some sort of parent and family intervention is employed. This can range from parent groups to individualized family sessions. Residential treatment and inpatient hospitalization also incorporate graduated home visits for the child until discharge. Those programs that do not emphasize a parent and family component may be setting up a situation for relapse. It is logical to believe that, if the child returns to a family situation that has not changed, he or she may revert to previous behaviors and functioning. The interested reader should consult Chapter 5 for a description of parent and family skills training.

The Pelham and Hoza (1996) summer treatment program provides an illustration of how effective intervention components are provided to children in a restrictive setting. Children attend the program for 8 weeks during the summer, Monday through Friday, 8:00 A.M. to 5:00 P.M. They participate in academic classrooms with licensed teachers for 3 hours a day and take part in various recreational/sports and social programming activities throughout the day. A point system is utilized to shape adaptive behavior. Staff utilizes positive reinforcement and effective commands to promote social skills and compliance behaviors in children. Noncompliance in children is dealt with using time-out procedures. A brief social skills program occurs each day. Much of the day is spent prompting and reinforcing children to utilize the social skills they learn. Children also participate in a buddy system that pairs children to assist each other in intervention-related activities. A daily report card is sent home to parents regarding the child's behavior. Medications are utilized for those children where they are clinically indicated. This type of programming could be delivered in other restrictive settings.

Follow-Up Services

Too often little or no follow-up services are in place upon a child's discharge from a restrictive treatment setting. Of course, poor follow-up makes it more likely that a child will regress and/or relapse. It is therefore imperative that outpatient treatments and other school- and community-based services be in place for the child and family upon discharge. This includes helping the child and family access child and family support services such as those explained in Chapter 10 of this volume. If this is successfully accomplished, it would reduce the level of stress for the child and family upon discharge and possibly prevent serious problems from redeveloping.

Summary

Table 6.5 provides a summary of best practices for restrictive treatments. Given the cost of restrictive treatments and the mixed evidence about the

TABLE 6.5. Summary of Best Practices for Restrictive Settings

Procedures	Best practices
Making a careful decision to place a child in a restrictive treatment setting	Restrictive treatment placements should be reserved for children with severe problems or for children who are a potential danger to self or others.
Incorporating effective intervention components into the restrictive treatment setting	Best practices in assessment/diagnosis, medication treatment, behavior management, social competence training, academic skills building, and parent and family skills training should be emphasized.
Follow-up services	Make sure that outpatient mental health services and other school- and community-based services are in place upon discharge.

long-term benefits of very restrictive services like residential treatment, it behooves practitioners to adhere to these best practices.

CONCLUSION

Mental health treatments are designed for children with diagnosed psychiatric disorders such as ODD, CD, ADHD, and other comorbid conditions. These treatments can be most helpful in reducing symptoms and building the strengths of children and families if effective intervention components are utilized within the mental health setting. This chapter described research and best practices for a continuum of mental health treatments ranging from medications to clinic therapy to restrictive treatments. In our opinion, mental health treatments should be considered for many children with ACP. Effective mental health services can potentially enable children with ACP to profit from other interventions described in this book.

PART IV

CONTEXTUALLY BASED INTERVENTIONS

CHAPTER 7

School Interventions for Academic Engagement and Skill Building

As we noted in Chapter 1, academic problems are common among children with ACP, and likely play a significant role in the many negative long-term outcomes they experience. Children with ACP often struggle with active participation in learning activities, also referred to as academic engagement. In addition, they have problems with academic skills, such as focusing on tasks and completing work, that are required to develop knowledge in academic content areas like math and reading. Academic achievement, the goal of academic engagement and academic skills, is defined and measured in various ways. This variability has contributed to confusion over the effectiveness of different interventions. Measures used to determine academic achievement range from the number of correct responses on daily work and scores on classroom tests to grades on report cards, scores on standardized achievement tests, and grade-level placement.

Many teachers view children with ACP as the most difficult to teach and as the least likable (Kauffman & Wong, 1991). Children with ACP have been described as emotionally variable, fearing failure, slow to develop trust in teachers, and difficult to keep engaged in the learning process (Coleman & Vaughn, 2000). They tend to have high rates of off-task behavior, poor academic and work-related skills, splinter skills in basic academic areas, and low achievement (Walker et al., 1995). Many of the characteristics associated with children exhibiting ACP listed in Table 1.3 interfere with academic functioning. Academic interventions for children with ACP must address these issues if they are to have success in improving academic functioning.

We suggest that effective academic engagement and skill building interventions reduce risk factors and promote protective factors in the child and contextual life domains (see Tables 2.3 and 2.4 in Chapter 2). Specifically, these interventions reduce academic problems and ineffective/harmful school responses. Protective factors that are promoted include academic skills/success and involvement with an effective school.

In this chapter we focus on empirically supported interventions used to improve the academic skills of children with ACP. There is an extensive literature on effective academic interventions (Brophy & Good, 1986; Elliot, Busse, & Shapiro, 1999; Gettinger & Stoiber, 1999; Kavale & Forness, 1999), yet limited reporting on academic interventions specifically focused on children with ACP (Coleman & Vaughn, 2000; Gagnon & Conoley, 1997; Gunter & Denny, 1998; Hinshaw, 1992b; Maguin & Loeber, 1996; Ruhl & Berlinghoff, 1992; Walker et al., 1995). As a result, research involving children with ACP, as well as children at risk for ACP (e.g., children with ADHD, learning problems, or low SES), will also be reviewed here.

We present a wide variety of interventions addressing the academic functioning of children with ACP. All these interventions share the distal goal of increasing academic achievement, but differ in their proximal goals. In the first section we focus on interventions targeting self-management skills in children. In the second section we present teacher practices that influence academic achievement by increasing child engagement in learning activities. In the third section we offer some interventions that promote effective parent involvement in the educational process. Each of these sections begins with an overview of the research and then presents best practices.

OVERVIEW AND RESEARCH EVALUATION OF SELF-MANAGEMENT TRAINING

Interventions targeting children's self-management of academic behaviors commonly focus on increasing on-task behavior, work-completion rates, and accuracy of academic work. This can be especially helpful for children with ACP who are disengaged or only passively involved in the learning process. These interventions help children develop skills that increase their engagement in learning activities and result in greater learning.

Self-management training involves teaching children skills in self-monitoring, self-evaluation, and sometimes self-reinforcement. Children are trained to observe and objectively record their own behavior (self-monitor), compare their behavior to a set standard (self-evaluation), and administer a reward if they determine they have met the standard (self-reinforcement). For example, a child might monitor the number of correct responses on a math worksheet, compare the number correct to the expected standard (e.g., 20 correct responses), and administer the reward (e.g., free time on the computer) if the standard is achieved.

Self-management techniques have produced positive effects on academic behaviors for children with behavior problems (Carr & Punzo, 1993; Levendoski & Cartledge, 2000; McQuillan, DuPaul, Shapiro, & Cole, 1996; Nelson, Smith, Young, & Dodd, 1991) and children with learning disabilities (Reid, 1996). A review of 16 studies using self-management techniques with children who were behaviorally disordered found "moderate to large effects" on social and academic behaviors (Nelson et al., 1991). The academic behaviors included on-task behavior and accuracy of work. One aspect of self-management, self-reinforcement, has been found to be more effective than teacher-administered reinforcement with children manifesting ADHD (Ajibola & Clement, 1995). Based on a review of the research, Reid (1996) concluded that for children with learning disabilities, self-monitoring has been shown to produce a "pronounced" effect on on-task behavior and a positive effect on academic productivity. The effect on accuracy of work has not been well studied.

Despite the positive results reported for self-management techniques, limitations with this intervention have been noted. There are concerns with generalization (Brigham, 1992; Carter, 1993; Cole & Bambara, 1992; Pfiffner & Barkley, 1998), lack of long-term effects (Carter, 1993), limited value of the targeted behaviors (Braswell, 1998), and insufficiency of self-monitoring and self-evaluation as stand-alone interventions (Evans & Sullivan, 1993). In addition, limited effectiveness has been noted with children exhibiting ADHD (Abikoff, 1991; Braswell, 1998; Pelham & Waschbusch, 1999; Pfiffner & Barkley, 1998). Pfiffner and Barkley (1998) concluded that for children with ADHD, continued teacher monitoring is necessary, as complete management of the self-monitoring program by the child him- or herself is not realistic.

To summarize, self-management interventions have yielded short-term improvements on variables such as attention to task and number of correct responses, but not on measures of academic achievement such as grade placement or scores on standardized achievement tests. As a result, self-management would seem to be a strategy that should be used as one component of a more comprehensive intervention for children with ACP.

BEST PRACTICES FOR SELF-MANAGEMENT TRAINING

We will use Carter's (1993) nine-step process as the framework to present best practices for self-management training. We derived best practices from the following sources: (1) Bloomquist's (1996) review of skills training procedures for children with behavior disorders; (2) Braswell's (1995) presentation of cognitive-behavioral approaches in the classroom; (3) Cole and Bambara's (1992) discussion of self-management interventions in schools; (4) Elliott and colleagues' (1999) techniques for intervening with academic performance problems; (5) Evans and Sullivan's (1993) presentation on the use of self-management with children; and (6) Skinner and Smith's (1992) discussion of the use of self-management to increase academic performance.

Before the classroom teacher implements a self-management program, it should be determined that it is appropriate for the child and the classroom. The child should be motivated to cooperate with the program, able to learn and follow the procedures, and capable of making the judgments required by the plan. The teacher should have the knowledge, skills, and motivation to train the child and consistently monitor the program.

Selecting a Target Behavior

One advantage of self-management training is that a variety of behaviors can be targeted, including behaviors related to academic and behavior management goals. Examples of targeted behaviors include completing work, staying in one's seat, paying attention to work, and doing accurate work. The targeted behavior should not be overly difficult to manage or aggressive/dangerous. The behavior monitored should be observable so the teacher can determine that the child is implementing the procedure, correct the child's mistakes, and reinforce the child when he or she observes the correct behaviors. If the problem behavior occurs when a child is upset and has reduced control over the behavior, it may be useful to target a behavior prior to the emotional arousal that may prevent the escalation. A replacement behavior should always be selected and the teacher may want the child to self-manage the replacement behavior rather than the problem behavior. For example, if a child has trouble calling out comments and answers, the child might monitor the number of times he or she raises his or her hand and waits to be called on. A common procedure is to first bring a behavior under control by using a teacher-managed contingency plan and then to maintain that positive behavior with a self-management procedure.

If the goal is improved academic functioning, it is recommended that academic behaviors be targeted rather than general classroom behavior, with the expectation that this will improve academic functioning. A related issue is whether targeting attention to task or targeting accuracy and productivity will result in greater academic progress. Targeting attention to task does not always result in increased academic functioning. While no firm conclusion is possible, targeting accuracy and productivity may have some advantages (Reid, 1996; Skinner & Smith, 1992). If attention to task is targeted, data on academic progress should also be collected to ensure that learning is taking place.

Defining the Target Behavior

The second step is to operationally define the target behavior and assist the child in clearly identifying it. Providing the child with specific examples of behaviors that fit and do not fit the definition is helpful. Clearly defined behaviors are important for success, as they will promote more accurate self-observation and easier matching of the child's observations with the teacher's observations. For example, if the child's work completion is being monitored, what the assignment consists of (e.g., number of items) and what constitutes "completion" should be clearly defined. Examples of completed work (e.g., showing the steps for math problems or the length of responses for written work) and noncompleted work (random responses or phrases instead of sentences) should be shown to the child.

Designing the Data-Recording Procedure

The type of data recorded and the recording form will vary depending on the type of behavior being self-monitored. A sample self-monitoring recording form is presented in Figure 7.1. Levendoski and Cartledge (2000) successfully used this recording form with 9- to 11-year-old children labeled EBD. The children were to record whether they were doing their work during math class when a bell was sounded at 10-minute intervals. Further information on recording procedures and recording forms can be found in Chapter 8.

Teaching the Child to Use the Recording Form

Before teaching the child how to use the recording form, the teacher should explain the rationale for the program to elicit the child's cooperation. The teacher then demonstrates the recording procedure while verbalizing each step. For example, using the recording form in Figure 7.1, the teacher might demonstrate working on a task and say, "I am working on a math problem and the bell rings. I read 'At this exact second am I doing my work?' Yes, I am doing my work so I will put an 'X' under the 'Yes' for the first bell on Day 1." The teacher would also demonstrate behaviors that would receive a "No" rating. Next, the child practices using the recording form while getting feedback from the teacher. The child must be able to demonstrate a high level of accuracy prior to initiating independent self-monitoring.

Using a Strategy to Ensure Accuracy

A strategy is needed for promoting accurate child recording. The most common strategy is to match the child's ratings with the teacher's ratings. Both the child and the teacher complete the recording form on the child's performance and then they compare ratings at the end of the recording period. The child

Name: _____

Date: _____

*At this exact second am I doing my work?

Day	Yes 1st Bell	Yes 2nd Bell	No 1st Bell	No 2nd Bell
1			X	X
2	X			X
3		X	X	
4	X	X		
5		X	X	
6		X	X	
7	X	X		
8	X	X		

FIGURE 7.1. Student self-monitoring form. From Levendoski and Cartledge (2000). Copyright 2000 by the Council for Children with Behavior Disorders. Reprinted by permission.

earns rewards for accurate matches. Since the recording form in Figure 7.1 only requires two ratings per period, both the child's ratings would likely have to agree with the teacher's ratings to earn the reward. On recording forms that potentially require many ratings per period (e.g., talking without raising hand), the child's total may be expected to be within one of the teacher's. In some programs, the child will start out only earning points for matching the teacher's ratings. In other programs, the child can earn points for reaching the criterion and bonus points for matching the teacher's ratings. Once the child's ratings are consistently accurate, the matching can be gradually reduced so that only spot checks are conducted.

Establishing Goals and Contingencies

To this point, the focus of self-management training has been on self-monitoring (self-observation and self-recording). To complete the process, the child must also be capable of self-evaluation (comparing one's behavior to a standard) and self-reinforcement (rewarding oneself if the standard has been met). To begin this process, goals and contingencies are identified. Specific criteria are set so the teacher and the child can determine when the goal has been met. Using the recording form in Figure 7.1 as an example, the goal may be to have two Yes's in a period. Over the course of a week, the goal may be to have seven Yes's in 5 days. The time frame (e.g., over the course of a subject period, a morning, a day) needs to be determined. The optimum length of the self-management period will vary. Shorter time periods are recommended for younger children, for children with ADHD, and for all children while they are learning the self-management process. The level of success (e.g., all items completed, 90% completed, 75% completed) also needs to be determined. The goal should be attainable, yet challenging for the child.

If self-reinforcement is utilized, the child has access to a reward (e.g., use of the computer) and administers it when appropriate. It is best for the child to be involved in the selection of the rewards. A reinforcement menu may be used to determine the child's preferences and help in identifying effective rewards (see Figure 8.2 in Chapter 8). In selecting contingencies, rewards should be used prior to mild punishments. For example, the program may begin with the child earning extra computer time or lunch with the teacher. If the use of rewards proves to be ineffective, mild punishments such as completing work during recess can be added.

Reviewing Goal and Child Performance

The teacher and the child need to meet on a regular basis to discuss the child's performance, the helpfulness of the procedure, and progress toward the final goal. The child and the teacher monitor the child's functioning. As it improves, they modify the expectations and goals to match the child's improvement. For example, if the child has achieved the goal of completing 75% of daily work for a week, they can discuss whether 90% work completion would be a realistic goal. If the goal has not been consistently achieved, the teacher and the child evaluate the goal, the plan, or factors affecting the child's performance and make needed changes. This meeting can also be used to give the child support and discuss factors related to motivation for improvement.

Planning for Reducing Self-Recording Procedures, and Promoting Generalization and Maintenance

When the final goal is reached, it is recommended that the self-management procedure not be abruptly stopped. The procedure should be gradually withdrawn and a plan put in its place to maintain performance and support generalization to other behaviors and settings. Reducing the frequency of rewards or extending the time period over which the behavior is monitored can support maintenance. For example, rather than monitoring a behavior during one class period, it might be monitored over the whole day. It can also be helpful to transition to naturally occurring contingencies such as grades and social reinforcement. Finally, self-management procedures can be used in other settings, at other times of the day, and for other behaviors.

Summary

Table 7.1 provides a summary of best practices for training in self-management. Self-management can be an effective intervention for academic problems. However, for most children with ACP it does not have sufficient power as a stand-alone intervention, so it is best used in combination with other strategies.

OVERVIEW AND RESEARCH EVALUATION OF INSTRUCTIONAL STRATEGIES

Children with ACP bring many behaviors and qualities to the classroom that make teaching and learning difficult. In selecting instructional strategies, teachers should consider two questions. First, has the strategy been demonstrated to effectively increase academic achievement? Second, does the strategy address the behaviors or problems children with ACP bring to the classroom? In this section, increasing the academic success of children with ACP is targeted through teacher instructional strategies. More specifically, academic achievement is promoted by teachers using strategies that increase children's engagement in learning activities.

The interventions discussed in this section consist of instructional strategies such as teachers using a high level of interaction with children, allowing for frequent responding, and providing work that permits a moderate to high level of success. In addition to general categories of strategies, specific interventions such as peer tutoring, cooperative learning, and direct instruction will be presented. Methods for assessing how instructional time is utilized are presented, as well as factors involved in selecting an effective academic intervention.

A prerequisite for effective instruction is a *positive and supportive cli-*

TABLE 7.1. Best Practices for Self-Management Training

Procedures	Best practices
Selecting a target behavior	Consider selecting behaviors brought under control by teacher-managed contingency plan, identify and select replacement behaviors, select overt behaviors.
Defining the target behavior	Operationally define target behaviors, provide examples of behaviors that fit and do not fit the definition.
Designing the data-recording procedure	Specify the type of data to be recorded, begin program with frequent recordings and reduce frequency as program progresses.
Teaching the child to use the recording form	Explain the rationale, model the recording procedure, have child practice with the teacher providing feedback.
Using a strategy to ensure accuracy	Match child ratings to teacher ratings, provide rewards for accurate ratings.
Establishing goals and contingencies	Set specific criteria for the goal, determine the time frame, determine the level of success needed to earn reward, involve child in selection of contingencies.
Reviewing the goal and child performance	Meet regularly with child to evaluate progress, modify expectations as needed to keep the goal challenging but reachable.
Planning for reducing self-recording procedures, and promoting generalization and maintenance	Gradually withdraw plan by reducing the frequency of the reward or extending the time period; substitute naturally occurring contingencies; utilize self-monitoring procedures in other settings, at other times, or with other behaviors.

mate and *effective management of behavior.* School climate has been demonstrated to effect academic achievement (Haynes, Emmons, & Ben-Avie, 1997), and is believed to be an especially important variable for low-income and minority children (Esposito, 1999; Haynes et al., 1997; Pierce, 1994). In their review of research on effective teaching, Brophy and Good (1986) concluded that "low-SES-low-achievement children" benefit from increased control and structure in the classroom, as well as from increased teacher warmth, support, and encouragement. Similarly, climate and classroom management issues have been supported as important for the academic success of children considered EBD (Wehby, Symons, Canale, & Go, 1998). Factors related to school climate and behavior management are presented in Chapter 8.

Child engagement in learning tasks has been identified as an important factor in academic progress. In their extensive review of research relating teacher behavior to academic outcomes, Brophy and Good (1986) observed that a common theme in the research is the importance of the amount of time children are engaged in appropriate learning tasks. More recently Greenwood (1996) has hypothesized that instructional factors affect achievement through their impact on engagement time.

Effective strategies for children with mild handicaps (e.g., learning disabilities and EBD) promote child engagement and enhance classroom climate and management. Christenson, Ysseldyke, and Thurow (1989), in their review of critical instructional factors for children with mild handicaps, compiled a list of 10 essential factors for positive instructional outcomes:

1. Classrooms are managed effectively and efficiently.
2. There is a sense of "positiveness" in the school environment.
3. There is an appropriate instructional match between child and task characteristics.
4. Goals for child performance are clearly stated and understood.
5. Lessons are presented clearly and follow specific instructional procedures.
6. Adequate instructional support is provided for the individual child.
7. Sufficient time is allocated to instruction and the time is used efficiently.
8. Opportunity to respond is high.
9. Teachers actively monitor child progress and understanding.
10. Child performance is evaluated appropriately and frequently.

Direct instruction is a teaching approach that calibrates work to a child's academic level, provides for a high level of teacher–child interaction, and promotes a high level of child responding. The term direct instruction is used in the literature in different ways, but commonly refers to a structured approach to instruction that incorporates the following six critical features (Gersten, Carnine, & Woodward, 1987):

1. An explicit step-by-step strategy.
2. Development of mastery at each step in the process.
3. Strategy (or process) corrections for child errors.
4. Gradual fading from teacher-directed activities toward independent work.
5. Use of adequate, systematic practice with a range of examples.
6. Cumulative review of newly learned concepts.

Direct instruction has been demonstrated to be effective at increasing academic achievement for a wide variety of children, including low-income and learning-disabled children (Becker & Carnine, 1980; Forness, Kavale, Blum, & Lloyd, 1997; Gersten, Woodward, & Darch, 1986; Swanson & Hoskyn, 1998). Forness and colleagues (1997) reviewed meta-analytic studies of special education interventions and found that direct instruction was one of the effective interventions. Swanson and Hoskyn's (1998) meta-analytic review of interventions with children with learning disabilities also found that direct instruction was one of the most effective academic interventions.

Cooperative learning is an instructional strategy that involves children working together in small groups with an emphasis on both the group process and individual accountability. Cooperative learning has received much research support (Antil, Jenkins, Wayne, & Vadasy, 1998; Johnson, Johnson, & Stanne, 2000). However, outcomes for children with learning or behavioral problems have been inconsistent. Some have concluded that cooperative learning cannot be recommended for all children with handicaps (Tateyama-Sniezek, 1990). Others have stated that it holds promise, although current research does not support its widespread use with children labeled EBD (Sutherland, Wehby, & Gunter, 2000). How cooperative learning is used in the classroom very likely impacts its effectiveness (Johnson & Johnson, 1999; Slavin, 1999). Antil and colleagues (1998) found that most teachers (76%) did not use the individual accountability factor (each child's performance and contribution to the group goal is assessed) that is recommended by many experts.

Peer tutoring involves children working in pairs with one functioning as a tutor and the other as a tutee. It has been found to have positive academic effects for both the tutor and the tutee (Garcia-Vázquez & Ehly, 1995). Peer tutoring has resulted in increased academic engagement and performance for children with ADHD (DuPaul & Eckert, 1998), increased academic performance for children with behavior problems (Cook, Scruggs, Mastropieri, & Casto, 1985–1986; Gagnon & Conoley, 1997), improved reading skills in children that are EBD (Coleman & Vaughn, 2000), and improved long-term academic achievement with low-SES children (Greenwood, Delquadri, & Hall, 1989; Greenwood, Terry, Utley, Montagna, & Walker, 1993). With children exhibiting ADHD, behavioral change with peer tutoring has not been shown to generalize to other classroom activities (DuPaul & Eckert, 1998).

In summary, research has identified several effective instructional strategies. There is much less research available specifically on effective instructional strategies for children with ACP. As a result, more research is needed to better define best practices. Much of the research on instructional strategies for children with ACP focuses on short-term outcomes with rather modest goals. The currently available research tends to support the importance of classroom climate and behavior management, interventions promoting engagement in academic tasks, peer tutoring, and direct instruction.

Support for cooperative learning with children manifesting ACP is less clear, yet it is a promising approach with such children if utilized in an effective manner.

BEST PRACTICES FOR INSTRUCTIONAL STRATEGIES

The instructional strategies utilized by teachers are important determinants of academic progress for children with ACP. The strategies we present in this section for promoting child engagement were selected because they have been demonstrated to increase academic achievement and address the challenges brought to the classroom by children with ACP. These best practices were derived from (1) Christenson and colleagues' (1989) review of critical instructional factors for children with mild handicaps; (2) Elliott and colleagues' (1999) techniques for intervening with academic performance problems; (3) Gettinger's (1995) presentation of best practices for increasing academic learning time; (4) Gettinger and Stoiber's (1999) review of instructional and environmental variables involved in effective teaching; (5) strategies for working with children exhibiting ADHD (Jones, 1999; Pfiffner & Barkley, 1998; Welch, 1999); (6) Skinner, Fletcher, and Henington's (1996) procedures for increasing child response rates; (7) Walker and colleagues' (1995) work on effective school strategies for children with antisocial behavior; (8) Wehby and colleagues' (1998) teaching practices in classrooms for children with emotional and behavioral disorders; and (9) Zentall's (1995) suggestions on modifying classroom tasks and environments. We begin this section with information on how to assess the amount of time children are engaged in learning activities. Then we discuss strategies for promoting child engagement in learning activities and factors in selecting an effective academic intervention.

Assessing Time Engaged in Learning Activities

The first step in increasing time engaged in learning activities is to assess the current level of engagement. The assessment process can verify effective use of school time, identify problems with low levels of engagement, provide a baseline against which improvement can be measured, and increase awareness of academic engagement. To help teachers assess their use of classroom time, Gettinger (1995) recommended calculating four types of time usage: (1) opportunity time (total length of the school day), (2) instructional time (opportunity time minus time for lunch, recess, transitions, nonacademic tasks, etc.), (3) engaged time (time children are actively engaged in learning activities), and (4) academic learning time (time children are engaged in learning activities with 80% accuracy).

Instructional time can be determined in a number of ways. Teachers can estimate the amount of time spent in learning activities or keep a log of learning times, or an observer can record the amount of learning time.

Academic engagement time is more difficult to calculate. Walker and colleagues (1995) provide a method for calculating academic engagement time for individual children. First, it must be decided what behaviors indicate academic engagement. Typical behaviors would include looking at the teacher during instruction times, working on worksheets, reading, and discussing the topic with others. Next, an observer keeps track of how long a child is academically engaged by clicking on a stopwatch when a child is engaged and clicking it off when the child is not so engaged. The percent of academic engagement time is calculated by dividing the time on the stopwatch by the total observation time and multiplying by 100. This should be done a number of times and the percentages averaged.

Teachers do not control the length of the school day, but they do control the instructional time. Instructional time can be increased by reducing classroom time spent on transitions, organizing materials, and preparing materials. Teachers have less control over engagement time, but they can maximize the probability of children being engaged in learning activities through the instructional practices they use. These practices are discussed below. Teachers control success rate by managing the difficulty of the work and providing effective instruction. However, we recognize that modifying materials for varying ability levels in the classroom presents a major challenge.

Utilizing a High Level of Teacher–Child Interaction

Children are more engaged in learning activities when there is a high level of teacher–child interaction. This starts with teachers welcoming children individually in the morning and proceeds through the school day. Teacher–child interactions take many forms and include questions, discussions, cues or reminders, feedback, praise, and supportive comments. The use of behavior-specific praise can increase on-task behavior for children that are EBD (Sutherland, Wehby, & Copeland, 2000). Feedback is most effective if it is specific and includes information on the correctness of the response, the expected outcome, and the steps needed to reach the expected outcome. *Cueing*, or reminding children to attend to work, to utilize appropriate strategies, and to focus on goals, can increase engagement in learning activities. Cueing can be done verbally or by using predetermined physical cues such as raising a flag or stopping a timer used to record time on task. Teacher awareness of child behavior and work progress, and frequent interactions with children to demonstrate this awareness, promotes children's engagement in learning activities. A teacher's physical proximity and eye contact are also conducive to child engagement.

A common time for behavior problems and poor academic engagement is during extended periods of independent seatwork. These are times when there generally are not high levels of teacher–child interactions. Extended periods of seatwork can be limited by utilizing a variety of instructional approaches, varying how information is presented, and varying how children respond. Skills can be practiced in small groups rather than individually. Interspersing other activities such as instruction or group work can reduce the length of independent seatwork periods. Training children in self-management skills, closely monitoring and cueing children, and frequently interacting with children by giving feedback and individual help can maximize academic engagement during seatwork.

Allowing for a High Level of Child Responding

Allowing for a high level of child responding and active involvement in activities is conducive to child engagement in learning activities. Class discussions and frequent questioning of children increases child involvement. Group and physical responding allow for all children to respond and be involved. Examples of group responding include choral responding, children standing for correct responses and sitting for incorrect responses, holding up a green flag if the answer is true and a red flag if the answer is false, or children giving a thumbs-up or thumbs-down to answer true/false questions. Children can respond physically by acting out parts of stories or by role-playing situations related to the topic of instruction. Using manipulatives for math lessons is a form of active involvement in learning activities. Children can also be used as aides to present topics, write information on the board, collect papers, and so on.

Allowing for a Moderate to High Rate of Success

As we discussed earlier, a moderate to high rate of correct responding increases a child's academic engagement and learning. It has the added benefit of increasing a child's sense of efficacy with academic tasks. Work that is too easy can lead to boredom and lack of interest; work that is too difficult can lead to frustration and discouragement. Calibrating the difficulty of assignments to match children's ability levels is extremely important but also difficult. It requires frequent monitoring of child progress and adjustment of assignments.

One instructional approach that is commonly recommended for children with ACP and utilizes strategies to ensure appropriate rates of success is direct instruction. This approach emphasizes how teaching is conducted and what is taught. Skills and concepts are broken down into their component parts and are taught in a step-by-step manner. Teachers are actively involved in instruction, which often takes place in small groups. Daily lessons are scripted, directing the teacher in what to do and what to say. Mastery is achieved at each step and there is frequent feedback to the child. There are also frequent assessments that serve to ensure mastery, confirm that the instruction is at the appropriate level for the child, and make sure the child will experience a high level of success.

Promoting Child Interest in the Topic

Promoting interest in the subject being taught is especially important for children whose interest in learning may be marginal. Interest can be increased by relating topics to previously learned topics, relating topics to the children's lives, explaining why the topic is important, and explaining why they are being asked to learn the topic. The use of real-world examples and problems and allowing children some choices in learning activities often increases their interest in a subject. For example, children may be allowed to choose from a list of topics for an assignment or may be allowed to select their own topic as long as it matches certain guidelines. Choices can be offered for how skills or knowledge will be demonstrated (e.g., a written test, an oral test, a presentation, or a project). Child engagement and interest are also commonly promoted by allowing choice in nonacademic matters such as determining group or individual rewards, selecting free-time activities, or planning how to celebrate holidays.

One criticism of direct instruction is that the focus on isolated skills may result in children not seeing the value of the learning, which could interfere with their interest and motivation. Also, by focusing excessively on lower level skills, too little focus may be put on the application of the skills to real-world problems. As a result of these problems, Schulte, Osborne, and Erchul (1998) suggested that a combination of direct instruction and indirect instructional strategies could prove to be a very effective way of helping children with mild academic deficits. Indirect approaches focus on teacher–child and child–child dialogue related to complex and authentic learning tasks. Schulte and colleagues (1998) cited studies that successfully combined these two approaches.

Utilizing Small-Group Activities

Small-group activities are another approach to increasing child engagement in learning activities. This strategy allows children to respond more frequently. Moreover, the social component can increase motivation for many children. Small groups can be utilized for learning activities in many ways. Two approaches to small-group learning are cooperative learning strategies and peer tutoring.

Cooperative Learning

It is often pointed out that effective cooperative learning is more than just having children work together in groups. There are numerous approaches to cooperative learning (Nastasi & Clements, 1991), but effective cooperative learning is thought to require both positive interdependence (i.e., children must work together to accomplish a goal) and individual accountability (i.e., each child's performance and contribution to the group goal is assessed) (Antil et al., 1998). In one form of cooperative learning, team learning (Nastasi & Clements, 1991), children assist each other in learning the assigned material. Each child on the team is assessed to determine what was learned. The team earns a reward based on the sum of the team members' individual scores.

To be used in an effective manner with children exhibiting ACP, cooperative learning requires much teacher time and energy to facilitate the cooperative group process. Teachers need to first assess ACP children's levels of cooperative behavior and ability to work in a group and then provide training to address any skill deficits (Gillies & Ashman, 1997; Nastasi & Clements, 1991; Pomplun, 1997; Sutherland et al., 2000). The behavior of children with ACP should be closely monitored in cooperative learning groups (Sutherland et al., 2000).

To promote the collaborative skills needed for children to be successful with cooperative learning, Nastasi and Clements (1991) suggested that teachers do the following:

1. Emphasize the importance of social support among children for the goal of all children learning.
2. Teach communication skills such as active listening, asking and answering questions, and providing explanations.
3. Provide children with feedback and social reinforcement, teach children to give feedback, and model appropriate interactive behavior.
4. Teach and model conflict resolution skills such as negotiation, compromise, and cooperative problem solving.
5. Encourage perspective taking.

Peer Tutoring

A second form of small-group learning strategies is peer tutoring. As with cooperative learning, there are a number of models of peer tutoring (Fantuzzo, King, & Heller, 1992; Fuchs, Fuchs, Phillips, Hamlett, & Karns, 1995; Greenwood et al., 1989). DuPaul and Eckert (1998) define peer tutoring as "any instructional strategy wherein two children work together on an academic activity, with one child providing assistance, instruction, and feedback to the other" (p. 61). All forms of peer tutoring share characteristics known to improve the attentional functioning of children with ADHD, including one-on-one work with a child, the pace of the work is determined by the child, continuous prompting for academic responses, and frequent and immediate feedback (DuPaul & Eckert, 1998). The effective implementation of a peer tutoring program requires a skilled teacher and much time (Elliott et al., 1999), as well as training and monitoring of the children (Garcia-Vázquez & Ehly, 1995).

In one form of peer tutoring, Classwide Peer Tutoring (Greenwood et al., 1989), children are either randomly assigned to tutoring pairs or paired based on ability level, depending on the subject. Tutoring pairs work together for 20 minutes at a time. The child selected as the tutor dictates one item at a time and the tutee responds by writing and saying the answer. If the response is correct, the tutor awards two points. If an incorrect response is given, the tutor gives the correct response and awards one point when the tutee repeats the correct response three times. After 10 minutes the two children switch roles and repeat the process for the next 10 minutes. The class is divided into teams and individual point totals are calculated for each team.

Increasing Awareness and Motivation
for Engagement and Effort

Increasing awareness and motivation for engagement in learning activities can be achieved by acknowledging and praising individual children or the entire class for being engaged in learning activities. The class can earn rewards for remaining engaged in a learning activity for a certain length of time. Charting classroom engagement time and setting goals can also increase awareness and interest in academic engagement.

A concept related to engagement is effort. If children believe that putting effort into learning makes a difference, they are more likely to become engaged in their learning activities. Children who attribute learning or academic problems only to their own ability or to teacher skill will be less likely to put effort into learning. Teachers can promote effort by talking about the importance of effort, acknowledging child effort, and rewarding child effort. It is helpful to point out examples of increased effort resulting in increased learning or success.

Selecting an Academic Intervention

Selecting or designing an intervention that will be effective with a particular child is an important step in the intervention process. Elliott and colleagues (1999) offered four factors to consider when selecting an academic intervention. First, the intervention should have empirical support for its effectiveness and be of sufficient "strength" to accomplish the goal. For example, instituting a peer tutoring program in a math class for 6 weeks may have the strength to increase math test scores for those 6 weeks, but is unlikely to have the strength to impact long-term math achievement.

Second, the intervention should be acceptable to both the child and the people implementing it. Factors related to acceptability include the teacher's knowledge and skills with the type of intervention being considered, approach to instruction and classroom management, attributions concerning the child, beliefs about causes of the behavior, and beliefs about the efficacy of the intervention.

Treatment integrity (i.e., whether the intervention will be implemented as intended) is the third factor to consider. Reducing the complexity of the intervention, the time involved in implementing the intervention, and the number of people involved in the intervention can increase treatment integrity. In addition, increasing the motivation of those implementing the intervention, using reminders and integrity checks (i.e., monitoring program implementation through observation, interviews, review of charts or forms, etc.), and using treatment protocols that specify procedures in detail also boost treatment integrity. Each participant's responsibilities should be clearly specified, and, if needed, participants should receive training to ensure they have the skills and knowledge to accurately implement the intervention. Treatment integrity can be improved by providing participants with support (e.g., assistance with problem solving if problems occur), encouragement, and acknowledgment for accurate implementation. The availability of resources will affect how accurately an intervention will be implemented. School resources that should be considered include availability of teachers' time, availability of teachers' aides, type and amount of social rewards, and training for teachers and teachers' aides. Including the participants in the selection or design of the intervention will assist in addressing many of these issues.

The fourth factor in selecting an academic intervention is whether the effects of the intervention will generalize to other situations and be maintained over time. Elliott and colleagues (1999) recommended that methods to promote generalization and maintenance be programmed into the intervention. This can be accomplished by selecting target behaviors that will be supported by natural contingencies (e.g., peer support, grades), targeting behavioral change across settings, including self-management techniques, and withdrawing intervention procedures systematically (e.g., gradually reducing the frequency of rewards).

In addition to the four factors related to the intervention and its implementation, factors related to the child and the environment should be considered. Numerous authors have noted the variability among children with ACP and ADHD and the variability of their responses to interventions (DuPaul, Eckert, & McGoey's, 1997; Greene, 1996; Hinshaw, 1992b; Maguin & Loeber, 1996). Greene (1996) argued that the target for intervention might vary depending on the characteristics of the child, the teacher, the learning context, the classroom environment, and the task. He recommended the incorporation of these factors into intervention decisions. For example, peer tutoring may be more appropriate than self-management training for a child who is focused on socializing, but has limited motivation for doing academic work. Self-management may be more productive than peer tutoring with a child who is motivated to learn, but tends to be disruptive and belligerent in peer interactions.

Effectively matching the intervention to the child and the context is an important factor in achieving successful outcomes. DuPaul and colleagues (1997) recommended that functional assessment be used to select interventions for individual children. Penno, Frank, and Wacker (2000) successfully used functional assessment (see Chapter 3) with adolescents manifesting severe emotional or behavioral disorders to make instructional accommodations that resulted in improved academic productivity and accuracy. Jolivette, Wehby, and Hirsch (1999) used an academic strategy identification procedure to identify academic strategy interventions for individual elementary-age children considered EBD. Interventions based on the results of this procedure were successful at increasing the accuracy of math responses.

Summary

Table 7.2 provides a summary of best practices for engaging children with ACP in learning activities. A positive and supportive climate and effective classroom management are essential preconditions for the effective use of these strategies. Teachers who use these strategies are likely to be more effective at promoting academic engagement and progress.

OVERVIEW AND RESEARCH EVALUATION OF HOME–SCHOOL ACADEMIC INTERVENTIONS

Schools control only some of the factors that affect academic achievement—for example, school climate, instructional approach, and in-school behavior management. By involving parents in the educational process, they are able to influence a greater number of factors. If parents and schools are able to work together effectively, it greatly increases the chances of successful academic outcomes for children.

Family status and family process variables have been found to be associated with school success. Family status variables such as socioeconomic status, level of parents' education, and family structure are not readily impacted by interventions. Family process variables such as parenting practices, family communication, and family relationships are more modifiable.

TABLE 7.2. Best Practices for Instructional Strategies

Procedures	Best practices
Assessing time engaged in learning activities	Calculate opportunity time or length of the school day, time allocated to learning activities, time children are actively engaged in learning activities, and time engaged in learning activities with 80% accuracy on their work.
Utilizing a high level of teacher–child interaction	Use greeting, questioning, discussing, cueing, praising, and giving feedback and encouragement; limit extended periods of independent seat work.
Allowing for a high level of child responding	Utilize discussing material, answering questions, group responding, physical responding, role playing, and functioning as teacher's aide.
Allowing for a moderate to high rate of success	Calibrate difficulty of work to child ability level, frequently monitor child progress and adjust assignments, utilize direct instruction.
Promoting child interest in the topic	Relate topic to previously learned topics or to the lives of children, use real-world examples, explain why children are learning about the topic, allow children choices in learning activities.
Utilizing small-group activities	Allow for frequent responding and social interaction, utilize cooperative learning and peer tutoring approaches.
Increasing awareness and motivation for engagement and effort	Acknowledge and reward individuals and class for engagement, set goals and chart engagement time, emphasize the importance of effort, acknowledge and reward effort.
Selecting an academic intervention	Select an intervention that has empirical support, is acceptable to participants, can be implemented as designed, and allows for generalization and maintenance of effect; match the intervention to the characteristics of the child, setting, and people implementing the intervention.

However, many family process variables are not typically a direct focus of school-based interventions. One type of family process variable, parent involvement in the education process, is modifiable to a greater extent by school-based interventions. Parent involvement is targeted by the interventions in this section. Much research supports the relationship between the proximal target of parent involvement in school and the distal goal of increased academic achievement. Interventions in this section promote parent involvement by targeting the removal of barriers to parent participation, attitudes and beliefs about parent involvement in education, communication and problem solving between school and home, and involvement of parents in their children's learning activities.

After reviewing the research, we identify barriers to parent involvement and then discuss factors that promote effective home–school collaboration. Interventions include a process for parents and teachers to work collaboratively to solve problems involving individual children, a common and effective strategy for school–home communication, and a program that trains parents to work with their children on reading skills.

Parent involvement in their children's education has been demonstrated to be a significant factor in academic achievement (Christenson & Buerkle, 1999; Christenson, Rounds, & Franklin, 1992). This has been found to be especially true for children in disadvantaged families (Raffaele & Knoff, 1999). Parent involvement in school is related to improved grades, higher achievement test scores, better reading and math achievement, higher rates of homework completion, and greater participation in classroom learning activities. Research has also found parent involvement to be associated with fewer placements in special education, greater enrollment in postsecondary education, higher attendance rates, and lower dropout rates (Christenson & Buerkle, 1999).

In families of high-achieving children there tends to be frequent dialogue between parents and children, strong parental encouragement of academic pursuits, warm and nurturing interactions, clear and consistent limits, and consistent monitoring of how time is spent (Clark, 1983). In addition, parents feel responsible for helping their children learn, communicate regularly with school staff, and are involved in school activities. These findings have been replicated with children and families across socioeconomic levels, ethnic backgrounds, and grade level (Christenson, Hurley, Sheridan, & Fenstermacher, 1997).

The three specific parent involvement interventions we present in this section have demonstrated positive effects on academic variables. First, a form of parent–teacher problem solving, conjoint behavioral consultation, has resulted in improvements for children with academic problems (Galloway & Sheridan, 1994). Second, daily report cards have been shown to improve children's on-task behavior, productivity, and accuracy (Kelley & McCain, 1995). Third, Dialogic Reading, the reading component of Arnold and colleagues' (1999) parents reading with preschoolers program, has demonstrated a positive effect on children's language development (Arnold, Lonigan, Whitehurst, & Epstein, 1994; Whitehurst et al., 1988).

In summary, there is strong research support for the positive effect of parent involvement on academic functioning. However, many questions remain concerning parent involvement. The relative value of different types of parent involvement is not clear (Dimmock, O'Donoghue, & Robb, 1996; Feuerstein, 2000; Marcon, 1999; Powell-Smith, Shinn, Stoner, & Good, 2000). Marcon (1999) raised a number of questions in her study that are relevant to much of the research on parent involvement in schools. She noted that questions remain concerning dose effects (i.e., both how much parent involvement and how many different kinds of parent involvement are needed to bring about the desired effect) and the underlying mechanisms by which parent involvement produces academic gains.

BEST PRACTICES FOR HOME–SCHOOL ACADEMIC INTERVENTIONS

Home–school collaboration has the potential to significantly increase academic success for children with ACP. We reviewed research-supported strategies from the following sources to determine best practices for home–school interventions: (1) Christenson and colleagues' (Christenson, 1995; Christenson & Buerkle, 1999; Christenson et al., 1992, 1997) reviews and discussions of home–school collaboration; (2) Epstein's (1992) discussion of the role of school psychologists in school and family partnerships; (3) authors who have described the use of daily report cards (Bloomquist, 1996; Elliott et al., 1999; Pelham & Waschbusch, 1999; Pfiffner & Barkley, 1998); (4) Raffaele and Knoff's (1999) work on home–school collaboration with disadvantaged families; and (5) Walker and colleagues' (1995) strategies for working with children who exhibit antisocial behaviors in schools.

Removing Barriers to Home–School Cooperation

Most people support home–school collaboration as a good idea, yet many factors interfere with effective communication and cooperation between parents and schools. Both family factors and school factors can contribute to this problem. Some parents do not experience schools as welcoming institutions. As children themselves, some parents experienced school as a frustrating, punitive place that failed to support them. Thus they may have trouble trusting schools when they return to them as parents. Others may approach school with a sense of inadequacy related to a history of school failure. Some parents have already had negative experiences with schools as parents; they have felt unwelcome, ignored, or blamed at school. Economic or cultural differences between the family and the majority of school staff can result in parents feeling uncomfortable in schools. Language differences can clearly interfere with parent involvement. Other factors that can interfere with successful home–school cooperation include a lack of knowledge about school procedures, a lack of knowledge about how to help with schoolwork, and practical factors such as transportation, child care, and work schedules. Finally, some parents want to be involved in school, but are overwhelmed with personal, emotional, or economic concerns.

Schools too can be responsible for barriers to home–school cooperation. Some schools will talk about home–school collaboration, but have a limited commitment to the process and fail to effectively promote parent involvement. School staff can at times focus on family problems and view parents as dysfunctional, uninvolved, or unhelpful with their children's academic success. Communication with parents is often crisis-oriented or negative. There is limited training for teachers in how to work with parents as partners and a lack of clarity about parents' and teachers' roles and responsibilities. Finally, effective collaboration between teachers and parents takes time. With multiple responsibilities and demands on their time, it is difficult for teachers to attend adequately to all these needs.

To remove barriers to home–school cooperation, the school must make a commitment to parent involvement. The commitment needs to go beyond moral support to a willingness to allocate time and resources. A successful parent involvement program requires a needs assessment, planning, the establishment of procedures for parent involvement, training for staff and parents, and monitoring and ongoing support of the implementation of the program (see Raffaele & Knoff, 1999). Removing practical barriers may involve providing transportation, arranging for or providing child care, and scheduling meetings in the evenings. This is unlikely to happen unless a school is firmly committed to parent involvement.

Another factor in addressing barriers to home–school cooperation is the school taking a proactive approach. Engaging parents should begin long before there is the need for a cooperative relationship to solve a problem. If a parent's input is only sought when his or her child has a problem, and when most communication is negative, it will be difficult for the teacher and parent to work effectively as a team. A parent will be a more cooperative and effective collaborator following a problem if the parent has previously been taught the importance of home–school collaboration; has talked to the teacher about classroom rules, expectations, curriculum, and the parent's own goals for his or her child; and has been notified of his or her child's positive school achievements. This is especially true for parents who have historically had minimal involvement with schools. With some parents, changing attitudes and involvement in school will be a long-term process that cannot be accomplished at the time of problems or crises.

Promoting Belief in Shared
Responsibility for Academic Success

Promoting the belief that school success is the responsibility of both the school and the family is important. Christenson (1995) pointed out that "home–school collaboration is an attitude, not simply an activity" (p. 253). At the core of this attitude is the belief that school staff and parents are active partners in successfully educating children. Christenson and Buerkle (1999) made a distinction between what they called the "traditional approach" to family involvement in school and the "partnership approach." In the traditional approach, parents and teachers have separate roles and responsibilities, there is limited contact between parents and teachers, degree of parent involvement is determined by the school, and parents are passive recipients of one-way communication from the school. In addition, family issues and conditions are often not taken into account when working with parents, which can leave parents feeling uninvolved. In the partnership approach to parent involvement, there is a shared responsibility for the child's education and socialization. The communication is two-way with a collaborative interaction between the school and the family. There is a focus on building and maintaining the relationship between home and school. The knowledge and skills of both teachers and parents are respected and valued.

An effective strategy for promoting a belief in shared responsibility for academic success is to train school staff and parents. Training involves learning the value of shared responsibility and learning how to carry it out. We discuss the training of school staff and parents in the next section.

An example of the practical application of shared responsibility for academic success is a parent joining with a teacher to solve a child's school problems. There are numerous models for parents and teachers working together to solve problems (Christenson & Buerkle, 1999; Sheridan & Kratochwill, 1992; Walker et al., 1995). The first step in a parent–teacher problem-solving process is to set the stage for a collaborative approach. A number of models utilize a facilitator (e.g., a school psychologist or a behavioral consultant) to guide the problem-solving process. The facilitator will acknowledge the expertise of both the parents and the school staff and talk about the advantages of working together to solve the problem. An effort is made to create shared ownership of the problem and the solution and to eliminate blaming.

Once a cooperative atmosphere is established, the problem and its controlling factors need to be specified. It is important that both the parent and the school staff provide their own perspectives. If there is not sufficient information provided by the parent and the teacher (and the child, if appropriate) to define the problem and its controlling factors, further information will need to be collected before an effective intervention can be designed. This may involve direct observation in the problem area, charting of behaviors, or input from others familiar with the child. A more complete review of this process is contained in Chapter 3.

Once the problem is defined and its controlling factors are understood, possible solutions need to be generated and a final plan agreed to by all participants. This process should include agreement on what data will be collected to assess effectiveness. It should also include a clear delineation of people's roles in carrying out the plan and a date for the parent and teacher to meet again to review the plan. During implementation of the plan it is often necessary for the facilitator to be involved in training, monitoring, and supporting those who are carrying out the plan. If the plan has been successful, the follow-up meeting can be used to discuss how to fade out the plan to promote maintenance of behavioral gains. This meeting can also be used to set up a procedure for ongoing communication between school and home. If the plan was not successful, the problem-solving process can be used again to modify the plan or to design a new plan.

Parent–teacher problem solving may not be a useful option in all cases. Sheridan and Kratochwill (1992) suggested that conjoint behavioral consultation, a form of parent–teacher problem solving, requires that both parents and school staff be willing and able to participate in the process. They must have the time available, the process must be acceptable to them, and they must have the personal skills needed to make the process work. Severe family dysfunction or a teacher's low level of self-efficacy may interfere with successful problem solving. Also, the facilitator needs to have sufficient training and skills or his or her effectiveness may be compromised.

Training School Staff and Parents
for Effective Collaboration

Both the school staff and parents need to be trained in the importance of parental involvement, types of parental involvement, and how to work effectively with each other. As part of this process, school staff and parents should discuss their roles and responsibilities in the education process. Roles and responsibilities may vary from one school to another depending on the needs, values, and goals of the school, families, and community. Training should also take place to help school staff and parents better understand each other's cultures, attitudes, and beliefs; how these differences affect the educational process; and how these differences affect the home–school relationship. This allows for better perspective taking, which can contribute to effective collaboration. School personnel are better able to effectively involve parents if they understand the fears, anger, mistrust, beliefs, and pressures parents may bring to their school involvement. School personnel also have to be sensitive to the varying needs of parents. Some parents will only need information to increase their involvement in school; others will need both information and ongoing support to be involved in their child's education.

Parents also need to increase their knowledge and awareness. Parents should understand the multiple demands and expectations placed on teachers and their time and how this can effect their work with children and parents. It is also helpful for parents to understand the differences between working with a child in the context of a family and working with a child in the context of a classroom. Parent and teacher training can be accomplished through written materials, workshops, parent–teacher committees focused on increasing parent involvement in school, or individual problem-solving meetings that include a facilitator who can promote mutual understanding.

Promoting Effective Communication between School and Home

Multiple methods should be used to communicate with parents. Options include orientation nights at the beginning of the year, parent–teacher conferences, school open houses, teacher phone calls to parents concerning their children's positive achievements and problems, newsletters, workshops, and home visits. Teachers should provide parents with information concerning classroom rules and expectations, curricula, and how their child is performing. It is also helpful for parents to be told how they can promote educational progress. This includes information on how to help children do homework, how to read with children to promote reading skills, and educational activities parents can share with their children. In addition to teachers providing parents with information, parents need to provide information to teachers on their goals for their child, home factors affecting school performance, and home factors affecting the parent's involvement in school.

Utilizing Daily Report Cards

The use of daily report cards is one strategy that is used to increase communication and cooperation between school and home. Daily report cards are useful because they can target many different behaviors, can be easier to implement in the classroom than other behavioral interventions, and provide regular feedback to children and parents. In addition, the rewards and mild punishments available in the home generally have greater variety and potency than those available in school. Daily report cards share many common components with contracts and token/point systems (see Chapter 8). Pelham and Waschbusch (1999) suggested that daily report cards are an essential component of school-based treatment of children with ADHD.

The first step in using daily report cards is an assessment to better understand and define the problem behavior. Following the assessment, general goals are selected. Specific behaviors that will lead to achieving the goals are then identified. For example, if the goal is to increase academic performance, specific behaviors may include having the necessary materials, completing assigned tasks accurately, and completing and returning homework. The number of behaviors monitored may vary from one to seven, with three to five behaviors typically being included. It may be helpful at the start to include one or two positive behaviors that the child regularly exhibits so the child will experience some initial success. The behaviors monitored should be quantifiable. If descriptive ratings are used (e.g., good, fair, poor), they should be objectively defined (e.g., "good" means 90% to 100% of work completed, "fair" means 50% to 89% of work completed, and "poor" means less than 50% of work completed). The child's behavior should be monitored and the child given feedback on a regular basis during the day (e.g., after each class or subject).

Criteria must be set by which to judge successful performance. The criteria should be challenging, yet achievable. For example, if a child is completing 25% of the expected schoolwork, an initial goal may be to increase work completion to 50%. If there is a high frequency of problem behaviors, it may be helpful at the start of the program to monitor behavior for only a portion of the day. The criteria should be reviewed frequently to ensure they remain appropriate as progress is made.

The child will generally be responsible for bringing the report card home. Oppositional behavior or disorganization can interfere with this important component of the program. If the card is not brought home, it should be responded to as if the child had received poor ratings. Some problem solving may be needed to increase the frequency with which the card is brought home. If it is a matter of organization, the child can be taught a strategy for remembering the card or the teacher can check to be sure it is in the child's backpack. If the problem is the result of resistance, rewards and mild punishments can be utilized.

The final step is to assist parents in setting up rewards the child can earn for positive ratings. One option is to use privileges that previously did not have to be earned, such as television or video games. It is helpful to have a menu of rewards divided into several levels so the child can earn smaller rewards for improvement short of the final goal. An example of a daily report card is provided in Figure 7.2.

When the child is consistently achieving the goal, generalization and maintenance are addressed. If other behaviors are problematic, the behaviors monitored can be changed. To support maintenance of the improved behavior, the frequency of the monitoring can be reduced, rather than abruptly ending the program. This can be achieved by reducing the frequency of the monitoring during the day (e.g., from each class period to once in the morning and once in the afternoon) or reducing the frequency with which the report cards are sent home (e.g., from daily to weekly).

There are some limitations to the use of daily report cards. Both the teacher and the parents must have an understanding of the principles of behavior modification. They also must be capable of implementing the program on a consistent basis. Daily report cards may not be effective for children who live in highly dysfunctional families. While daily report cards can be used alone, they are commonly used as one component of a treatment package.

Child's name: _____ Date: _____

	Special		LA		Math		Reading		SS/Science	
Follows class rules with no more than 3 rule violations per period.	Y	N	Y	N	Y	N	Y	N	Y	N
Completes assignments within the designated time.	Y	N	Y	N	Y	N	Y	N	Y	N
Completes assignments at 80% accuracy.	Y	N	Y	N	Y	N	Y	N	Y	N
Complies with teacher requests (no more than 3 instances of noncompliance per period).	Y	N	Y	N	Y	N	Y	N	Y	N
No more than 3 instances of teasing per period.	Y	N	Y	N	Y	N	Y	N	Y	N

OTHER

	Special	
Follows lunch rules	Y	N
Follows recess rules	Y	N

Total number of Yeses: _____

Teacher's initials: _____

Comments: _____

_____

_____

FIGURE 7.2. Sample daily report card. From Pelham and Waschbusch (1999). Copyright 1999 by Kluwer Academic/Plenum Publishers. Reprinted by permission.

Providing Multiple Options for Parent Involvement

Schools will be more successful at involving parents if there are multiple ways for parents to be involved. Options include attending school functions, attending parent–teacher conferences, volunteering in the classroom or school office, taking part in advisory or planning committees, and being actively involved with helping their child practice or learn new skills. The type of parent involvement promoted will depend on the established goals. Raffaele and Knoff (1999) illustrated that the type of parent involvement activity will vary depending on which parents the school is focused on: all parents, parents at risk of being disengaged from school, or parents who already are disengaged from school. Within each of these categories, the parent involvement activity will vary depending on the goal: increased parent awareness, increased parent cooperation, or increased parent collaboration. For example, if the school wants to increase awareness for parents in general, the school can send home handouts on child development, school policies, and so on. If the school wants to target parents who are disengaged or at risk of being disengaged, school staff may need to conduct home visits to increase awareness.

An important type of parent involvement is the planning of efforts to improve home–school collaboration. Parent input is important so the perspectives and needs of parents are adequately addressed. If parents are to be true partners in the educational process, they need to be partners in deciding how they can most effectively be involved.

Another form of involvement is parents engaging their children in learning activities. An example of this type of parent involvement is provided by a program to teach parents how to read to their preschoolers (Arnold et al., 1999). This program was selected as an example because of its focus on low-income families and its use of empirically supported interventions. The program combined two research-supported interventions to promote positive development in high-risk children.

Arnold and colleagues' (1999) project involved preschoolers, their parents, and their preschool teachers from a low-income community. The parents and teachers met in separate groups for 2-hour sessions for 8 weeks. Parents and teachers were given homework assignments based on the material covered in each group. Teachers were encouraged to read to their children in groups of three to five so they could use the interactive approach recommended in the Dialogic Reading Program (Arnold et al., 1994). A new book was provided each week for 12 weeks and children were encouraged to bring books home to read with their parents. Parents were encouraged to read as often as possible with their children, but at least three times a week.

The academic portion of the program involved the Dialogic Reading Program (Arnold et al., 1994). This program uses videotaped training for parents to teach them interactive techniques to use when reading picture books with their children. The first of two videos teaches parents to ask "what" questions, follow answers with questions, repeat what the child says, help the child as needed, praise and encourage the child, shadow the child's interests, and have fun. The second video focuses on asking open-ended questions and expanding on what the child says. Along with Dialogic Reading, this program used a videotape behavior management program developed by Webster-Stratton (1994).

Summary

In Table 7.3 we provide a summary of strategies for promoting effective home–school collaboration. Research strongly supports the involvement of

TABLE 7.3. Best Practices for Home–School Academic Interventions

Procedures	Best practices
Removing barriers to home–school cooperation	Identify barriers, commit resources and time, implement interventions proactively.
Promoting a belief in shared responsibility for academic success	Promote the value of schools and parents working as partners in educating children, two-way communication, a focus on building a relationship between school and home, and respecting the knowledge and skills of teachers and parents; parent–teacher problem solving is one strategy for implementing shared responsibility.
Training school staff and parents for effective collaboration	Train school staff and parents in the importance of parent involvement, types of parent involvement, how schools and parents can effectively work together, and the need for schools and parents understanding each other's cultures, attitudes, and beliefs.
Promoting effective communication between school and home	Use multiple methods to communicate; teachers provide information on classroom rules and curriculum, child functioning, and parent involvement in learning activities; parents provide information on their child's needs and home factors affecting school functioning.
Utilizing daily report cards	Select quantifiable behaviors to monitor, determine goals, rate child on the behaviors, assist child in bringing card home, utilize rewards in the home for successful performance.
Providing multiple options for parent involvement	Offer multiple ways for parents to be involved; type of involvement will depend on the goals selected; parent involvement in learning activities is one form of parent involvement.

parents in the educational process. As pointed out by Epstein (1992), however, parent involvement by itself will not increase academic achievement. Parent involvement needs to be used in combination with other interventions, such as effective instructional practices, to be most successful in raising academic achievement.

CONCLUSION

Empirically supported and promising interventions exist for improving academic functioning in children with ACP. We reviewed some of these interventions in this chapter, along with issues related to their successful implementation. Much more research is needed to better define effective academic interventions for children with ACP. In addition, there is a need for research to better specify for whom academic interventions are most effective and the factors that influence positive outcomes. Finally, most of the reviewed interventions were effective at improving some measure of academic achievement. Despite this, we are still limited in our ability to consistently bring about long-term academic success for children with ACP. What are needed are comprehensive and long-term programs with sufficient power to change academic outcomes for this challenging population.

CHAPTER 8

Schoolwide Interventions to Promote Positive Behavior

Due to the large amount of time children spend in school and the important role school plays in their socialization, school contextual factors play a major role in interventions with children exhibiting ACP. In the previous chapter we focused on children's academic functioning. In Chapters 8 and 9 we emphasize children's behavior and social development. For organizational purposes, we have separated interventions targeting academic functioning and interventions targeting behavioral and social functioning. In practice, however, these interventions would not be separated. Many interventions have both academic and behavioral effects. Thus the interventions discussed in these chapters should be used together to promote successful outcomes.

Experts recommend that schools implement a comprehensive, three-level approach to interventions involving children with ACP (Dwyer & Osher, 2000; Sugai, Sprague, Horner, & Walker, 2000). The first level is a schoolwide foundation that supports positive behavior and skills for all children. This foundation level is sufficient for promoting positive behavior for approximately 80% of children. The second level is early interventions for children at risk for academic or behavioral difficulties. The second level will meet the needs of an additional 15% of children. The third level of more comprehensive and individualized interventions focuses on the approximately 5% of children experiencing significant difficulties. Children with ACP commonly require interventions at all three levels. In this chapter we focus on interventions at the first level; in the following chapter we present interventions that cover all three levels.

Schoolwide interventions to promote positive behavior and social development are applied throughout the school and involve all students. They include a broad array of procedures. The interventions are designed to reduce risk factors and promote protective factors in multiple domains including child, social/peer, and contextual life domains (see Tables 2.3 and 2.4 in Chapter 2). Specifically, the interventions we discuss in this chapter promote effective school responses to the behavioral and academic needs of children, bonding with school and adults within the school, adaptive social interactions among children, and social and emotional skills in individual children.

Following an overview and review of the research on schoolwide interventions, we describe procedures for implementing schoolwide programs for promoting positive behavior. Next, we present the content areas that should be addressed. We conclude this chapter with a description of an effective peer mediation program, which is a common component of schoolwide programs to promote positive behavior.

OVERVIEW AND RESEARCH EVALUATION OF SCHOOLWIDE INTERVENTIONS TO PROMOTE POSITIVE BEHAVIOR

An important aspect of the interventions presented in this chapter is that they not only attempt to decrease ACP behaviors, they also have a specific focus on defining and promoting positive behavior. The interventions described here are universally applied, meet the behavioral needs of most children in the school, and provide a necessary foundation for the interventions with children at risk for or already experiencing ACP problems. The specific targets of these interventions include children's knowledge of appropriate behaviors, rule-following behavior, and respectful interactions with peers and adults.

Schoolwide programs to promote positive behavior are implemented by everyone in the school setting, including administrators, teachers, nonteaching staff, parents, and children. The process of designing and guiding the interventions is best managed by a team of school staff members and parents, often with the assistance of a consultant who has knowledge of the relevant research and program implementation procedures. The interventions focus on multiple aspects of a school's functioning, including how people interact with each other, rules and procedures, monitoring of behavior, acknowledgment and reward of positive behavior, and response to problem behavior.

Numerous studies have demonstrated the effectiveness of schoolwide interventions that promote positive behavior, including the Bullying Prevention Program (Olweus, 1991; Olweus, Limber, & Mihalic, 2000), the Child

Development Project (Battistich, 2000; Battistich, Watson, Solomon, Schaps, & Solomon, 1991), and a schoolwide program for children with behavior problems described by Nelson (1996). The Bullying Prevention Program used schoolwide, classroom, and individual level interventions to reduce bully/victim problems in schools. Based on self-reports, reductions were noted in the level of bully/victim problems and in general antisocial behavior (e.g., vandalism, theft, truancy). Two factors related to the effectiveness of the Bullying program may have implications for other interventions. Extensive media coverage at both the national and the local level in Norway may have contributed to the effectiveness of the program (Roland, 2000). Also, the program had limited long-term effects, which was attributed to difficulties in maintaining the interventions in the schools (Roland, 2000).

A 3-year follow-up study of the Child Development Project, a schoolwide intervention program, found positive effects on children's educational aspirations, academic self-esteem, sense of efficacy, and involvement in positive youth group activities (Battistich, 2000). Children reported a reduced frequency of misconduct at school, teachers rated children as being better students, and children received higher course grades and higher achievement test scores.

Nelson (1996) evaluated a multicomponent schoolwide program focused on increasing elementary schools' ability to successfully educate children with disruptive behaviors. The program resulted in a decrease in expulsions, suspensions, and emergency removals. Improvement was found in teacher ratings of behavioral adjustment and academic performance for children with behavior problems.

Research has demonstrated a relationship between school climate and self-concept, behavior, absenteeism, rate of suspension, and achievement in children (Haynes et al., 1997). School climate refers to the quality and consistency of interpersonal interactions in a school setting (Haynes et al., 1997). It is believed to be an especially important variable for low-income and minority children (Esposito, 1999; Haynes et al., 1997; Pierce, 1994). The Comer School Development Program provides a structure and a procedure for schools to improve their climate. Cook, Hunt, and Murphy (2000) evaluated the effectiveness of the Comer School Development Program in 10 inner-city Chicago schools over 4 years. They found that the Comer schools improved in reading and math at a greater rate than the control schools. Children reported improved social climate, decreased acting out and anger, and beliefs about what constitutes misbehavior that were more "mainstream."

In summary, outcome studies of schoolwide interventions have demonstrated their effectiveness. There are many common components among the interventions that help to define best practices. We must note that while demonstrating positive outcomes, many of the results are rather modest and the overall impact on individual children is not known. Also, given the multicomponent nature of the interventions, it is not known which components contribute to the effectiveness of many interventions.

BEST PRACTICE MODELS
FOR SCHOOLWIDE INTERVENTIONS

To define best practices for schoolwide programs, we identified common procedures from empirically supported programs. We included implementation procedures and content from the following programs: (1) the Child Development Project (Battistich, 2000; Battistich et al., 1991); (2) Project PREPARE (Colvin, Kameenui, & Sugai, 1993); (3) the Comer School Development Program (Comer, 1980; Comer, Haynes, Joyner, & Ben-Avie, 1996; Cook et al., 1998); (4) Safeguarding Our Children: An Action Guide (Dwyer & Osher, 2000); (5) Nelson's (1996) schoolwide program for children with disruptive behavior; (6) the Olweus Bullying Prevention Program (Olweus, 1991; Olweus et al., 2000); (7) Project ACHIEVE (Knoff, 2000); and (8) Walker and colleagues' (1995) description of schoolwide behavior management programming.

BEST PRACTICES FOR SCHOOLWIDE INTERVENTIONS:
PROGRAM IMPLEMENTATION

In this section we present nine steps involved in effectively implementing a schoolwide program to promote positive behavior. This involves procedures that school staff would utilize to set up, deliver, and maintain a schoolwide intervention program. The content of schoolwide interventions is presented in the following section.

Assembling a Schoolwide Team

The implementation of an effective schoolwide program to promote positive behavior requires much planning and work. Most effective programs recommend formation of a coordinating team to implement the program. The makeup of the team varies, but it commonly includes teachers from different grade levels, school administrators, and parents. Sometimes community representatives are included to provide additional expertise, be a voice for community values and goals, help coordinate the school program with community programs, and increase community support for the program. Team members should have diverse and complementary skills and should be willing and able to put time and effort into the program. The coordinating team must develop a vision, a procedure for making decisions, and sufficient trust and confidence in each other to function as an effective group.

Assessing the Needs of the School

Once a schoolwide team is in place, it needs to assess the effectiveness of the school's current approach to promoting positive behavior and the extent of current behavior problems. This assessment process is important in establishing the need for a program, building support among stakeholders, and effectively targeting the intervention program on vital school needs. The Bullying Prevention Program provides one example of how this is done. Before the program is initiated, the Olweus Bully/Victim Questionnaire (Olweus, 1996) is administered to children. This is an anonymous child survey that asks questions about bullying at the school. The survey includes questions about the type of bullying, its frequency, its location, and the response of adults. The results can be used not only to demonstrate the need for intervention, but also to help design aspects of the intervention. For example, if children identify the playground as a specific problem area, interventions focused on the playground can be included in the program. Teachers and parents can also be surveyed to determine their level of concern with child behavior, their awareness of current rules and procedures, and their views on the effectiveness of current procedures.

Setting Goals

Before interventions can be selected or designed, the coordinating team needs to determine the desired outcome or goal. Walker and colleagues (1995) recommended that the team design both a school mission statement and a statement of purpose for the behavior program. The mission statement should be designed with input from school staff, children, and parents, and express the broad goals and values of the school. This includes goals such as helping all children to reach their potential and develop the skills they need to function successfully in society. The statement of purpose for the behavior program is more specific and sets goals that support the school's mission. This generally includes goals related to increasing positive behavior, decreasing problem behavior, and creating a supportive learning environment.

Selecting/Designing Intervention Components

There are a number of factors to consider in selecting interventions. First, the interventions should focus on the specific goals determined by the school. Second, the interventions must be consistent with the structure, values, and resources of the school. Third, it is best if the interventions emphasize proactive and positive strategies as opposed to reactive and punitive strategies. Fourth, the interventions need to have empirical support, preferably from controlled studies. It is helpful for the school team to have a member who is knowledgeable about research on effective behavior programs; if not, the team should consider hiring a consultant who has this knowledge. Finally, the strength of the interventions need to be sufficient to achieve the desired goals. For example, a peer mediation program may be one component of an effective violence prevention program, but by itself is unlikely to significantly reduce violence in a school. Numerous experts have concluded that short-term, single-component interventions cannot be expected to result in long-term changes in ACP behavior (Durlak, 1995; Kazdin, 1995; Mulvey et al., 1993). For school-based interventions, Walker and colleagues (1995) suggested that the magnitude of the effect is determined by four factors: (1) the comprehensiveness of the intervention, (2) the intervention being applied according to empirically supported standards and guidelines, (3) the intervention being of sufficient intensity, and (4) the length of the intervention being sufficient to produce enduring effects.

Establishing Support for the Intervention

A common factor highlighted by successful schoolwide programs is the importance of establishing a broad base of support. The effectiveness of the schoolwide program is dependent on it being implemented consistently, broadly, and accurately. To achieve this, it is necessary to obtain the support of all stakeholders, including teachers, nonteaching school staff, school administrators, parents, children, and community leaders. Teachers implement the majority of the interventions, so their full support is essential for consistent and broad implementation. Teachers have many different beliefs about effective behavior interventions. As a result, it may take much discussion and presentation of evidence to build consensus and demonstrate to teachers how the program can work effectively in the school and in their classrooms.

The strong and visible support of the school's administration is of vital importance. Effective implementation often requires policy changes, the reallocation of financial resources, staff time, and administrative backing for staff implementing the program. The principal is a key figure in providing both moral and practical support. In addition to teachers and administrators, many programs also involve lunchroom and playground monitors, food service and office staff, bus drivers, and custodians. Their behavior very much affects school climate and a school's consistent response to child behavior. As a result, they too must be willing and able to implement the program.

Training School Staff

Another critical aspect of schoolwide programs is effective training for the staff. Colvin and colleagues (1993), in discussing Project PREPARE, noted how difficult it is to change teacher behavior. They cited three principles proposed by Guskey (1987) that should be taken into account when designing staff development programs: (1) change for teachers is a slow and gradual process; (2) it is helpful for teachers to receive regular feedback on child outcomes; and (3) ongoing support is necessary. They also noted that the training should address teachers' sense of efficacy (teachers' belief concerning their ability to effectively impact child behavior) and collegiality (the process by which teachers effectively work together). The training they proposed, in which a team of teachers is trained to guide and support other teachers in the intervention process, is a gradual process that takes place over the course of a year.

The training of teachers and other school staff must not only teach them the intervention procedures, but also assist them in incorporating the interventions into their daily practice. To accomplish this, school staff should be provided information on the rationale for the intervention along with detailed information on how to implement it. To help them in understanding how the procedures are implemented, the staff can watch an actual implementation of the intervention on video or via a live demonstration and role-play implementation themselves. Once the intervention is being used in the classroom, staff should be observed and offered supportive feedback. A support person should be available to help staff problem-solve when difficult situations are encountered. Intervention procedures should be reviewed periodically and the staff provided with regular information on the positive effects of the intervention in the school.

Coordinating and Monitoring Accurate Implementation

The coordinating team needs to be actively involved in the direction, coordination, and monitoring of the program and its various components. A high-quality program that is not implemented as planned, or that is only partially implemented, is unlikely to have the desired effects. Therefore a process needs to be in place to determine whether the school staff is properly implementing the program, as well as a procedure to correct deficiencies. Monitoring of implementation can be done by observation of implementation, meetings to discuss program implementation, and the review of paper work generated by program implementation. There are many reasons why a program may not be implemented properly, including the need for more training, the staff not having sufficient time to implement the program, or the staff questioning the efficacy of the program. The team must determine why there are implementation problems and design corrective actions.

The quality of program implementation and the effectiveness of the program are affected by the amount of assistance provided to the staff implementing the program. The school administration must allow the staff sufficient time to properly implement the program. Often new programs and responsibilities are added on top of existing responsibilities, with the result being that the staff has inadequate time to attend to their various duties. This can compromise the accurate implementation of the program and build resentment among the staff. In addition to sufficient time, it is helpful for staff members who are effectively implementing the program to receive recognition for their work. Adequate assistance should be available so that when problems arise staff members are not left on their own to manage them. Problems can be quickly identified and resolved if a feedback system is in place.

Assessing Intervention Effectiveness

A data collection system is needed to determine the effectiveness of the program. The data collected should be determined by the goals of the program. For example, if one of the goals is to reduce aggression on the playground, office referrals from the playground can be monitored, playground supervisors can periodically complete rating forms on the amount of aggression, or observers can periodically record the amount of aggression. If the program is not producing the desired effects, modifications need to be made and/or other interventions considered. Data supporting the effectiveness of the program is essential for maintaining the program. Data demonstrating the success of the program can increase the staffs' sense of efficacy and motivation; bolster the support of the school administration, parents, and the community; and help to maintain funding.

Maintaining the Program over Time

A problem that is often overlooked is how to maintain a program after the initial enthusiasm and excitement wanes (Roland, 2000). Changes in school administrators and teachers, other issues that compete for attention and resources, and complacency can reduce the commitment and resources given to the program and erode its effectiveness. If the program is to have lasting power, there needs to be a structure in place to support and maintain it. The coordinating team should be actively involved in ongoing implementation, monitoring, and problem solving. This involves continued training for new and veteran staff members. Data collection and discussion with school staff are essential to keep the program focused on current behavioral issues. As we previously noted, data collection can demonstrate effectiveness, which is helpful in maintaining support and funding. Keeping parents and community members informed and involved serves the dual purpose of ensuring that the program will continue to respond to community concerns and keeping community members and parents informed of the effectiveness of the program. Both of these factors will help maintain support for the program.

Summary

Table 8.1 provides a summary of best practices for procedures used to implement schoolwide interventions promoting positive behavior. Attending

TABLE 8.1. Summary of Best Practices for Schoolwide Interventions: Program Implementation

Delivery procedures	Best practices
Assembling a schoolwide team	Include teachers from all grade levels, school administrators, parents, and possibly community representatives.
Assessing the needs of the school	Assess current approach and unmet needs by surveying children, school staff, and parents.
Setting goals	Develop mission statement, then base intervention goals on mission statement.
Selecting/designing intervention components	Select components that address goals, emphasize proactive and positive strategies are empirically supported, and have sufficient strength to achieve goals.
Establishing support for the intervention	Elicit support from all stakeholders and participants, provide for sufficient administrative and financial support.
Training school staff	Provide information on intervention rationale, detailed description of procedures, and how procedures are implemented; observe implementation and offer supportive feedback; provide ongoing support and review.
Coordinating and monitoring accurate implementation	Develop procedure for monitoring implementation and correcting problems; provide adequate support to those implementing interventions.
Assessing intervention effectiveness	Collect data to demonstrate program effectiveness or need for modifications.
Maintaining the program over time	Develop structures and procedures to maintain program support, implementation, and effectiveness; utilize ongoing training; keep staff, parents, and community members informed of program results.

to the effective implementation of schoolwide interventions is essential if the desired results are to be attained. We present the content of effective interventions in the next section.

BEST PRACTICES FOR
SCHOOLWIDE INTERVENTIONS: PROGRAM CONTENT

In this section we present four common content areas addressed by effective schoolwide programs designed to increase positive behavior and reduce aggressive and noncompliant behavior. School staff members use the previously discussed implementation procedures to bring about changes in these content areas. All four areas should be addressed in schoolwide programs.

Creating a Positive School Climate

A school climate characterized by low academic and behavioral expectations, reactive approaches to behavior management, and coercive relationships between staff and children can increase children's aggression, defiance, and alienation from school. Children with ACP often receive limited praise and many reprimands and have few positive interactions with school staff members. They begin to formulate beliefs about the staff such as "they are mean," "they are unfair," and so on. This results in the school environment becoming aversive for both the child and the staff. Being sent out of the classroom, suspended, or missing school becomes reinforcing for the child.

A positive and supportive climate is a necessary foundation for effective promotion of positive behavior. The climate of a school is affected by many factors, including academic instruction, classroom and schoolwide behavior management, and parental involvement, as well as by relationships among teachers, school administrators, nonteaching staff, children, and parents. Successful programs such as the Comer Child Development Program (Comer, 1980) and the Child Development Project (Battistich et al., 1991) put a heavy focus on creating a supportive community within the school that will promote positive behavior and development.

The establishment of a supportive, cooperative, positive, and respectful climate begins at the start of the school year. It can be promoted by scheduling schoolwide and classroom activities that encourage a sense of community. One approach is to hold schoolwide assemblies involving staff, parents, and community leaders that focus on respect and cooperation. Open houses, dinners, and recreational activities can also nurture a sense of community and cooperation. In classrooms, teachers can utilize cooperative games, class meetings, and lessons focused on respect and cooperation.

Interpersonal relationships are an important aspect of a positive school climate. It should be expected that everyone at school, adults and children, treat each other with respect. This is especially important for children with ACP. It is not unusual for children with ACP to have a history of coercive and negatively toned relationships with adults. To prevent this from occurring in school, the school staff has to actively work on developing positive and productive relationships with children manifesting ACP. One strategy for doing this is to demonstrate interest in individual children. Becoming familiar with a child's interests, skills, history, and situation away from school can add to a positive relationship and help the teacher to better understand the child and his or her behavior. Another strategy is to increase the use of positive statements and decrease the use of negative statements. Teachers can monitor the ratio of their positive to negative statements by recording them on a chart. In addition, little things like greeting children individually in the morning, acknowledging successes either verbally or in a note, and occasionally interacting with children around nonacademic topics can help promote positive relationships.

Defining Behavioral Expectations

Schools should have a small set of clearly stated rules with which all children and staff members are familiar. There should be both general, schoolwide behavioral expectations and specific behavioral expectations for different locations (e.g., lunchroom, playground, hallways, the library). Four or five schoolwide expectations should be stated in simple, positive terms (Walker et al., 1995). Examples of schoolwide expectations are "respect the property of others" and "treat others respectfully." Children should be taught these behavioral expectations and given specific positive and negative examples so they have a clear understanding of what is expected of them. Behavioral expectations for specific settings also need to be established. Behavioral expectations for hallways might include "always walk," "use a quiet voice," and "keep hands and feet to yourself." Multiple strategies can be used to teach children these behavioral expectations, including school assemblies, classroom reviews, letters to parents, and posters throughout the school.

Supporting Positive Behavior

Following the establishment and teaching of behavioral expectations, positive behaviors should be monitored, supported, cued, and reinforced. The monitoring of behavior is important, especially during common problem times (e.g., transitions from one class to another) and in common problem locations (e.g., the lunchroom and the playground). Monitoring should be most intense during the time when the expectations are being learned. Once the expected behaviors are well established, the level of monitoring can be reduced. Monitoring by itself though is not sufficient. The supervising staff must intervene quickly and effectively when they see problems. Procedures for doing this are presented below. The focus should not just be on intervening with problem behavior, but also acknowledging and rewarding expected behavior.

It is helpful for schools to have both informal and formal procedures for acknowledging positive behavior. Informal acknowledgment and praise from school staff can help to increase the focus on positive behavior. More formal systems are also productive, such as set criteria (based on the established behavioral expectations) for earning certificates, acknowledgment at school assemblies, tickets for a school lottery, letters acknowledging positive behavior to parents, photos of children posted on a bulletin board, and lunch with the principal or other school staff. These rewards can be earned either by individual children or by whole classrooms.

Verbal reminders and review of behavioral expectations are proactive and effective interventions. This is especially helpful before common problem times. For example, Colvin, Sugai, Good, and Lee (1997) successfully used precorrection (verbal reminders and behavioral rehearsal) prior to transition times, plus active supervision, to reduce problem behavior when children were entering the school, going to lunch, and leaving the school. Before transitions, children were reminded to walk, keep hands and feet to self, and talk in a quiet voice.

Many schoolwide programs focused on promoting positive behavior teach not only behavioral expectations, but also skills such as conflict resolution and anger management that assist children in using positive behavior. These interventions are used not only on a schoolwide basis, but also on a classroom or small-group basis (see Chapter 9).

Utilizing a Consistent and Effective Response to Problem Behavior

Developing a positive climate and teaching positive behavior are important, yet not sufficient by themselves, for effective schoolwide interventions. Schools need effective approaches for managing problem behavior. Walker and colleagues (1995) proposed four steps for setting up schoolwide procedures for responding to problem behavior.

Defining Categories of Problem Behaviors

School staff members need to define different categories of problem behaviors. Minor problem behaviors are those that are disruptive to the learning process, such as talking in class or not having materials ready for class. Serious problem behaviors are violations of significant school rules and social norms, such as sustained noncompliance, verbal abuse toward staff, and physical aggression. Some schools will consider repeat minor problem behavior as a serious problem behavior. For example, three time-outs in the classroom in one day may automatically result in a referral to the office. Illegal behaviors are those that violate the law, such as theft, assault, or vandalism. The exact criteria will differ from school to school, but it is important that children and staff know what the criteria are and that they be applied consistently. All problem behaviors should be categorized, and this information should be distributed to all school staff, children, and parents. Once behaviors are categorized, schools need to establish a clear policy on how staff will respond to behaviors in each category. Options for responding include managing the behavior in the classroom, referring the child to an administrator or behavior management specialist, involving parents, suspending the child, or referring the child to law enforcement officials. These responses are discussed in the following sections.

Defining a Procedure for Responding to Minor Problem Behaviors

A standard procedure is needed for staff members to respond to minor problem behaviors. An attempt should be made to first deal with the behavior in a positive and nonpunitive manner. One option is to withdraw attention from the child and acknowledge a nearby child for exhibiting appropriate behavior. If the misbehavior continues, staff members can redirect the child to the appropriate behavior by stating the rule or the expected behavior. The child can also be asked to state the rule or expected behavior. If this is not successful, the child can be given a warning that indicates the consequence if the appropriate behavior is not chosen. Finally, the child is given the negative consequence in a matter-of-fact manner. Following any successful intervention, the previously misbehaving child should be quickly acknowledged for returning to appropriate behavior.

Developing a Procedure for Problem-Solving Meetings

It is helpful for schools to institute a procedure for holding regularly scheduled meetings to problem-solve when a child has repeated minor problem behaviors. This allows individual staff members to receive support and ideas on interventions from each other to more effectively respond to the problem behaviors. Staff members who work with the child in different settings should be included, as well as staff with expertise in managing behavior. A process similar to the parent–teacher problem-solving process can be used (see Chapter 7).

Developing a Response to Serious Problem Behavior

A consistent response to serious problem behaviors is necessary. The response should be written into school policy and used in a consistent manner. The response will typically involve a referral to the office with the consequence being handled by either an administrator or a behavior management specialist. It is important that everyone know what procedures will be followed when a referral is made. Common responses to serious problem behaviors include a parent conference, loss of school privileges, after-school detention, in-school suspension, and out-of-school suspension. In addition, a proactive intervention to help prevent recurrent problems should be employed. Proactive interventions include many of the interventions discussed in Chapter 9 such as child–teacher contracts and skills training.

For a school's response to serious problem behavior to be effective, the school needs to allocate sufficient staff to implement the procedure. Staff members are commonly needed to escort children to the office, supervise children while they are out of class, implement behavior plans used for children with repeat problems, and maintain records related to behavior referrals.

An office referral form should be developed that includes the teacher and the child involved, the date and time of the problem, a description of the problem behavior, and the action taken by the administration or behavior specialist. A sample behavior referral form is presented in Figure 8.1. Information on who was involved and the specific behavior can either be

---

Date:_____ Time: _____

Student/s: _____ Teacher: _____

_____   _____

_____   _____

Behavior (circle one):   Repeat minor problem behavior   Serious problem behavior

Describe:

_____

_____

_____

Office response: Plan:

Time-out _____   Return to class _____

Problem-solving process _____   Conference with teacher _____

Parents contacted _____   Conference with parent _____

In-school suspension _____   Behavior plan/contract _____

Suspension _____   Skills training referral _____

Time spent in office: _____

FIGURE 8.1. Sample behavior referral form.

written down by the teacher and sent to the office with the child or called into the office. The administrator/behavior specialist who works with the child writes in the action that is taken. Each school should individualize their behavior referral forms with the office responses and plans that are available at that school. It is helpful for the form to be in duplicate, with one being kept in the office and the other going to the student's teacher. A referral form promotes communication among staff concerning serious problem behaviors and allows for documentation. Documentation helps to ensure that procedures are being followed, provides a written record that is helpful in determining the need for further interventions, and helps to guide the interventions.

A procedure is needed to determine the school's response to children who are involved in repeated serious problem behaviors. This procedure will commonly involve a team of school staff members who will consider more intensive interventions. Options commonly include special education services and day treatment programs.

The importance of consistency cannot be overstated. Children need to know how school staff will respond to different types of behaviors. Consistent staff responses can be supported by ongoing staff training, regular discussion of behavior management practices, monitoring of both child behavior and staff implementation of behavior management procedures, and discussion of the effectiveness of the behavior management procedures. In addition, consistency can be promoted by the maintenance of staff morale, acknowledgment of effective staff behavior management, and allowing staff sufficient time in their schedules to fulfill their behavior management responsibilities.

Summary

Table 8.2 summarizes the content of effective schoolwide interventions promoting positive behavior. Schoolwide interventions are an essential component of effective school interventions for children with ACP and provide the foundation on which classroom and individual interventions are built.

OVERVIEW AND RESEARCH EVALUATION OF PEER MEDIATION PROGRAMS

Mediation and negotiation are problem-solving or conflict resolution processes in which disputants resolve a disagreement. Mediation differs from negotiation in that a neutral facilitator or mediator assists the problem-solving process (Crawford & Bodine, 1996). In schools, adults or children can conduct mediation. Peer mediation is a process in which a peer functions as a facilitator to assist disputants in resolving a conflict. It can be

TABLE 8.2. Summary of Best Practices for Schoolwide Interventions: Program Content

Content areas	Best practices
Creating a positive school climate	Plan activities that promote a sense of community; actively work on positive relationships with children with ACP by decreasing negative comments, increasing positive comments, and demonstrating interest in children's interests and activities.
Defining behavioral expectations	Develop a small set of general expectations and specific expectations for different school locations.
Supporting positive behavior	Closely monitor behavior, especially during common problem times; acknowledge and reward positive behavior; use reminders and reviews of behavioral expectations; train children in needed social skills.
Utilizing a consistent and effective response to problem behavior	Define categories of problem behaviors; use consistent procedures for responding to minor and serious problem behaviors; institute procedures for problem-solving meetings.

utilized as a stand-alone intervention or as one component of a more comprehensive schoolwide program. Many experts recommend that it be implemented with interventions that involve skills training for the entire student body (Crawford & Bodine, 1996). A distinction can be made between peer mediation programs that mediate disputes when they occur (on-line mediation) and those that take place at a later time (office mediation) (Cunningham & Cunningham, 1998). This section will focus on children being trained to mediate peer disputes when they occur.

Peer mediation interventions target ACP behaviors in school such as arguing, name calling, and fighting. These behaviors often arise as a result of conflicts or disagreements among children. Peer mediation targets these behaviors by providing children with assistance in achieving productive and nonaggressive resolution of their conflicts.

In peer mediation, a limited number of children are trained to use a problem-solving/conflict resolution procedure to help peers resolve disputes. The procedure involves the mediator setting the ground rules and then helping the disputants to state their concerns, suggest solutions, and select and implement a solution.

Many studies have reported a high rate of successful peer mediation in schools, yet most of these studies have had significant methodological limitations (Cunningham et al., 1998; Johnson & Johnson, 1996). In response to this, Cunningham and colleagues (1998) used a multiple-baseline design with three elementary schools to test the impact of the Collaborative Child Mediation Program on playground physical aggression. Decreases in observed aggression ranged from 51% to 65%. The program and the reduced levels of aggression were maintained over the course of 2 years.

Several authors have noted the limitations of conflict resolution strategies in schools. Olweus and colleagues (2000) pointed out that negotiation and mediation assume that the disputants have equal power and that both parties are partially right and partially wrong. In the case of bullying, neither of these assumptions is true. Since bullying involves the violation of another person's rights, Olweus and colleagues (2000) argued that negotiation and mediation are not appropriate responses. Similarly, McEvoy and Welker (2000) claim that conflict resolution may be helpful in resolving minor conflicts, but there is no evidence that it will have an impact on more serious and pervasive problems, such as bullying and gang violence. They argued that there is a need to consider the type of violence and the level of risk when considering an intervention. Johnson and Johnson (1996) noted that mediation tends to be unsuccessful if there is a high level of hostility, the mediator is distrusted, there is a lack of resources, disputants are uncommitted to mediation, the conflict involves general principles, disputants have unequal power, or there is significant psychopathology in the disputants' relationship.

In summary, there is a need for more rigorous research to better define the effectiveness of peer mediation. The available research suggests it can be effective, but methodological problems limit the conclusions that can be drawn. In addition to establishing its efficacy, future research needs to better specify with whom and with what types of conflicts peer mediation can be most effective.

BEST PRACTICES FOR PEER MEDIATION PROGRAMS

Peer mediation programs are a very popular form of conflict resolution intervention in schools. There are many peer mediation programs to choose from. Multiple programs are described and a list of resources is provided by Crawford and Bodine (1996). Unlike most other programs, the Collaborative Child Mediation Program has been demonstrated effective in reducing aggression in a methodologically rigorous study (Cunningham & Cunningham, 1998). As a result, we present this program as an exemplary model of peer mediation. Information on the Collaborative Child Mediation Program was obtained from Cunningham and Cunningham (1998) and Cunningham and colleagues (1998).

Preparing for a Peer Mediation Program

Whether peer mediation is used alone or in combination with other interventions depends on the goals the school hopes to achieve. If the goal is to reduce misbehavior in one specific area, such as the playground, a well-designed and implemented peer mediation program may be sufficient (Cunningham & Cunningham, 1998). If the goal is a schoolwide reduction in child risk and violence, a peer mediation program would likely need to be only one component of a more comprehensive program.

Cunningham and Cunningham (1998) recommend that before an effective child mediation program is implemented, parents, teachers, administrators, and children should be informed and consulted to elicit their support. It is helpful for the school to establish a number of organizational and policy directives. Teachers, parents, and children should agree on what behaviors are to be targeted by mediation. Mediation is a voluntary process, so it is important for the school to have a policy on how to handle conflicts when mediation is refused. Children will be reluctant to serve as mediators or to intervene in certain situations if they do not feel safe and actively supported. Consequences must be established for children who harass or threaten mediators.

Recruiting and Training Mediators

The successful recruitment of mediators will have an impact on the effectiveness of the program. Recruitment can be promoted by having parents, administrators, and community leaders make a presentation to the children that describes the program. Mediators can volunteer or be nominated by the school staff. There should be sufficient mediators to monitor all areas of the playground, handle simultaneous disputes, allow for rotation of mediators, and allow for backup mediators. Most schools need at least three teams of 8 to10 mediators. Research by Cunningham and colleagues (1998) suggested that an insufficient number of mediators reduces the impact of the program.

The training of mediators utilizes cognitive–behavioral procedures. Complex strategies are broken into small steps, with each step being mastered before proceeding to the next step. Training begins with simple conflicts and moves on to more difficult conflicts as the mediators' skills and confidence increase. The trainers model each step and provide prompts to assist mediators in rehearsing the steps properly. Mediators carry a clipboard and self-monitoring sheet with the steps involved in the mediation process as an aid to accurate implementation. Finally, mediators rehearse resolving conflicts similar to those they are most likely to encounter on the playground.

Child mediators must be trained to understand the concepts of mediation, master the component skills, identify conflicts quickly, and intervene confidently. Cunningham and Cunningham (1998) trained fourth- and fifth-grade children as mediators. Modifications may need to be made for training children of different ages. Complete training of mediators takes approximately 12 hours and follows a nine-phase process. Through this process children master the 18 component skills involved in the mediation procedure (see Table 8.3).

TABLE 8.3. Component Skill Checklist for Student-Mediated Conflict Resolution Program

Step	Component skill
1	Mediators in assigned playground position before students arrive.
2	Mediators in ready position, clipboard in hand, watching all students with special attention to high-risk areas or groups.
3	Mediator approaches disputants, asks whether problem has occurred.
4	Mediator asks whether disputants want to solve the problem.
5	Mediator finds quiet area, seats disputants, and sits between disputants.
6	Mediator introduces self and asks names of disputants.
7	Mediator states rules and secures agreement on each of the following: • Disputants must remain with mediator. • Mediator is neutral and won't take sides. • Disputants must listen without interrupting. • Disputants must tell the truth. • Disputants must treat each other respectfully. • Disputants must solve the problem. • Disputants must abide by their agreement.
8	Mediator asks disputant 1 to tell story.
9	Mediator summarizes disputant 1's story.
10	Mediator asks disputant 2 to tell story.
11	Mediator summarizes disputant 2's story.
12	Mediator asks disputants to suggest solutions.
13	Mediator summarizes each suggestion.
14	Disputants review pros and cons of each suggestion.
15	Disputants choose a solution.
16	Disputants plan when and how they will implement their solution.
17	Mediator asks if each disputant is satisfied.
18	Mediator closes mediation (students to shake hands).

Note. From Cunningham and Cunningham (1998). Copyright 1998 by The Guilford Press. Adapted by permission.

In Phase I of the training process, children meet the workshop leaders, the two teachers serving as the school's mediation program champions, interested parents, and the other child mediators. The principal talks about the importance of the child mediation program and the responsibilities of the mediators. In Phase II an overview of the mediation process is given, and in Phase III the children master the component skills. This is accomplished through presenting the skill, modeling it, and the child role-playing it. In Phase IV the children master the complete set of skills by rehearsing the resolution of increasingly complex disputes. Phase V involves responding to common problems such as children refusing to mediate or being unable to agree on a solution. In Phase VI children work on building communication skills and develop rationales supporting each step of the mediation process. In Phase VII children practice detecting situations that warrant mediation. In Phase VIII they master the mediation of simulated disputes. Phase IX involves the implementation of the program and the successful demonstration of the mediation process on the playground.

Implementing the Program

In implementing the program, mediators complete a checklist during each dispute mediation procedure. They check off each step of the process as it is completed and record the outcome. Completion of the checklist serves to remind mediators of the steps and supports the accurate implementation of the process. It also provides documentation of the effectiveness of the program.

Ongoing support is needed to maintain the mediation program. It is recommended that there be two playground supervisors to monitor and support the mediators. In addition, two teachers functioning as "mediation program champions" conduct weekly mediator meetings, support the mediators, recruit mediators, and run the training program. Other supports such as a mediator bulletin board and daily mediator announcements are helpful.

Making Modifications for Children with ACP

Modifications may need to be made in the peer mediation program for children with ACP. Older and more influential mediators can be assigned to areas where the more difficult or chronic problems occur, or two mediators can be used to conduct mediation involving children with ACP. The goal of successfully utilizing mediation can be added to the behavioral contract or daily report card of children with ACP. Another option is to include a limited number of children with ACP as mediators. The mediators with ACP may require additional training, monitoring, and support.

Playground peer mediation may not be sufficient to resolve some chronic, complex, intense, or group conflicts. In these cases, office mediation can be used. In office mediation, more time can be put into the mediation process, advanced mediation strategies can be used, and contracts can be written involving children, teachers, and the principal. Finally, in working with children exhibiting ACP, a child mediation program should be only one component in a comprehensive intervention plan. Child mediation should be combined with other interventions such as social skills training and parent training.

Summary

Table 8.4 provides a summary of the Collaborative Child Mediation Program. When implemented as described, peer mediation can reduce playground aggression. If the goal is to reduce schoolwide ACP problems, peer mediation is best combined with other interventions presented in this chapter.

TABLE 8.4. Summary of the Collaborative Child Mediation Program

Preparing for a peer mediation program

- Elicit support of parents, teachers, administration, and children.
- Specify goals and target behaviors.
- Institute policies to support the mediation procedure and to handle problem behaviors when mediation is refused.

Recruiting and screening mediators

- Recruit sufficient number of mediators.
- Utilize effective training procedures such as dividing complex skills into component parts and proceeding from simple to difficult conflicts.
- Train mediators to understand the concepts of mediation, master the component skills, identify conflicts quickly, and intervene confidently.

Implementing the program

- Mediators complete a checklist during each mediation procedure.
- Playground supervisors monitor and support mediators.
- Teachers functioning as "mediation program champions" recruit and train mediators, conduct weekly meetings with mediators, and support mediators.

Making modifications for children with ACP

- Use older and more influential mediators or two mediators for conflicts involving children with ACP.
- Add the goal of utilizing mediation to contracts for children with ACP.
- Utilize "office mediation" for difficult situations.
- Use other interventions in addition to peer mediation for children with ACP.

CONCLUSION

For schools to successfully target behavioral, social/emotional, and academic goals, they must have in place schoolwide programs and strategies to create a positive climate, promote positive behavior, and manage problem behavior. It is important that schoolwide programs attend not only to the content of their interventions, but also to how they are developed and implemented. The foundation of an effective schoolwide system focused on proactive interventions and positive behavior supports the successful implementation of classroom and individual interventions needed to address the needs of children who are at risk or already experiencing ACP behaviors. These interventions will be addressed in the following chapter.

CHAPTER 9

Classroom and Individual Interventions to Promote Positive Behavior

*I*n addition to using the schoolwide interventions presented in the previous chapter, schools will be most successful with children exhibiting ACP if they also employ effective strategies in the classroom. These strategies consist of both classroomwide interventions that focus on all children in the classroom and targeted interventions that focus on individual children. The classroom teacher will implement the majority of the interventions described in this chapter.

The interventions in this chapter address the same risk and protective factors as the schoolwide interventions we discussed in Chapter 8. They are designed to reduce risk and promote protective factors in the child, social/ peer, and contextual life domains (see Tables 2.3 and 2.4 in Chapter 2). Specifically, the interventions promote effective school responses to the needs of children, adaptive interactions among children, bonding with school and adults in the school, and the development of social and emotional skills in children.

After reviewing research on the effectiveness of classroom interventions, we present classroom interventions that have been found to be effective at promoting positive behavior and social development. These interventions focus on managing antecedents in the classroom, teaching children conflict resolution skills, effectively utilizing rewards and mild punishments, and intervening effectively with angry and acting-out behavior. First we discuss classroomwide strategies, then interventions for individual children. We conclude the chapter by discussing contracts and token/point systems.

OVERVIEW AND RESEARCH EVALUATION
OF CLASSROOM INTERVENTIONS
TO PROMOTE POSITIVE BEHAVIOR

Classroom interventions that are successful at promoting positive behavior use proactive strategies, include a focus on positive behavior and group interventions, and combine effective instructional techniques with effective behavior management. The promotion of positive behavior is a common component of programs designed to reduce aggressive behavior and make schools safer and more effective for all children (Battistich, 2000; Dwyer & Osher, 2000; Huesmann et al., 1996; Kamps, Kravits, Rauch, Kamps, & Chung, 2000; Knoff, 2000; Nelson, 1996; Olweus et al., 2000).

The classroom interventions we present target four areas of children's functioning. First, they promote positive behaviors such as compliance and following established procedures. Second, the interventions prevent problem behaviors such as talking at inappropriate times and fighting. Third, they teach social and emotional skills such as conflict resolution and problem solving. Fourth, the interventions prevent the escalation of angry/acting-out behavior. As with schoolwide interventions, the focus is on the behavior of all children in the classroom, not just those exhibiting ACP behaviors.

We present a variety of classroom interventions to address the four targeted areas of children's functioning. First, we discuss the teaching and monitoring of classroom rules and procedures. Next we present strategies for promoting positive behavior during common problem times and teaching social and emotional skills using classroom curricula. Then we address approaches for the effective use of rewards and mild punishment. Finally, we discuss strategies to prevent the escalation of angry/acting-out behavior.

The effectiveness of school-based interventions in managing disruptive and ADHD behavior is supported by meta-analytic research. Stage and Quiroz (1997) conducted a meta-analysis of 99 studies of interventions to decrease disruptive classroom behavior. These interventions were found to be effective, with group contingencies, self-management, and differential reinforcement being the most effective. They noted that there was large variability in the response of individual children. Aggressive children and children with conduct disorders benefited from the interventions, but as a group were the least likely to respond in a positive manner. DuPaul and Eckert (1997) conducted a meta-analysis of 63 school-based intervention studies for children and adolescents with ADHD. They found positive effects on behavior in the moderate to high range. Contingency management and academic interventions were more effective than cognitive–behavioral interventions in improving classroom behavior.

Positive results have been demonstrated for behavioral interventions in classrooms. Based on the criteria proposed by a task force of the American

Psychological Association (see Lonigan et al., 1998), the use of behavioral interventions in classrooms is a well established treatment for children with ADHD (Pelham et al., 1998). Pelham and colleagues noted that in addition to the large number of supportive studies of children with ADHD, there are also many studies supporting the use of behavioral classroom interventions with children described as "disruptive." Further support for the effectiveness of behavioral interventions comes from Bear's (1998) review of school discipline. However, Bear reported that despite their demonstrated effectiveness, there is evidence that behavioral interventions do not produce long-term changes in behavior and that generalization to other settings is often lacking.

The effectiveness of proactively managing antecedents to reduce behavior problems in the classroom is also widely acknowledged (Bear, 1998; Gettinger, 1988; Martens & Kelly, 1993; Munk & Repp, 1994; Wehby et al., 1998). Interventions at the beginning of the school year have been demonstrated to be important for establishing effective behavior management in classrooms (Gettinger, 1988; Martens & Kelly, 1993).

The effectiveness of classroom management techniques is also suggested by multicomponent school interventions. Numerous studies have found positive results when incorporating classroom management as one component of comprehensive interventions (Battistich, 2000; Huesmann et al., 1996; Kamps et al., 2000; Knoff, 2000; Nelson, 1996; Olweus et al., 2000).

Curriculum-based procedures for promoting social and emotional skill building and conflict resolution skills often increase children' knowledge, but have demonstrated only a modest effect on behavior (Grossman et al., 1997; Hausman, Pierce, & Briggs, 1996; Howard, Flora, & Griffin, 1999). For example, in a controlled study, Second Step: A Violence Prevention Curriculum demonstrated a moderate decrease in observed physical aggression with second and third graders (Grossman et al., 1997). Controlled studies evaluating the effectiveness of the PATHS curriculum have found reductions in peer ratings of aggression and hyperactive-disruptive behavior, as well as improvements in observer ratings of classroom atmosphere (Conduct Problems Prevention Research Group, 1999a). PATHS has also demonstrated improvements in emotional understanding and efficacy beliefs concerning the management of feelings (Greenberg et al., 1995). A study of the Resolving Conflict Creatively Program, which combines curriculum and peer mediation approaches, found that children exposed to a high number of lessons showed significantly slower growth in aggression-related processes and less of a decrease in competency-related processes (Aber, Jones, Brown, Chaudry, & Samples, 1998).

In summary, there is strong research support for the effectiveness of managing antecedents and consequences in promoting positive behaviors and decreasing problem behaviors. These interventions often require a high level of knowledge and skill on the part of school staff and much time to implement. Future research will need to address these practical issues to increase the utilization of these effective strategies. Conflict resolution curricula appear to hold promise, but would benefit from further work to strengthen effects on behavior. Areas to explore include refining the content or training procedures, improving methods for integrating skill use into the school and home environments, and combining conflict resolution training with other interventions.

BEST PRACTICES FOR CLASSROOM INTERVENTIONS TO PROMOTE POSITIVE BEHAVIOR

In this section we will describe common features and empirically supported aspects of effective classroom behavior management. The following sources were used to derive best practices because of the empirical support for their strategies: (1) Aber and colleagues' (1998) description of the Resolving Conflict Creatively Program; (2) Bear's (1998) review of school discipline; (3) the Conduct Problem Prevention Research Group's (1999) and Greenberg and colleagues' (1995) descriptions of the PATHS curriculum; (4) Crawford and Bodine's (1996) and Henrich, Brown, and Aber's (1999) reviews of violence prevention/conflict resolution programs; (5) Frey, Hirschstein, and Guzzo's (2000) and Grossman and colleagues' (1997) descriptions of Second Step: A Violence Prevention Curriculum; (6) Gettinger's (1988) methods of proactive classroom management; (7) Jones and Jones's (1995) procedures for comprehensive classroom management; (8) Keller and Tapasak's (1997) strategies for classroom management; (9) Martens and colleagues' (Martens & Kelly, 1993; Martens, Witt, Daly, & Vollmer, 1999) presentations on the use of behavior analysis in schools; (10) Mayer's (1995) strategies for preventing antisocial behavior in schools; (11) Pfiffner and Barkley's (1998) strategies for working with children with ADHD in school settings; (12) Rathvon's (1999) effective school interventions; (13) Striepling's (1997) presentation on the low aggression classroom; (14) Walker and colleagues' (Walker, 1979; Walker et al., 1995) strategies for working with behavior problems in schools; and (15) Wehby and colleagues' (1998) presentation on teaching practices in classrooms for children labeled EBD.

To effectively promote positive classroom behavior, teachers must utilize a comprehensive approach that goes well beyond a consistent response to misbehavior. In Table 9.1 we list 11 components of effective classroom management. Some of these components have been addressed elsewhere in this book and will not be discussed again here. Creating an accepting and supportive climate is an essential foundation for the effective implementation of other classroom interventions (see Chapter 8). The use of effective

TABLE 9.1. Components of Effective Classroom Management

1. Create an accepting and supportive classroom climate.
2. Utilize effective instructional practices.
3. Promote social and emotional skills.
4. Effectively manage common problem times: transitions and seatwork.
5. Establish and teach clear rules and procedures.
6. Involve parents.
7. Monitor child behavior.
8. Utilize rewards effectively.
9. Utilize mild punishment effectively.
10. Respond to mild problem behavior with a consistent procedure.
11. Effectively manage angry/acting-out behavior.

instructional techniques is an important factor in classroom management (Gettinger & Stoiber, 1999; Walker et al., 1995; see Chapter 7). Effective teaching can reduce aggression in children by reducing feelings of frustration and failure, which are potential antecedents to aggressive behavior, and by increasing academic engagement, which is incompatible with aggressive behavior (Keller & Tapasak, 1997). The involvement of parents and having a consistent response to mild problem behavior are also important factors in promoting positive behavior in the classroom (see Chapters 7 and 8).

Establishing and Teaching Rules and Procedures

How classroom rules and procedures are established, stated, monitored, and enforced is an important factor in classroom behavior management, especially for children with ACP. Striepling (1997) offered six "rules for making rules": (1) keep them few in number (three to six), (2) negotiate them with the children, (3) state them behaviorally and positively, (4) make a contract with the children to adhere to them, (5) send a copy of the rules home to parents, and (6) post them in the classroom. Once established, the rules should be frequently reviewed with the class. Examples of classroom rules include "Use a quiet voice," "Listen when others are speaking," "Keep hands and feet to yourself," and "Use respectful words."

As with classroom rules, classroom procedures need to be established and clearly stated, explicitly taught, closely monitored, and consistently followed. Procedures need to be established for activities such as entering the classroom in the morning, obtaining help from the teacher or other children, using the bathroom, asking questions, transitioning from one activity to another, and handing in work.

The beginning of the school year is the most important time to work on rules and procedures. Effective classroom managers tend to spend more time at the beginning of the year establishing and teaching rules and procedures. They need to be taught just as academic subjects are taught. This can be accomplished by stating the rule or procedure, modeling it, and having the children practice it. Teachers should also provide examples of behaviors that do and do not comply with the rules and procedures. To maintain compliance with the rules and procedure, they should be posted in the classroom, regularly monitored by the teacher, and frequently reviewed. Also, children should be cued to follow them prior to potential problem times.

A systematic and consistent response to children following or not following rules is essential. It is important that children receive acknowledgment and reinforcement for following rules and procedures. They should be given corrective feedback (e.g., by identifying the classroom rule that is not being followed or by asking the child to identify the behavior he or she is supposed to be engaged in), and, if needed, mild punishment, when they fail to follow rules and procedures. Consequences for following and not following rules and procedures need to be established and taught at the beginning of the school year.

Managing Common Problem Times:
Transitions and Seatwork

One common time for behavior problems in the classroom is during transitions. These times require special attention from teachers. The use of proactive approaches can prevent many problems. Behavior during transitions can be improved by reducing the length of transitions, establishing clear procedures for transitions and practicing them, reminding children of appropriate behavior prior to the transition, and closely monitoring behavior during transitions. One strategy for reducing the length of transitions is to use a stopwatch to time children and then reward them when their transition times drop under a certain length of time.

Independent seatwork is another common problem time. Academic engagement tends to be lower during independent seatwork and behavior problems are more common. Effective approaches include using instructional strategies that limit independent seatwork, closely monitoring behavior during seatwork, training children in self-monitoring strategies, frequently interacting with children during seatwork, and using incentives for successful seatwork (see Chapter 7). Teachers can also set goals and rewards for the entire class related to the number of children completing the assigned work during a period, the length of time without disruptive behavior, or the total length of time the class as a whole is engaged in work. For example, one strategy is for the teacher to keep a stopwatch running when everyone is working and stop it when someone is not working or is disruptive. The teacher has a green flag in a stand on the desk when the watch is running. This is changed to a red flag when the watch is stopped. The class earns a reward for accumulating a certain number of quiet working minutes.

Promoting Social and Emotional Skills

One factor that contributes to ACP behavior is the lack of skills needed to successfully manage personal and interpersonal problems in school. Helping children to develop the needed social and emotional skills can promote positive behavior and reduce ACP behavior. Hundreds of classroom curricula have been designed to promote emotional/social skill development and violence reduction (Howard et al., 1999). These curriculum-based interventions are described by a number of labels, including violence prevention, conflict resolution, and social/emotional skills training. In addition to curriculum-based programs, schools will often utilize peer mediation to assist children in resolving conflicts. In peer mediation, a limited number of children are trained to use a problem-solving/conflict resolution procedure to help their peers resolve disputes (see Chapter 8).

Classroom teachers present most curriculum-based programs. Training is provided to teachers, generally in the form of a 1- to 3-day workshop. Ongoing supervision and support is often provided. In addition to training teachers, some programs offer training for noninstructional staff, administrators, and parents. Wider training helps to provide consistency throughout the school and between school and home. For example, the Second Step program involves a 1-day workshop for teachers and a half-day workshop for other school staff members. A videotape introduction is provided for parents, as well as six video-based instruction modules. After receiving instruction in the philosophy of the program, teachers are provided with the opportunity to discuss and practice instructional strategies. They are taught how to effectively conduct the lessons and modify the classroom environment to promote the use of the skills.

There is much overlap in the knowledge and skills taught in the various curriculum-based programs designed to prevent aggression, resolve conflicts in nonaggressive ways, or develop social and emotional skills. These programs commonly include information and skills related to communication, positive or prosocial behavior, expression and management of feelings, and problem solving or strategies for resolving conflicts. In many of the programs, the content is adjusted for children of different ages. For example, the Second Step program has separate programs available for preschool, elementary, and middle school/junior high children. Table 9.2 provides a list of the lesson titles for first-grade children in the Second Step program.

The number and frequency of lessons vary from program to program and from age to age. A typical program includes about 50 lessons that are

TABLE 9.2. Lesson Titles for Second Step, Grade 1

Empathy	Impulse control (problem solving)	Anger management
Introduction to empathy training	Introduction to problem solving	Introduction to anger management
Identifying feelings	Identifying the problem	Anger triggers
Looking for more clues	Choosing a solution	Calming down
Similarities and differences	Evaluating a solution	Self-talk
Feelings change	Is it working?	Reflection
Predicting feelings	Ignoring distractions	Keeping out of a fight
Communicating feelings	Interrupting politely	Dealing with name calling and teasing
	Dealing with wanting something that's not yours	

Note. From Frey, Hirschstein, and Guzzo (2000). Copyright 2000 by PRO-ED, Inc. Reprinted by permission.

taught from once a week to three times a week. Some programs have more frequent lessons at the beginning of the year with lesson frequency decreasing as the year progresses.

Programs generally use multiple methods to teach children the knowledge and skills. The methods include classroom instruction, worksheets, videos, classroom and small-group discussions, role playing, and modeling. The methods are often interactive and experiential, with children practicing the skills they learn. Real classroom issues are used in the training to maintain interest, demonstrate the relevance of the skills, and help with the generalization of the skills.

Most programs include procedures to promote utilization and generalization. Nonteaching staff, administrators, and parents are sometimes trained to help the children use the skills outside the classroom. A number of programs include posters that can be hung up around the school to promote the use of program skills. Generalization of skills is promoted by recommending that school staff create classroom and school environments that support the use of the learned skills. This is done by the school staff modeling valued behaviors; cueing, coaching, encouraging, and reinforcing skills; and when appropriate, allowing for child decision making.

Using Rewards Effectively

While the proactive management of antecedents and the development of skills are important for the effective promotion of positive behavior in classrooms, they are not sufficient for many children with ACP. The use of consequences is also important and effective in the short-term control of classroom behavior. For children with serious behavior problems, the use of both rewards and mild punishment will be needed. Rewards and mild punishments can be used on both a classwide and an individual basis.

A prerequisite for the effective use of rewards is the close monitoring of behavior. Without being aware of behavior in the classroom, a teacher cannot respond in a consistent manner. While closely monitoring children's behavior is a challenge because of the many demands on teachers' time, positive behavior will be promoted if children know that their teacher will notice both their positive behavior and their problem behavior.

Three types of rewards are commonly used in school settings: activities or privileges (e.g., recess, games, parties, computer time), social rewards (teacher praise, peer recognition, notes home to parents), and material rewards (stickers, certificates). Despite the proven effectiveness of using rewards, many teachers have concerns with "bribing" children and its effect on the child's intrinsic motivation. Some researchers too have suggested that external reinforcement may be damaging to intrinsic motivation (Deci, Koestner, & Ryan, 1999; Schwartz, 1990). But others (Cameron & Pierce, 1994) have concluded that the negative influence is minimal and limited to situations in which tangible rewards are given for simply doing a task, without concern for its quality. Verbal praise has been shown to increase intrinsic motivation. We view rewards as an essential component of promoting positive behavior; however, they are only one of many factors that need to be considered when working with motivation and behavior. Teachers can utilize external rewards and still be sensitive to promoting intrinsic motivation.

Selecting the reward is very important. It must effectively function as a reinforcer, that is, the child must increase desirable behavior when it is paired with the reward. Care must be taken to select rewards that are practical enough to be used repeatedly. Children can be informally questioned about what they would find reinforcing, or a more structured approach can be used. Reinforcement menus, such as the one suggested by Rathvon (1999), can be used to determine useful rewards (see Figure 9.1). Reinforcement menus should be used periodically, as children's preferences will change. Further options for reinforcement menus, such as using open-ended questions or multiple-choice formats, are presented by Raschke (1981).

Rewards can lose their reinforcing quality if used repeatedly. This reduced effectiveness, or satiation effect, can be addressed in a number of ways (Rathvon, 1999). Children can be given a role in determining rewards, rewards can be varied, or the selection of the reward can be made unpredictable (e.g., by picking a reward out of a hat). Social rewards tend to be less susceptible to losing their reinforcing quality and therefore can be helpful in reducing satiation effects.

Directions: Below is a list of possible rewards our class could earn. Please circle the number that matches your level of interest in each reward. Your ratings will be used to help select the rewards.

Possible rewards	Level of interest		
	Low	Middle	High
Extra recess	1	2	3
Good note home	1	2	3
Classroom games	1	2	3
Special art project	1	2	3
Free time	1	2	3
Watching a video	1	2	3
Listening to tapes	1	2	3
Homework pass	1	2	3
Class computer time	1	2	3
Trip to school computer lab	1	2	3
Media center time	1	2	3
School supplies	1	2	3
Class field trip	1	2	3
Class party	1	2	3
Group games in gym	1	2	3

FIGURE 9.1. Reinforcement menu. From Rathvon (1999). Copyright 1999 by The Guilford Press. Reprinted by permission.

Social rewards can be very effective and have the added value of potentially increasing positive interactions and relationships within the classroom. Social rewards include the child interacting with the teacher, other adults in the school setting (other teachers, administrators), peers, parents, and people outside the school setting. Examples of social rewards involving the school staff include verbal praise, public praise, having lunch with a staff member, and helping a staff member during or after school. Social rewards with peers can include reading with a friend, playing a game with a friend, and being able to sit next to a friend. Outside of school, social rewards can include activities with parents or others, sleepovers, and outings with friends.

Praise is an effective social reward. Despite its effectiveness, praise is generally used at a low rate, especially in classes for children with behavior problems (Wehby et al., 1998). For praise to be effective, its use should be contingent on the performance of appropriate behavior, be related to specific behavior, and be believable to the child being praised (Rathvon, 1999). Walker and colleagues (1995) suggested that it be immediate, frequent, enthusiastic, descriptive, varied, and involve eye contact. Praise should identify the specific behavior being praised (e.g., "You did a nice job of sharing with your partner."). Walker and colleagues recommended that the ratio of praise to reprimands be at least 4:1.

Using Mild Punishment Effectively

The purpose of mild punishment is to reduce inappropriate behavior. Mild punishments in school settings commonly include reprimands, response cost procedures, and time-outs (described in Chapter 5). Reprimands can be effective, but loose their effectiveness if overused. They are most effective when they are brief, made in a quiet manner, and presented when the teacher is in close proximity to the child. For example, a teacher walks over to a student, makes eye contact, and says in a quiet voice, "William, stop talking."

Response-cost procedures involve the removal of a reinforcer following inappropriate behavior. This generally consists of the loss of a pleasurable activity or of a previously earned reward such as recess, free time, or classroom fun activities. When used with a token system, it involves the loss of earned points or tokens.

Walker and colleagues (1995) presented guidelines for the use of response-cost programs. First, the response cost system is carefully explained to the child. The child should know what behaviors will result in losing privileges or points. It is recommended that response-cost plans include the use of rewards, with the child's positive behavior being consistently praised. A delivery system needs to be designed that will inform the child when the response cost has been applied, for which behavior, and what was lost (what privilege or how many points). One option is to tape a card to a child's desk on which the teacher puts a mark whenever previously identified behaviors are observed (see Figure 9.2). The system used in Figure 9.2 applies different point values to different behaviors. The points lost for the day/period are totaled. If the number of points lost exceeds a preset number, a privilege is lost. It is important that the response cost be implemented immediately after the target behavior and every time the behavior occurs. Verbal interaction should be kept to a minimum when implementing the response cost and the teacher should not argue with the child about whether a response cost was appropriate.

The use of negative consequences is a common and important part of effective classroom management, yet is problematic and less effective when it is the only or primary technique. Bear (1998) noted that teachers are more likely to use punitive techniques than positive techniques. The least effective teachers tend to manage hostile-aggressive children using a combination of negatively focused strategies such as warnings, punishments, scoldings, and contacting authorities. Effective classroom managers used these strategies less often and combined them with more positive strategies.

| | Point value | | | Days | | |
		M	T	W	Th	F
Out of seat	2					
Talk outs	2					
Nonattending	1					
Noncompliance	3					
Disturbing others	2					
Foul language	4					
Fighting	5					

FIGURE 9.2. Response-cost delivery/feedback form. From Walker (1979). Copyright 1979 by Allyn & Bacon. Reprinted by permission.

When a child begins receiving many negative consequences, it is a sign that an individual intervention plan may be needed. The process for designing individual interventions is presented in a later section.

Effectively Managing Angry/Acting-Out Behavior

Teachers need specialized skills to respond effectively to children with ACP when they are upset. Ineffective responses can result in situations escalating and children exhibiting more dangerous or destructive behaviors. Walker and colleagues (1995) presented a seven-phase model to describe the escalation of acting-out behavior and strategies for managing behavior in each of the phases (see Table 9.3). This chapter, along with Chapter 8, focuses mainly on proactive strategies utilized in the first two phases. If these procedures are used effectively, escalation of angry behavior can often be avoided.

No matter how skilled the teacher, though, children with more severe ACP problems will at times proceed to further stages of the acting-out cycle. When this happens, teachers need the skills to help children calm down by using strategies such as empathic comments, allowing the child space and time, and allowing independent or relaxation activities. Teachers should remain calm, engage the child in a respectful manner, and avoid power struggles. If the behavior continues to escalate, the teacher should state the expected behavior, the consequence for not engaging in the expected behavior, and then disengage from the child. If the behavior becomes aggressive or destructive, the child or the other children should be removed to isolate the child. Schools should clearly define when and how this should happen. The use of physical restraint should be minimized, with the procedure clearly defined and staff well trained in when and how to im-

TABLE 9.3. Phases and Strategies for Managing Anger/Acting-Out Behaviors

Phases	Angry/acting-out behavior	Strategies
Calm	Emotionally stable, productive behavior and interactions with others	Use predictable routines, structures, rules, and expectations; clear communication, quality instruction, attention to positive behavior, and promote social skills development.
Triggers	Those situations and/or circum-stances that begin the cycle (e.g., conflicts, disagreements, pressures, mistakes, stressors, etc.)	Use problem-solving, conflict resolution, and stress management strategies.
Agitation	Unresolved problems/situations result in emotional arousal (e.g., angry, upset, depressed, worried, frustrated, etc.) and unfocused/off-task behavior (e.g., staring, poor eye contact, withdrawal, short speech utterance, etc.)	Use calming strategies such as recognizing others' feelings (e.g., "I see you look upset"; "I'm sure this makes you frustrated/angry," etc.). Allow space and time to calm (e.g., separate, temporarily stop talking about problems, walk around, etc.) and temporarily do distracting activity (e.g., something fun or interesting).
Acceleration	Escalating behaviors that engage others in conflict (e.g., questioning and arguing, defiance, provoking comments, complaining, whining, threats, attempting to leave, verbal abuse, etc.)	Avoid escalating verbal statements (e.g., power struggles, blaming, etc.); stay calm, respectful, and detached; present the expected behavior and the consequence if not followed (plan consequence ahead of time); and follow through with consequence.
Peak	Serious threats to safety of self and/or others (e.g., destruction of property, assaultive, self-abusive, tantrumming, hyperventilating, etc.)	Isolate and remove others from the angry/acting-out individual; get help; and, if needed, restrain (physical guidance to a safe place or complete restraint) the child.
Deescalation	Reduction in agitation with uncooperative behavior (e.g., confusion, withdrawal, blaming, denial, avoidance of discussion, possible responsiveness to directions, etc.)	Isolate and supervise the child, allow time to cool down, have child engage in independent work, and restore the environment (e.g., pick up and clean up anything resulting from incident).
Recovery	Return to calm, but may be subdued; eagerness to return to a task or activity	Resume normal routines, follow through with consequences, develop a plan for next incident, and communicate expectations for behavior.

Note. From Walker, Colvin, and Ramsey (1995). Copyright 1995 by Thomson Learning. Adapted by permission.

plement it. All of these situations should be well documented and reviewed so plans can be made to prevent future occurrences.

Summary

Table 9.4 provides a summary of best practices for promoting positive behavior and reducing problem behavior in the classroom, teaching social and emotional skills, and preventing the escalation of angry behavior. These procedures will be most effective if there is consistency between the expectations and strategies utilized in the classroom, the school as a whole, and the home.

OVERVIEW AND RESEARCH EVALUATION OF INDIVIDUAL INTERVENTIONS TO PROMOTE POSITIVE BEHAVIOR IN SCHOOL

For many children with ACP, schoolwide, classroom, and skill-building interventions will be essential, but often not sufficient, to promote positive

TABLE 9.4. Summary of Best Practices for Classroom Interventions to Promote Positive Behavior

Procedures	Best practices
Establishing and teaching rules and procedures	Focus on rules and procedures at the beginning of the school year; state, model, practice, and post rules and procedures; monitor and establish consistent responses when rules and procedures are followed and not followed.
Managing common problem times: transitions and seatwork	Establish, train, and monitor procedures; manage and limit seatwork by utilizing varied instructional strategies, monitoring, training children in self-management, and using incentives.
Using rewards effectively	Monitor behavior; select rewards that are effective, practical, and resistant to satiation effect; focus on social rewards and praise.
Using mild punishment effectively	Utilize time-outs and response cost; effectiveness is reduced if used excessively or not combined with rewards.
Effectively managing angry/acting-out behavior	Remain calm, engage child in a respectful manner, and avoid power struggles; state expectation, state consequence, and disengage; establish procedures for when and how to isolate and restrain children.

behavior. Teachers individualize academic and behavioral interventions on a daily basis. When these informal modifications fail to bring about the desired results, a formal procedure can be helpful. This often involves a consultative or collaborative problem-solving process including the teacher and other school staff members with expertise in working with children's behavior. This section focuses on individual interventions to promote positive behavior with children manifesting ACP.

Individual interventions target the same child behaviors and skills as classroom interventions: increasing positive behaviors, decreasing problem behaviors, and increasing social/emotional skills. The difference is that now the interventions are designed specifically to match the needs and situation of the individual child. As with classroom interventions, antecedents, consequences, and social/emotional skill building are utilized.

This section is divided into two parts. First we describe a process for individualizing interventions. This involves the identification of factors affecting the child's behaviors and the selection of interventions to target these factors. In the second part of this section we describe the use of contracts and token/point systems.

Research support for the effectiveness of individualized interventions for children comes from a number of sources. Many of the studies verifying the effectiveness of interventions to decrease disruptive behavior in schools have used individualized interventions evaluated with single-case designs (Stage & Quiroz, 1997). Rathvon (1999) reviewed studies addressing the effectiveness of a form of school consultation called Intervention Assistance Programs (IAPs). IAPs involve individualizing interventions to meet the needs of individual children. Rathvon cited research on IAPs that demonstrated a reduction in special education referrals, improved teacher attitudes toward diverse learners, and improved child performance.

Functional behavioral assessments are used to design individual interventions for students. Interventions based on these assessments have successfully reduced problem behavior and/or increased positive behavior with students with behavior problems (Heckaman et al., 2000) and ADHD (Ervin et al., 2000). Another source of modest support for individualizing interventions comes from research on special education outcomes. Children in special education are required to have a plan that individualizes school interventions. Reviews of the effectiveness of special education services have generally found modest positive outcomes (Kavale & Forness, 1999; Schulte et al., 1998).

In summary, individual interventions can be effective for children with ACP. More research is needed on factors that can limit their effectiveness and utilization. Effective individual interventions are generally time-consuming to design and implement and require a certain level of skill. The development of efficient and standardized procedures for designing and implementing individual interventions could reduce the time and skill level required.

BEST PRACTICES FOR INDIVIDUAL
INTERVENTIONS TO PROMOTE
POSITIVE BEHAVIOR IN SCHOOL

The productive use of individual interventions is an important component of schools' work with children with ACP. We reviewed information from the following sources to derive best practices for individual school interventions to promote positive behavior: (1) the Center for Effective Collaboration and Practice's (1998) recommendations for addressing child problem behavior; (2) DuPaul and colleagues' (1997) approach for individualized assessment and intervention with children exhibiting ADHD; (3) Dwyer and Osher's (2000) guide for reducing violence and other problem behaviors in schools; (4) Greene's (1996) presentation on matching interventions for children with ADHD to individual and contextual factors; (5) Kratochwill, Elliott, and Rotto's (1995) approach to school-based behavioral consultation; (6) Martens and colleagues' (1999) discussion of behavior analysis in educational settings; (7) O'Neill and colleagues' (1997) procedures for functional assessment and intervention for problem behaviors in schools; (8) Rathvon's (1999) procedures for effective school interventions; and (9) Zins and Erchul's (1995) work on school consultation. After discussing individual interventions, we will explain the use of contracts and token/point systems.

Individualizing Interventions

Individualizing interventions involves an assessment of the child and contextual factors, selection/design of the intervention, and implementation of the intervention. This process begins with accurately defining the problem behavior. Information is obtained on what the behavior consists of, when and where it occurs, how often it occurs, its intensity, and its duration. Child, teacher, classroom, school, family, and peer factors affecting the behavior are determined. This may involve a formal functional behavioral assessment (see Chapter 3) or a briefer assessment to obtain similar information.

Once the problem behavior is defined and variables affecting it identified, an intervention is designed/selected to target the factors affecting the behavior. Individualized interventions utilize strategies similar to those used in schoolwide, classroom, and skill-building interventions. The advantage of individualized interventions is that they can target specific factors affecting the child rather than general variables targeted by schoolwide and classroom interventions. The specific variables targeted are determined by the assessment. In selecting/designing the intervention, empirical support for the intervention, the acceptability of the intervention to participants, and the ability to implement the intervention as designed should be considered (see Chapter 7 for details).

Interventions can target antecedents, child skills and beliefs, family factors, and consequences. For example, if a problem behavior occurs more frequently when the child misses breakfast or has trouble on the bus, these antecedents are targeted. If the problem behavior generally occurs during extended periods of independent seatwork, intervention options could include reducing the amount of seatwork by the use of varied instructional techniques (e.g., peer tutoring), reducing the length of seatwork periods, introducing a self-monitoring program, or writing a child–teacher contract targeting behavior during independent seatwork (see Chapter 7 for further details).

If the assessment identifies a skill deficit, interventions focused on skill building or teaching appropriate behaviors can be used. It is not uncommon for problem behaviors to be present because a child just isn't aware of other, more appropriate responses. Teaching children alternative behaviors that will result in their desired outcome (e.g., attracting peer attention) can reduce problem behaviors. Once aware of alternative behaviors, children must develop the skills that allow them to use the behaviors even in difficult and stressful situations. For example, increasing a child's anger management or social skills will allow the child to manage social problems in a more adaptive manner. Skill-building interventions can be administered through schoolwide or classroomwide training programs, or through small-group or individual training sessions. Further details on skill-building interventions are contained in the previous section and in Chapter 4.

Increasing parent involvement can be an effective strategy for reducing problem behaviors in individual children. Common interventions include joint parent–teacher problem solving and the use of daily report cards (see Chapter 7). These interventions improve parent–teacher communication, assist in identifying factors effecting behavior, promote the coordination of strategies between home and school, and increase the variety and potency of consequences used to manage school behavior.

Assessments commonly identify consequences that are associated with the problem behavior and outcomes that are meaningful to the child. Problem behaviors in school often have reinforcing outcomes such as more peer attention or avoidance of work. The goal of the intervention is to have the consequences of the desired behavior be more reinforcing than the results of the problem behavior. Interventions should reduce the reinforcing outcomes for the problem behavior (e.g., reduce peer encouragement or the avoidance of work) and increase the reinforcing results of the desired behavior (e.g., praise or the child's recognition of success). An attempt should also be made to decrease the negative outcomes associated with the desired behavior (e.g., boredom or reduced peer contact). For example, reduced talking in class results in less peer contact during class. If peer contact is motivating for the child, the reward for reduced talking may involve more opportunities for peer interaction once work is completed. Further details on the use of rewards and mild punishments were presented earlier in this chapter.

It is not uncommon for the assessment to identify factors associated with the problem behaviors that are beyond the direct control of the school. Through collaboration with, or referral to, community agencies, many of these factors can be addressed. Interventions such as mentoring, after-school programming, and case management can complement the services provided by the school (see Chapter 10). Options for mental health interventions include psychotherapy, medication, hospitalization, day treatment, and residential treatment (see Chapter 6).

Utilizing Contracts and Token/Point Systems

Contracts and token/point systems establish structured approaches for providing rewards and response costs. They are commonly used to promote both behavioral and academic goals, and can be utilized with an individual child or an entire classroom. Contracts are agreements (generally written) between a teacher and a child that specify what the child will do, what the teacher will do, and what will happen if the contract is or is not honored. They specify the expected behavior, how it will be monitored and recorded, and the rewards/mild punishments that will be earned. Contracts will sometimes involve token/point systems. Depending on the age and ability of the child, it is helpful to negotiate the contract with the child. It is important that the child view the contract as fair and reasonable.

Token/point systems entail a child being given tokens/checkmarks/points following a targeted behavior, with the number of tokens/checkmarks/points determining the reward or response cost. They can target one behavior or multiple behaviors. For example, a child might receive a token each time the child raises his or her hand before responding to a question, and lose a token/point for responding without raising his or her hand. A token/point system for multiple behaviors might involve a child receiving two token/points for each completed assignment, three tokens/points for staying in his or her seat for an entire period, and five tokens/points for not arguing with the teacher during the day. Tokens are generally used for younger children, checkmarks or points for older children. Further details on token/point systems are presented in Chapter 5.

Contracts and token/point systems share many common features. Six steps are involved in setting up both systems. The first step involves setting a goal or defining a target behavior. A simple plan would monitor one behavior, such as swearing, staying in one's seat, or raising one's hand and waiting to be called on. A more complex plan might identify a general goal such as not being sent out of the room, and then monitor behaviors related to this goal, such as not swearing, staying in one's seat, keeping hands and feet to one's self, and following directions. The behaviors monitored should be observable, quantifiable, and clearly defined. For example, if following directions is targeted, it should be specified whether the child has to comply the first or second time a command is given, how long the child has to comply (e.g., 3 seconds or 10 seconds), and whether the child will be given any warnings. The child should be given examples of behaviors that fit the definition and behaviors that do not. If descriptive ratings such as "good," "fair," or "poor" are used, they should be objectively defined. For example, "good" means following all directions, "fair" means following directions all but one or two times, and "poor" means not following directions three or more times.

Once the target behavior is selected, the second step is deciding on the period of time the contract or point/token system will be in effect and how frequently behavior will be evaluated. Options for the time period covered by the contract include one subject period (e.g., every day during math), one type of activity (e.g., all transition times during the school day), the total school day, or a full week. Contracts and token/point systems will sometimes begin using a short period of time (e.g., one class period) until the child achieves mastery, and then extend the time period (e.g., all class periods). How often the target behavior is evaluated or recorded will vary depending on the behavior. Behaviors such as work completion are recorded once at the end of each period or each day. When the frequency of a behavior is being monitored—for example, how may times someone is out of his or her seat, or how often he or she swears—the behavior is recorded whenever it occurs.

The third step is determining the expected level of performance. To set the beginning expectation, monitor the behavior for a week to establish a baseline level of performance. The initial expected level is then set high enough above the baseline level to be challenging, yet at a level still low enough to allow for moderate success. For example, if the child is out of his or her seat an average of five times during the baseline period, the initial goal may be for the child to be out of his or her seat three or fewer times.

The fourth step is determining the reward and/or response cost. This is an important step because if the reward and response cost are not motivating for the child, or if they cannot be maintained by the teacher, the contract will not be effective. Further information on rewards and response cost is presented in a previous section.

The fifth step is designing a procedure for monitoring and recording the child's performance. Because of the many demands on teachers' time, it is important that a method be devised that is not disruptive or excessively time-consuming. The recording form or chart used will vary depending on the number of behaviors targeted (one or multiple behaviors), the frequency of ratings (whenever cued, whenever the behavior occurs, once a period, once a day), the length of time covered (one period, 1 day, or 1 week) and the type of data recorded. The type of data recorded can include the frequency of a behavior (e.g., talking without raising hand), the presence or absence of a behavior (e.g., fighting), or ratings of a behavior (e.g., followed directions all the time, most of the time, or some of the time). Examples of recording forms are contained in Figure 7.1, Figure 7.2, and Figure 9.2.

Different strategies can be used to record frequently occurring behaviors. One option is for the teacher to mark a chart that can be on the teacher's desk, on a clipboard so the child can bring it from class to class, or on the child's desk. Other options include making a hash mark on a piece of tape on the teacher's wrist, moving tokens from one pocket to another, or moving tokens into or out of a container. At the end of the monitoring period the total is written on a recording form or chart.

The sixth step is setting a date to review the results and to plan for generalization and maintenance. This step is commonly neglected. The results should be reviewed at least weekly to ensure the contract or token/point system is working and that the expected level of performance is appropriate. Generalization can be promoted by expanding the behaviors monitored, using the plan in multiple settings, or extending the length of the monitoring period. When the final goal has been reached, the contract or token/point system should be slowly faded to support maintenance of the effect. This can be achieved by reducing the frequency of the monitoring, reducing the frequency of the rewards, or changing to and emphasizing naturally occurring contingencies such as social rewards and grades.

Summary

Table 9.5 provides a summary of best practices for individual school interventions. These interventions focus on specific factors identified by the as-

TABLE 9.5. Summary of Best Practices for Individual Interventions to Promote Positive Behavior in School

Procedures	Best practices
Individualizing interventions	Determine location, time, intensity, and duration of behavior; assess child, classroom, school, peer, and family factors effecting the behavior; design/select an intervention to target identified factors, including antecedents, consequences, skill deficits, and family factors; refer to community agencies to target factors beyond the control of the school.
Utilizing contracts and token/point systems	Identify and define target behavior, decide on time frame and frequency of data recording, set expected level of performance, determine reward/response cost, develop recording system and form, set a review date and plan for generalization and maintenance.

sessment that are associated with the targeted behavior. They will be most effective when combined with schoolwide and classroom interventions.

CONCLUSION

Classroom and individual interventions for children with ACP can be effective in promoting positive behavior, reducing ACP behavior, and promoting social and emotional skills. When schools productively combine effective academic, schoolwide, classroom, and individual interventions, they can reduce ACP behaviors. However, consistently implementing effective interventions at all these levels is a challenging task. Despite the multiple options for intervention, many risk and protective factors for ACP are beyond the influence of schools. As a result, school interventions should be viewed as only one component of a comprehensive intervention for children with ACP.

CHAPTER 10

Community Interventions for Child and Family Support

Community interventions involve programs and services that provide support for children and their families. By addressing numerous risk and protective factors, they are an important component of comprehensive services for children with ACP. The interventions presented in this chapter are hypothesized to reduce risk factors and promote protective factors in the individual, parent/family, social/peer, and contextual domains (see Tables 2.3 and 2.4 in Chapter 2). Specifically, community interventions reduce family problems, decrease children's affiliation with antisocial peers, and indirectly reduce neighborhood problems. In addition, they enhance children's self-esteem and sense of self-efficacy, promote positive values and association with prosocial peers, strengthen bonds with prosocial institutions, and improve opportunities for positive community activities and access to community services.

In this chapter we present interventions focused on children and families at varying levels of risk. First, we provide information on mentoring and after-school programs that provide meaningful relationships with prosocial adults in the community and structured activities in safe, supervised settings. We then examine case management, a common component of support services for families who are at risk or who have children exhibiting ACP problems. Case management helps parents to access and coordinate services and develop needed skills such as advocacy and working with schools. In the final section of this chapter we discuss therapeutic foster care, a community-based program providing services to children who are experiencing significant ACP problems.

OVERVIEW AND RESEARCH EVALUATION
OF MENTORING PROGRAMS

Mentoring, a popular and expanding form of community intervention for at-risk children, involves pairing an adult with a child, who then engage in activities together on a regularly scheduled basis. Programs are based in a variety of organizations, including churches, colleges, community agencies, courts, and schools. Mentoring is being promoted, financially supported, and evaluated by the Juvenile Mentoring Program (JUMP), a federal program administered by the Office of Juvenile Justice and Delinquency Prevention (OJJDP; 1998). JUMP's goals are to reduce delinquency and gang involvement, improve academic performance, and reduce school dropout rates. It is believed that mentors can provide youth with meaningful social connections, supervision and guidance, skills training, career or cultural enrichment opportunities, knowledge of spirituality and values, a sense of self-worth, and goals and hope for the future (OJJDP, 1998).

The factors targeted by mentoring vary depending on the goals of the specific program. Most mentoring programs focus on exposure to prosocial norms and activities, a sense of social belonging, and a meaningful and consistent relationship with a positive adult role model. Some programs develop specific skills such as academic or leadership skills.

Most mentoring programs address these goals through a system in which an adult forms a relationship with a child and together they share pleasurable activities. Some programs expect mentors to address additional goals with children through guidance, monitoring, rewarding, teaching, training, and advocating for services.

While mentoring is generally presumed to be effective, limited research supports this conclusion (Grossman & Tierney, 1998; OJJDP, 1998). A number of narrative reviews concluded that noncontingent, supportive mentoring is not effective in reducing aggression and conduct problems (Catalano, Arthur, Hawkins, Berglund, & Olson, 1998; Reid & Eddy, 1997). Catalano et al. did find some support, however, for mentoring programs in which mentors used behavioral contracting and contingency management techniques. A study by McPartland and Nettles (1991) of a program in which adults served as mentors and advocates for middle school students found improved attendance and grades in English, but also found that the program by itself was not sufficient to eliminate academic risk.

A recent study by Grossman and Tierney (1998) found positive results in an evaluation of the Big Brothers Big Sisters of America (BBBSA) mentoring program using youth self-report information. Compared to a waiting-list control group, youth ages 10 to 16 with mentors were less likely to start using drugs or alcohol (males only), hit someone, or skip school (females only). They also were more confident about their school performance and reported getting along better with their families (males only). Using data from the Grossman and Tierney (1998) study, Rhodes, Grossman, and Resch (2000) found that mentoring had a direct effect on the youths' perception of their scholastic competence and school attendance. The effects on global self-worth, valuing of school, and grades were mediated through perceived improvements in parental relationships and scholastic competence.

In summary, the results of outcome studies with mentoring have been mixed. More research is needed to better define the appropriate goals for mentoring programs, with whom mentoring is effective, and the components of mentoring programs that are essential to produce positive outcomes. There is, however, sufficient research support to suggest that mentoring is a promising intervention.

BEST PRACTICES FOR MENTORING PROGRAMS

The BBBSA mentoring program currently has the most research support for its efficacy. As a result, it will be presented as an exemplary model. Information on the model was obtained from the following sources: (1) Grossman and Tierney's (1998) study of the BBBSA mentoring program; and (2) McGill, Mihalic, and Grotpeter's (1997) description of the BBBSA mentoring program.

Overview of the BBBSA Mentoring Program

BBBSA, a federation of more than 500 agencies providing services to children and adolescents, directs the largest mentoring program in the country. It provides mentoring to youth from ages 6 to 18, with the majority of them coming from single-parent homes. On a national level, BBBSA emphasizes positive youth development rather than specifically targeting the prevention of problems such as delinquency, chemical dependency, or pregnancy. It believes that supportive relationships with caring adults can promote healthy development in youth. As a result, the focus of the mentoring program is on the relationship and trust developed between the adult and the child and not on a set of prescribed activities. On a local level, individual goals for children may focus on specific issues. Two of the most common objectives reported by BBBSA staff are delaying antisocial behavior and improving academic functioning.

Mentors meet with a child for 4 hours at a time, two to four times a month. Mentors and children share developmentally appropriate activities such as attending plays, movies, or school activities; playing sports; cooking or eating out; visiting the library; or watching television. BBBSA recommends that the child take part in the decision making about activities. Case managers are used to screen, match, monitor, and support mentors. BBBSA has developed a set of core elements and standards that programs must follow. Both the national and the local offices provide training.

Screening and Supervision of Mentors

Local offices decide on the criteria for volunteer mentors. Generally they need to be at least 18 to 21 years old, have lived in the area for 3 to 6 months, have a stable means of support, and have transportation. Much effort is put into the effective screening of potential volunteers to maximize the chance that volunteers will be capable of developing healthy and supportive relationships with children and fulfill their commitments. Volunteers undergo an extensive interview, are subject to criminal background checks, and must provide references. They must attend an orientation that clearly spells out their expected time commitments. Volunteer mentors make a 1-year commitment to meet with their child. A significant proportion of volunteers screen themselves out of the process once informed of these expectations and requirements. Training is recommended for the mentors. BBBSA has a volunteer education and development manual that focuses on issues such as relationship building, communication skills, and child development.

Along with volunteer screening, much attention is given to the monitoring and supervision of the mentoring relationship. Case managers, who generally have bachelor or master's degrees in social work, perform this function. National standards require the case manager to have contact with the child, the parent, and the mentor within 2 weeks of the match, monthly contact the first year, and quarterly contact after that. Case managers help mentors identify and solve problems in the mentoring relationship. The case manager makes a written evaluation of the mentoring relationship on a yearly basis. It is believed that this close monitoring and supervision contributes to successful and long-lasting relationships.

Child Screening and Matching with Mentor

Children who are referred to the program also undergo a screening. The parent completes a written questionnaire and the parent and child are interviewed. Most programs will not accept children with severe disabilities due to the difficulty of locating and training appropriate mentors. Once the needed information is available, the case manager attempts to make a good match between the adult volunteer and the child. Factors that go into this decision include the needs of the child, the abilities of the volunteer, the preferences of the child's parent, and the capacities of the program staff.

Factors Thought to Affect Outcomes

Grossman and Tierney (1998) proposed four prerequisites for effective mentoring programs:

1. A thorough screening process for mentors to increase the chances that a mentor will follow through on the commitment and not pose a safety risk to the youth.
2. Mentor training that includes information on communication, limit setting, relationship building, and ways to best interact with a youth.
3. Procedures for matching mentors with youth that include a professional case manager determining the match and considers the preferences of the youth, the youth's family, and the mentor.
4. Intensive supervision and support by a case manager who has frequent contact with the youth, the youth's parent, and the mentor, and who provides assistance as difficulties arise.

The focus and goals of the mentor's relationship with the youth affects the longevity of the relationship and thus likely affects the outcome. McGill and colleagues (1997) cited a study (Morrow & Styles, 1995) that looked at different approaches to the mentoring relationship. One group of mentors focused primarily on developing a positive relationship with the child before introducing other goals. They respected the child's desire to have fun and allowed the child input into activities. The majority of these relationships persisted. Another group of mentors had high expectations for behavior change in the child and set the goals and ground rules for the relationship. The majority of these relationships "faltered" or discontinued.

Summary

Table 10.1 provides a summary of the BBBSA mentoring program that was presented as an exemplary program. We recommend following these guidelines when implementing a mentoring program. Future research is likely to better define best practices.

OVERVIEW AND RESEARCH EVALUATION
OF AFTER-SCHOOL PROGRAMS

For many children, the after-school period is a time of reduced supervision and structure. It is also when a high proportion of juvenile crimes are committed (Fashola, 1998). Historically, youth development organizations have tried to create an alternative to delinquent activities by providing recre-

TABLE 10.1. Summary of Big Brothers Big Sisters Mentoring Program

Overview

- Based on the belief that supportive relationships with caring adults promote healthy development in children.
- Mentors and children share developmentally appropriate activities for 4 hours, two to four times a month.
- Case managers screen, match, monitor, and support mentor.
- National standards are in place.

Screening and supervision of mentors

- Extensive screening of mentors is required.
- Mentors must make 1-year commitment.
- Training is provided on such issues as relationship building, communication, and child development.
- Case manager has periodic contact with mentor, child, and child's parent.

Child screening and matching with mentor

- Parent completes questionnaire and the child is interviewed.
- Case manager matches child with a mentor based on the needs of the child, mentor's ability, preferences of the parent, and capacities of the program staff.

Factors thought to affect outcomes

- Thorough screening procedures
- Mentor training
- Careful matching of mentor and child
- Intensive supervision and support
- Focus on developing a positive mentor–child relationship prior to introducing other goals.

ational opportunities in a safe setting. The focus of after-school and recreational programs has recently expanded, with a growing emphasis on the development of academic and other skills. The term "after-school programs" encompasses a broad array of activities and services that are more accurately described as "outside-of-school-hours programs." These programs meet before school, after school, on weekends, and even during vacations. They include many programs commonly referred to as "recreational programs."

After-school programming is provided by a wide array of institutions and agencies. Private, nonprofit social service agencies and schools are the largest providers for low- to moderate-income children (Halpern, 1999). National youth-serving organizations that sponsor after-school programs include Boys and Girls Clubs, YMCAs and YWCAs, police athletic leagues, Boy Scouts, Girl Scouts, 4-H, and Camp Fire Girls. Local agencies include community centers, settlement houses, youth sports organizations, and child-care centers. Park and recreation departments and religious organizations also sponsor after-school programs.

These programs differ in terms of the behaviors and skills targeted in the children they serve. Many focus on general social and personal development for children. Others attempt to reduce the opportunity for antisocial behavior by providing supervised and engaging activities. Many programs target skill development in the areas of academics, social skills, cultural activities, sports, and the arts.

The various goals of after-school programs are addressed by providing supervised recreational, social, and educational activities. The degree of structure varies from program to program. An important component of most programs is children's exposure to positive adult and peer role models. Some programs offer direct training in specific areas such as academics, sports, and the arts.

Currently, there is limited research on the effectiveness of after-school and recreational programs (Dryfoos, 1999; Fashola, 1998; Lovell & Pope, 1993; Mulvey et al., 1993), but several large-scale evaluation programs are underway that should provide increased information on the effectiveness of different programs and their components (Dryfoos, 1999; Walker, Grossman, & Raley, 2000). Based on the available outcome studies, Vandell and Shumow (1999) concluded that evidence for positive effects is strongest for low-income children, children in high-crime neighborhoods, younger children, and boys. Fashola's (1998) review concluded that there are a number of promising models, "many of which have encouraging but methodologically flawed evidence of effectiveness" (p. 39). Lovell and Pope (1993) suggested that recreational programs hold promise, but they should be viewed as only one aspect of a multicomponent approach to youth development. Peer involvement is a potentially important factor in the effectiveness of after-school programs (Mahoney, 2000). Based on a longitudinal study that followed individuals from childhood to ages 20 to 24, Mahoney (2000) found high-risk individuals were less likely to exhibit antisocial patterns if they and individuals in their social network participated in school extracurricular activities.

Evaluating after-school programs presents many challenges. Consequently, much of the research has significant methodological problems. Common limitations include high dropout rates and the lack of random assignment of subjects. This makes it difficult to separate the effects of the after-school program from the effects of other factors. A study by Posner and Vandell (1999) highlighted this concern. They followed low-income children's after-school activities and adjustment from third to fifth grades. Evidence was found for both a self-selection effect (third graders who were more successful at school tended to engage in more after-school academic and enrichment activities in fifth grade) and for a positive effect of after-school programming on fifth graders' adjustment.

In summary, research support for after-school programs is similar to that for mentoring. Some research suggests that after-school programs can have a positive impact on children, especially those at risk for ACP problems. More research is needed, though, to determine the specific effects of after-school programs, who is likely to benefit from them, and what components are needed for positive outcomes. A number of large-scale research programs are underway that will likely better define best practices for after-school programs.

BEST PRACTICES FOR AFTER-SCHOOL PROGRAMS

There is great variability in the quality of after-school programs (Dryfoos, 1999; Halpern, 1999). Despite the lack of methodologically sound research, factors thought to affect the quality of after-school programs have been identified. Information on best practices was drawn from the following sources: (1) Dryfoos's (1999) discussion of the role of schools in children's out-of-school time; (2) Fashola's (1998) review of the effectiveness of extended-day and after-school programs; (3) Halpern's (1999) presentation on after-school programs for low-income children; (4) Lovell and Pope's (1993) discussion of recreational interventions for gang and delinquency problems; (5) Quinn's (1999) presentation on youth development programs for early teens; (6) the U.S. Department of Education and U.S. Department of Justice's (1998) suggestions for effective after-school programming; (7) Vandell and Shumow's (1999) presentation on after-school child-care programs; and (8) Walker and colleagues' (2000) discussion of extended service schools. These sources suggest practices common to effective after-school programs.

Clarifing Goals and Activities

Historically, many after-school and recreational programs focused on promoting healthy child development. This goal continues to be emphasized, but there is a trend today toward adding additional components. In a survey of after-school programs administered by community-based organizations or community schools, Walker and colleagues (2000) found the top seven goals to be as follows:

1. Improve academic performance.
2. Foster positive relations with peers and adults.
3. Build partnerships between community organizations and schools.
4. Use youth out-of-school time safely and productively.
5. Involve parents more in their children's lives and schools.

6. Keep youth off the streets and out of trouble.
7. Enrich youth's lives with more athletic and cultural experiences.

It is important that after-school programs clarify their focus and goals. The goals need to be realistic given the resources of the agency and should match the needs of the community. Clearly defined goals help to focus the activities of the program and allow for meaningful evaluation. In determining goals, it is helpful to include staff, parents, and community members to ensure that the program is responsive to community needs.

The activities sponsored by after-school programs are determined by the established goals. Walker and colleagues (2000) found much consistency among programs in the types of activities provided, but differences in their content and instructional style. All the programs provided some form of direct academic support (e.g., homework help, tutoring, or academic enrichment) and cultural or creative programming. Many provided athletic, decision-making and leadership, community service or service learning, and free-time activities. Walker and colleagues provided a sample schedule of the after-school program in one elementary school. From 3:00 to 3:45 P.M. the children receive help with homework from high school youth functioning as group leaders and mentors. Following a snack, the children take part in structured activities from 4:00 to 5:00 P.M. The activities vary from substance abuse prevention education to arts and crafts. Various "clubs" are offered 1 to 2 days a week with programming focused on science, drama, hiking, art, and multicultural activities. Family math and reading clubs are also offered. From 5:00 to 5:30 P.M. children are given free time to read, color, or play board games until they are picked up.

Providing for a Quality Staff

High-quality staff is viewed by many as an essential component of effective programs. The staff needs to be committed, have appropriate experience, and relate to the children in a caring and supportive manner. Quality workers are able to form positive and supportive relationships with the children. They are available to the children during activities and provide individual attention and guidance to ensure that every child experiences support and success. They are capable of identifying and responding to individual needs. Low pay and part-time hours often result in frequent turnover and make it difficult for programs to attract qualified staff. The staff should receive ongoing training to develop and improve their skills. An effective training program can help in retaining qualified staff. Many programs utilize volunteers. Just as with paid staff, volunteers require supervision and training to work effectively with the children

Maintaining a Low Staff-to-Child Ratio

Appropriate staff-to-child ratios are important for quality programs. The recommended ratio is between 1:10 and 1:15 depending on the age of the children and the type of program (U.S. Department of Education & U.S. Department of Justice, 1998). The size of groups should also be limited and not exceed 30 children (U.S. Department of Education & U.S. Department of Justice, 1998). The size of groups should be determined by the age of the children and the activity, and should allow for a high level of positive staff–child interaction.

Developing Partnerships with Community Organizations

Partnerships are common for after-school programs, with schools and community organizations frequently working together. Dryfoos (1999) used a three-part typology to categorize school-based after-school programs. In school-administered programs, the school itself serves as the lead agency. These programs commonly involve extracurricular activities, extended-day programs, homework clubs, and child-care services (e.g., 21st Century Community Learning Centers) (Dryfoos, 1999). The second category is school-based after-school programs administered by a community organization. The community organization, in collaboration with the schools, offers programming in schools (e.g., Beacon and Bridges to Success programs) (Walker et al., 2000). In Dryfoos's third category, community schools, the classroom and after-school programs are integrated, with the school becoming a resource for the entire community. In this model, after-school programs are part of the health, mental health, social service, and recreation services brought into the school (e.g., the Settlement House in a School model [Coltoff, 1998]; and "CoZi" schools [Zigler, Finn-Stevenson, & Stern, 1997]).

Partnerships offer a number of advantages. They allow for community input into goals and activities, thus keeping the program focused on local needs. Partnerships expand programming through collaboration with other agencies and increase coordination of services. They also expand the expertise available to the program. In addition to partnerships with community agencies, after-school programs can develop links with the community by forming advisory boards of community members.

Involving Parents

The involvement of parents can help after-school programs work more effectively with children, promote healthy parent–child interactions, and focus the program on community needs. This involvement can be promoted through parent participation on advisory committees, volunteer opportunities, and family-oriented recreational and learning opportunities. Factors affecting family involvement should be considered, such as working parents' schedules, transportation, and the cost of programs. Procedures for engaging families are discussed in more detail in Chapter 12.

Coordinating Programming with Schools

After-school programs should attempt to support and supplement learning during the school day with interesting and challenging activities and experiences. Communication between after-school and school staff allows for the coordination of curriculum and activities. It also helps in planning for the social and academic needs of individual students.

Creating a Structured and Supportive Milieu

It is important that staff members establish, monitor, and enforce age-appropriate behavioral expectations in a firm but respectful manner. This creates a safe and controlled environment that allows for organized and successful activities. A good balance should be found between structure and flexibility. In addition to providing structure, the staff is also responsible for establishing a supportive climate. Staff members' ability to form positive relationships with the children is vital in developing a sense of support. This involves attending to each child individually, recognizing and responding to individual needs, and assisting all children to participate in the activities.

Implementing Evaluation Procedures

Quality after-school programs incorporate evaluation procedures to assess multiple factors. They periodically assess the degree to which they have maintained a focus on their established goals and whether their goals are consistent with community needs. They also evaluate the effectiveness of their programs at achieving these goals. In addition, they assess community, parent, and child satisfaction with the program. These evaluations help to identify areas in need of modification. Further information on program evaluation can be found in Chapter 12.

Summary

Table 10.2 provides a summary of recommended practices for after-school programs. Best practices have yet to be determined by methodologically sound research. The practices described here are those commonly utilized by quality programs.

TABLE 10.2. Summary of Best Practices for After-School Programs

Procedures	Best practices
Clarifing goals and activities	Set goals to reflect community needs and agency resources; utilize staff, parent, and community members help to define goals; design activities to support the goals.
Providing for a quality staff	Select staff members who are committed, experienced, able to relate to children in a caring and supportive manner, and identify and respond to children's individual needs; ongoing training is provided.
Maintaining a low staff-to-child ratio	Set staff-to-child ratio and size of groups that are appropriate for the age of the children and type of activity, and allows for a high level of staff–child interaction.
Developing partnerships with community organizations	Obtain community input into goals and activities through partnerships, coordinate services with other agencies, and expand expertise and programming.
Involving parents	Promote parent involvement with service on advisory committees, volunteer opportunities, family-oriented activities, and attention to factors such as working parents' schedules.
Coordinating programming with schools	Support and supplement school activities, communicate with school staff.
Creating a structured and supportive milieu	Establish, monitor, and enforce age-appropriate behavioral expectations; create a balance between structure and flexibility; establish a supportive climate by forming positive staff–child relationships and attending to each individual.
Implementing evaluation procedures	Assess program's focus on established goals, effectiveness, satisfaction with the program, and areas in need of modification.

OVERVIEW AND RESEARCH EVALUATION OF CASE MANAGEMENT SERVICES

In addition to community services targeting the needs of children with ACP, there is a need for services that support their families. The behaviors of children with ACP can severely challenge families. These families can benefit from services that help them to more effectively manage these problems and promote positive development in their children. A central component of many support programs for at-risk families, which includes many families of children with ACP, is case management. Case management is best described as a set of functions intended to mobilize, coordinate, and maintain the services and resources needed to meet an individual's needs over time (Stroul, 1995).

Case management services (also referred to as "service coordination" or "therapeutic case advocacy") for families with children exhibiting ACP target a variety of factors. Among these factors is the family's ability to manage stress, provide adequate structure and supervision for children, and provide nurturance and support for children. A family's ability to access needed services and build a social support network are also targeted.

Case management services provide, or assist families in accessing and coordinating, a wide range of support services. These services include advocacy, information and referral, support and self-help groups, education and training, respite care, and cash assistance or help with concrete needs such as transportation and day care. The function of case management differs from program to program, but commonly involves assessing needs, linking families to appropriate services, and coordinating services.

Most of the research on case management focuses on services for adults with severe mental illness. The results of this research are inconsistent, but it does find case management to be associated with reduced symptoms, improved quality of life, and reduced psychiatric hospitalization (Burns, Farmer, Angold, Costello, & Behar, 1996). Limited research has been conducted on the effectiveness of case management for children with serious emotional disturbances, which includes many children with ACP (Burns et al., 1996; Burns, Gwaltney, & Bishop, 1995; Rivera & Kutash, 1994). Results from the Fort Bragg Demonstration Project did not find improved clinical outcomes from service delivery changes that emphasized case management (Bickman, 1996; Bickman, Lambert, Andrade, & Penaloza, 2000). Identifying the results of case management is challenging due to the difficulty of separating its effects from the effects of other provided services. The effectiveness of case management is dependent on the utility of the services it coordinates. However, case management is an essential component of some effective programs, such as Multisystemic Therapy (Henggeler et al., 1998) and Multidimensional Treatment Foster Care (Chamberlain & Mihalic, 1998).

Burns and colleagues (1996) describe a study in which youth with serious emotional disturbances (77% with externalizing diagnoses) were randomly assigned to one of two conditions. Youth (ages 8–17) received services from a multiagency treatment team led by a case manager or a treatment team led by the primary mental health clinician. There were few differences in outcome measure, but the case management services did result in fewer days in the hospital and greater parental satisfaction with the services. Evans, Armstrong, and Kuppinger (1996) compared a treatment foster care program with Family-Centered Intensive Case Management (FCICM) for children ages 5 to 12 referred for treatment foster care. Children assigned to FCICM demonstrated a significant decrease in number of symptoms and significant improvement in behavior and mood. These results should be interpreted with caution as the study involved a small number of subjects and results consisted solely of treatment staff ratings.

In summary, the limited research on case management for children with emotional problems and their families is inconsistent. It is theoretically appealing, though, because it targets factors such as family stress and difficulty accessing services that interfere with families working effectively with their children displaying ACP. As a result, we support efforts to better define best practices and evaluate the effectiveness of case management with the families of children with ACP.

BEST PRACTICES FOR CASE MANAGEMENT SERVICES

Best practices are not well defined for case management services with families of children with ACP. The factors we believe should be considered when providing case management services were derived from the following sources: (1) Burns and colleagues' (Burns et al., 1995, 1996) study and review of case management; (2) Early and Poertner's (1995) presentation on approaches to case management for families with children who have serious emotional disorders; (3) Rivera and Kutash's (1994) review of case management services; and (4) Stroul's (1995) discussion of case management in a system of care. In the remainder of this section we describe issues that need to be considered in providing case management services.

Defining Case Management Functions

Case management for children with emotional and behavioral problems serves multiple functions. Burns and colleagues (1995) identified the following six functions common to many forms of case management:

1. Assessment: determine the strengths and needs of the child and the child's family.
2. Planning: develop a service plan to address the needs of the child and family.
3. Linking: refer child and family to needed services.
4. Monitoring: ensure that services remain appropriate and effective over time.
5. Advocacy: overcome barriers to the child and family obtaining needed services.
6. Support: provide supportive clinical services such as counseling.

The many forms of case management emphasize different functions and implement them in a variety of ways. For example, the linking function may be a central component for some case managers and only a minor task for others. It can be a passive process of providing the family with the name of an agency to contact, a more active process of arranging services for the family and providing it with transportation and support, or it can involve the case manager training the family in how to locate and access service itself. No one approach is best for all cases. Each will meet the needs of some families some of the time. For linking and the other functions of case management to be effective, the approach needs to be accurately matched to the family's needs and abilities.

While there is some consistency in the general function of case management services, there is little consistency in its form. When designing case management services for children with ACP, many different factors need to be considered. Unfortunately, there is limited research to help guide the design of these services. Multiple factors affect the type and quality of case management. These factors include who provides the case management services, where the services are located, what authority the case manager has, and what is the intensity of the services.

Selecting a Provider of Case Management Services

There are a number of options to consider when deciding who should provide the case management services. One strategy is to use an individual practitioner. Individuals can function solely as case managers or can provide case management in addition to other clinical services. Another strategy is to use a team to provide case management services. Different types of teams are involved. The team can consist of multiple case managers who share responsibility for a number of children and families. This approach has the advantage of more easily allowing for 24-hour availability; enhancing continuity of care through staff sickness, vacations, and turnover; and increasing support and consultation among staff. A limitation of this approach is that it requires the family to become comfortable with multiple case managers and may make it more difficult for them to form trusting and cooperative relationships. Teams can also be multidisciplinary or multiagency. An individual case manager generally organizes these teams. The case manager will facilitate the team performing many of the case management functions.

There is little agreement on, and great variability in, the qualifications, specialty area, and training of case managers. The level of education ranges from high school diplomas to doctoral degrees, with a bachelor degree being a common requirement. Individuals serving as case managers include social workers, mental health counselors, nurses, psychologists, and consumers of case management services. Rather than level or type of education, qualifications for a specific case management position should be determined by the skills needed to competently carry out the specific responsibilities of the position. Given the great variety of case management responsibilities, it is not surprising that there is great variability among the qualifications of case managers.

In some programs, families are trained to function as their own case managers. Parents can be trained to take on various case management roles, with professional case managers providing training and monitoring. This approach is consistent with strength-based approaches to case management that emphasize empowering families to meet their own needs.

Determining the Location of Case Management Services

Case management services can be provided by schools, social service agencies, court systems, mental health agencies, or interagency programs. Each location has strengths and weaknesses. The best location for a specific case management program will depend on the form and goals of the program, family needs, the relationship among agencies, and the availability of resources. For example, if the main goals of a program are to reduce truancy and improve academic and behavioral functioning in school, it may be most productive for the case management services to be based in the schools. While court, mental health, and social services may be involved, the school personnel would be in the best position to coordinate these services to maximize their effect on school-related variables.

Defining the Authority of the Case Manager

The amount of authority a case manager has to make decisions, access services, and influence agencies and providers varies widely. This factor likely influences the effectiveness of case management services. To fulfill common functions, the case manager needs to have a certain level of authority to make or influence decisions on types of service, the coordination of services, and access to services. A case manager's level of control over different services will vary. For example, a case manager may be able to authorize respite care or cash payments for transportation, a membership to the YMCA, or the fee for a summer camp. The case manager may have less control over placement in a therapeutic foster care program, but have the skills and knowledge to determine whether it is needed and to successfully advocate for the service. Case managers need the authority and skills to effectively coordinate court, school, after-school, and mental health services for a child with ACP.

The availability of needed programs and financial resources plays a major role in the effectiveness of case management services. If it is determined that a family needs respite or transportation services, but these services do not exist or are unavailable because of financial concerns, the effect of case management will obviously be diminished.

Deciding on the Intensity of Case Management Services

The intensity of services refers to the amount of time and resources provided to each child and family. The intensity of services, size of caseload, and functions of the case manager are all directly related. The caseload of case managers can range from 4 to 75 or more, with 5 to 15 commonly being suggested as the preferred number (Stroul, 1995). The optimal caseload is affected by the functions performed by the case manager, as well as by the level of needs of the children and families. Some families require daily contact, while others requiring only infrequent contact. Case management services can also differ in duration. Intensive, crisis-oriented services are often short term in nature.

Given the long-term nature of ACP problems, case management will generally be needed over an extended period of time. However, the intensity and type of services that will be beneficial will vary over time. During times of crisis, intense and comprehensive case management services will be needed to meet the needs of the family. For example, the family may require daily contact concerning stress and behavior management, locating and accessing mental health services, finding employment or day-care services, frequent respite, school advocacy, and transportation problems. In contrast, during more stable periods, only monthly contact might be needed to monitor child and family functioning, identify goals and needs, and assist the family with problem solving.

Family-Centered Intensive Case Management

Family-Centered Intensive Case Management (Abate, Brennan, & Conrad, 1995; Evans et al., 1994) is an example of a case management program for children with emotional and behavioral problems. Based on the strengths model of case management, its goal is to keep children in their "natural environments" (i.e., their family, school, and community). FCICM focuses on developing the family's social network while helping families develop the skills and social support needed to care for a child with serious emotional disturbance. It serves families with children between the ages of 6 to 12 who are at risk of being placed outside the home as a result of emotional or behavioral problems.

FCICM is a comprehensive program with case management being only one of many components (see Table 10.3 for a full list of program components). Case managers are required to have at least a bachelor degree in a human services field and experience working with children with serious emotional disturbances. They receive 10 days of case management training, ongoing training on a variety of child and family topics, supervision, regular contact with other case managers, and psychiatric consultation on specific cases. The case manager serves multiple functions. In conjunction with

TABLE 10.3. Program Components of Family-Centered Intensive Case Management

- Support from a parent advocate and family-centered intensive case manager (ICM) team.
- 24-hour-a-day/7-day-a-week response capability.
- Planned and emergency respite care.
- Parent skills training for natural parents.
- Parent support groups.
- Comprehensive family and child needs assessment.
- Case management and linkage to needed services and/or to develop new programs and services for the collective group of family-centered intensive case management clients.
- Home visits by the parent advocate and family-centered ICM, both scheduled and on an emergency basis.
- Client and system advocacy.
- Psychiatric consultation.
- Family recreation events.

Note. From Abate, Brennan, and Conrad (1995). Copyright 1995 by Paul H. Brookes Publishing. Reprinted by permission.

the family and parent advocate, the case manager assesses the needs of the family and develops a family service plan. The case manager links the family to needed services, coordinates planning meetings with the family service providers, and monitors needs and outcomes. Flexible service dollars are available for the case manager to use to meet the needs of the family. The case manager provides parent training, assists families in developing formal and informal support systems, and functions as an advocate for the family.

Some of the case management duties are shared with the parent advocate, who is the parent of a child with a serious emotional disturbance. The parent advocate assists the case manager in conducting home visits, advocates for the parents, trains respite providers, coordinates support groups, and provides parents with an open ear and an open mind.

Summary

Table 10.4 presents a summary of best practices for case management services. These services are relatively new for children with ACP and their families, with best practices still in the developing stage. The procedures described should be considered when designing and implementing case management services.

OVERVIEW AND RESEARCH EVALUATION
OF THERAPEUTIC FOSTER CARE

Therapeutic foster care is a commonly used out-of-home intervention for children with severe ACP behaviors. It is referred to by a number of terms, including "specialized foster care," "special foster care," "treatment foster care," "foster family-based treatment," "individualized residential treatment," "professional parenting," and "intensive foster care" (Rivera & Kutash, 1994). There is great variability among the different models of therapeutic foster care, with differences being found in treatment approach, amount of structure, level of intensity, and type of training and support provided to foster parents. They also share many common components, including special selection of foster parents, specialized training of foster parents, the establishment of a support system for the foster parents, and a higher than normal stipend. Other common components include placement of one child in a foster home at a time, small caseloads for program staff,

TABLE 10.4. Summary of Best Practices for Case Management Services

Procedures	Best practices
Defining case management function	Consider various functions including assessment, planning, linking, monitoring, advocacy, support; match the function and how they are implemented to the needs and strengths of the family.
Selecting a provider of case management services	Select individual case manager who provides only case management services or combines with other clinical services or case management teams consisting of multiple case managers, multidisciplinary teams, or multiagency teams; determine training and qualifications by the role and responsibility of the position.
Determining the location of case management services	Locate in school, social service agency, court system, mental health agency, or interagency program; location determined by the goal of the program, family needs, relationship among agencies, and availability of resources.
Defining the authority of case manager	Allow case manager sufficient authority to make or influence decisions on type of services, coordination of services, and access to services.
Deciding on the intensity of case management services	Allocate amount of time and resources based on the goals and needs of the family; determine case load by the functions of the position.

and provision of services to the family the child will return to as preparation for the transition home (Rivera & Kutash, 1994). Therapeutic foster care is believed to have a number of advantages over other forms of intensive treatment such as residential treatment or hospitalization. These advantages include keeping the child in the community and in a family environment. It also allows for flexibility and an individualized approach, as well as avoids the possible negative effects of placing the child with a group of children with ACP (e.g., in a residential treatment center).

Therapeutic foster care targets multiple areas of child and family functioning. Through appropriate supervision, structure, and support, a child's ACP behaviors, emotional skills, social relationships, and academic functioning are targeted. In addition, therapeutic foster care targets the parenting, family functioning, and social support systems in the family to which the child will return.

In therapeutic foster care a child with ACP is placed in a foster home with specially trained and supported foster parents. The central intervention consists of the behavior management and supportive parenting provided by the foster parents. Case management services are used to support the foster parents and to arrange and coordinate other needed services. These services may include social and emotional skills training, psychotherapy, academic interventions, and social and recreational interventions.

Due to the wide variability among therapeutic foster care programs, one must be careful in making general statements about its effectiveness. Based on a narrative review of outcome studies, Rivera and Kutash (1994) concluded that therapeutic foster care has generally been found to be effective. A major limitation of the research is that the majority of the studies have only looked at discharge rates as the outcome measure, with discharge rates to less restrictive settings ranging from 62% to 89%. The few studies that have looked at variables related to the child's functioning and adjustment have reported positive results. A meta-analysis by Reddy and Pfeiffer (1997) found a large positive effect on placement permanency (youth remaining in the same placement) and social skills. A medium positive effect was found for reducing behavior problems, improving psychological adjustment, and reducing restrictiveness of postintervention placement. Reddy and Pfeiffer commented on the poor methodological quality of most studies and the lack of agreement on what constitutes a successful outcome. They concluded that the research generally supports the effectiveness of therapeutic foster care, but the limited number of well-designed studies prevents a firm conclusion.

The effectiveness of Multidimensional Treatment Foster Care (MTFC) has been supported by several studies (Chamberlain & Mihalic, 1998). In a recent study, 79 male juvenile delinquents (ages 12 to 17) were randomly assigned to MTFC or a group-care program that involved individual, group, and family therapy (Chamberlain & Reid, 1998; Fisher & Chamberlain, 2000). At both 1- and 2-year posttreatment, boys in the MTFC group had significantly lower arrest rates than the boys in the group-care program. At 2-year posttreatment, significantly more boys in the MTFC group reported working at legal jobs, having positive relationships with parents, and refraining from unprotected sex. They also reported less drug use than the comparison group.

In summary, while methodological limitations prevent firm conclusions, therapeutic foster care does have some support as an effective intervention. MTFC is a well-defined intervention whose effectiveness with juvenile delinquents has been supported with methodologically sound research. It appears to require a high level of skill and commitment on the part of foster parents and a high level of supportive services. These could be limiting factors to its widespread use. Further research is needed to better define therapeutic foster care's specific effects, with whom it is most effective, and its essential components.

BEST PRACTICES FOR THERAPEUTIC FOSTER CARE

MTFC is an approach to therapeutic foster care that has been demonstrated effective in controlled studies, is designed for youth who have serious and chronic problems with delinquency, and includes many of the common components of therapeutic foster care. Although it targets children at the upper limit of the age range we cover in this book, we will present it as an exemplary program. Information presented in this section was derived from Chamberlain and colleagues' (Chamberlain, 1996; Chamberlain & Mihalic, 1998; Fisher & Chamberlain, 2000) studies and descriptions of MTFC.

In MTFC, foster parents are the primary intervention agents. Three mechanisms within MTFC are hypothesized to contribute to positive outcomes: (1) a proactive approach to reducing problem behavior; (2) a consistent, reinforcing environment for youth; and (3) separation and stratification of staff roles. The areas targeted by MTFC are listed in Table 10.5.

Selecting, Training, and Supporting of Foster Parents

MTFC parents are recruited in a number of ways, with word-of-mouth and newspaper advertisements being most effective. Applicants are screened by phone and then complete a formal application. Next, they receive a home visit to provide them with information on the program. The home visit also enables staff to evaluate the home environment. The parents must be able to take an active treatment perspective, to implement a daily structured program, and to work with a delinquent or troubled child. Important qualities in MTFC parents include being able to take the perspective of another

TABLE 10.5. Areas Targeted by Multidimensional Treatment Foster Care

- Reinforce normative and prosocial behaviors.
- Provide the youth with close supervision.
- Closely monitor peer associations.
- Specify clear and consistent limits and follow through on rule violations with nonviolent consequences.
- Encourage youth to develop positive work habits and academic skills.
- Support family members to increase the effectiveness of their parenting skills.
- Decrease conflict between family members.
- Teach youth new skills for forming relationships with positive peers and for bonding with adult mentors and role models.

Note. From Fisher and Chamberlain (2000). Copyright 2000 by PRO-ED, Inc. Reprinted by permission.

person, having a good knowledge of child development, and having a healthy sense of humor.

MTFC parents are provided 20 hours of preservice training that is both didactic and experiential. The program's policies and procedures are explained. The parents are taught how to analyze behavior, how to implement the program's individualized daily program, how to work with the child's biological family, and how to reinforce and encourage children. Much emphasis is placed on reinforcement and encouragement. Parents are discouraged from continuing if they cannot support this important aspect of the program.

Following completion of the training, a match is made between the MTFC parents and a child. After the MTFC parents are fully informed about the child, the case manager and the MTFC parents develop the individualized daily plan (described in the next section). MTFC parents are supported and supervised through weekly support meetings with program staff and other foster parents, daily phone calls from program staff to inquire about behavior, and weekly home visits from program staff during the early stages of treatment. Program staff is available to MTFC parents 24 hours a day.

Program Staff

An important aspect of the therapeutic process involved in MTFC is the separation and stratification of staff roles. Due to the often-opposing needs of the child, the biological family, the MTFC parents, and other involved individuals and service providers, it is believed that the effectiveness of "generalists" can be compromised by conflicts and multiple demands for support. Within MTFC, roles are clearly defined to minimize these difficulties. The treatment team consists of six separate individuals and roles: behavior support specialist (BSS), youth therapist, family therapist, consulting psychiatrist, Parent Daily Report (PDR) caller, and case manager/clinical team supervisor.

The BSS is trained in applied behavior analysis and the use of shaping procedures to teach new behaviors. The BSS is responsible for teaching the child problem-solving skills and prosocial behavior. The child is taught practical skills and behaviors in the community and school. The youth therapist serves as an advocate and support for the child in the MTFC family and the biological family. In some cases, the youth therapist will work with the child on issues related to past maltreatment. Rather than refer to community providers for medication evaluation and management, the MTFC program has found it helpful to have a consulting psychiatrist on the treatment team. A psychiatrist working with the team enables careful consideration of diagnoses and the effectiveness of medications.

The PDR caller is responsible for calling the foster homes daily and with the MTFC parent completing the PDR, a checklist of 40 items related to behavior problems. The foster parent indicates which behaviors occurred in the past 24 hours. This information is given to the case manager and is used to track progress and identify problems. Because the PDR is highly structured, the PDR caller needs good interpersonal skills, but not clinical experience.

The family therapist works with the child's biological parents or guardians on providing appropriate supervision, using fair and consistent discipline, providing encouragement, and promoting association with prosocial peers. The program recognizes that the child require parental support after they return home in order to maintain treatment gains. The family therapist first establishes a supportive and constructive relationship with the family and then begins parent training. As parents learn skills, they first use them in supervised visits at the treatment center. As skills improve, visits move to the family's home, and gradually proceed to overnight and then weekend visits. Parents are given practice assignments for the visits. Following reunification, the family therapist continues to work with the family for 1 to 3 months.

The case manager/clinical team supervisor is the primary advocate for the MTFC parent and is responsible for monitoring and integrating the activities of the team. The case manager typically has experience in other roles on the team and can assist with managing tensions that arise in providing effective treatment. Case managers carry small caseloads of 10 to 12 cases, which allows for intensive involvement in every case.

Behavior Management Program

A consistent, reinforcing environment is provided by developing an individualized, detailed behavior management program that is implemented in the foster home. The program is a three-level point system in which the child earns points for meeting clear behavioral expectations throughout the day. Points are earned for behaviors such as getting out of bed on time, doing homework, attending classes, and having a mature attitude. Points can be lost for rule infractions. A sample daily point chart is presented in Figure 10.1. In level 1, daily points are totaled for rewards the following day. In

School Days Level II			
Name:			
BEHAVIOR	DESCRIPTION	TIME	POINTS
UP ON TIME	Out of bed.		10
READY IN MORNING	Shower, teeth brushed, hair combed, wear clean clothes, eat breakfast.		10
MORNING CLEAN-UP	Bed made, dirty clothes put away, room neat, bath towel and wash rag put away, and dishes in sink.		10
GO TO SCHOOL	Attend school each day (all classes).		5
CARRY SCHOOL CARD	Carry card to each class and get signature from each teacher.		2 cl.
BEHAVIOR IN CLASS	Pay attention to tasks in class, cooperate with the teacher, and hand homework in on time.		5 cl.
READ AND STUDY	50 minutes reading/writing each day (not including letter writing).		20
CHORE	To be explained each day.		10
ATTITUDE/MATURITY	Being helpful, taking criticism well, being pleasant, not pushing limits, not being moody, accepting NO!		15 AM 15 PM
VOLUNTEERING	Volunteering to do extra tasks (Foster Parent will decide on Points).		2-10
EXTRA CHORE	Optional (Must be approved by Foster Parents).		5-10
BED ON TIME	IF you CAN buy BASICS. IF you CAN'T buy BASICS.	9:30 8:30	10

FIGURE 10.1. Sample daily point chart for Multidimensional Treatment Foster Care. From Chamberlain and Mihalic (1998). Copyright 1998 by the Center for the Study and Prevention of Violence. Reprinted by permission.

level 2, points are totaled over a week's time and rewards can be selected from an expanded list of privileges. Level 3 allows for even greater privileges that include community activities without direct supervision.

Summary

Table 10.6 provides a summary of best practices for therapeutic foster care as implemented in the MTFC program. While requiring much expertise and program support, MTFC can potentially result in positive behavioral changes for children with severe ACP problems.

CONCLUSION

In this chapter we reviewed a wide range of interventions targeting contextual factors in the community. These interventions are likely to be most effective when used in conjunction with interventions targeting individual

TABLE 10.6. Summary of the Multidimensional Treatment Foster Care Program

Foster parents

- Must be able to take an active treatment perspective and implement a daily structured program.
- Receive 20 hours of training on topics including behavior management and encouraging children.
- Supervised and supported through weekly meetings with program staff and other foster parents and daily phone calls.

Program staff

- Behavior support specialist: teachers child new behaviors and problem-solving skills.
- Youth therapist: provides support and advocacy for the child.
- Family therapist: provides parent training for the child's biological parents/ guardians in preparation for the child's move home.
- Consulting psychiatrist: manages questions of diagnoses and medication.
- Parent Daily Report caller: calls foster parents daily to complete behavior rating scale.
- Case manager/clinical team supervisor: monitors and integrates the work of the team.

Behavior management program

- Three-level point system.
- Points are gained and lost based on specifically defined behaviors.
- Rewards and privileges are earned.

and family factors so that a greater number of risk/protective factors are addressed. There is limited methodologically sound research on many of these interventions. As a result, best practices are not well defined and will likely evolve as further research better defines effective intervention components, intervention effects, and which children and families benefit from these interventions.

PART V

INTEGRATION AND CHALLENGES

CHAPTER 11

Comprehensive Multicomponent and Coordinated Services Programs

*I*t makes sense to combine two or more interventions to comprehensively address the wide range of problems faced by children with ACP and their families. More risk and protective factors can be addressed through comprehensive intervention approaches. Combining interventions increases the probability of changing the refractory condition of these children.

In this chapter we discuss multicomponent and coordinated services programs that bring separate interventions together into one comprehensive intervention package. Multicomponent programs are typically university-derived and are employed in clinical, school, and community settings. They bring together many of the intervention components that were discussed previously to address the multiple problems that are typical of children with ACP and their families. Often a research team organizes and orchestrates the delivery of multicomponent intervention programs. Coordinated services programs bring practitioners from "real-life" mental health, education, child welfare, juvenile justice, and community agencies together to assist families. Practitioners in each agency provide parts of an intervention that together comprise a comprehensive effort to address many family needs. Practitioners from these different agencies work together to coordinate service provision. Many of the multicomponent and coordinated services programs adhere to the concept of ACP being a "chronic" condition (Kazdin, 1995) and therefore provide intensive multi-year interventions.

These multicomponent and coordinated services programs are hypothesized to reduce risk factors and promote protective factors in the child, parent/family, social/peer, and contextual life domains (see Tables 2.3 and 2.4 in Chapter 2). The exact risk and protective factors addressed depends on which specific intervention components are combined in the overall program (see previous chapters about risk and protective factors and specific interventions). The more intervention components provided, the greater the likelihood of affecting many risk and protective factors.

Our presentation is divided into three sections. We begin by reviewing selected multicomponent intervention programs. Then we discuss selected coordinated services programs. The programs reviewed have shown promise in working with children identified as ACP and/or with multiproblem families. The multicomponent and coordinated services programs presented here could serve as models for practitioners intent on implementing these types of programs. In the last section we suggest best practices for delivering coordinated services to children and families. We chose to highlight best practices associated with coordinated services programs due to the practice orientation of this book. We make the point, however, that multicomponent intervention procedures can be incorporated into coordinated services programs.

We will employ a slightly different format from that used in preceding chapters. Since the selected models of multicomponent and coordinated services differ from each other in the types of interventions combined, we decided it would be best to present each model program and its own supporting research. Also, since we have already discussed specific intervention components (e.g., social competence training, classroom behavior management, etc.), we will not repeat practice parameters for specific interventions, but will highlight methods for coordinating them.

MULTICOMPONENT INTERVENTION PROGRAM MODELS

Multicomponent intervention programs provide two or more simultaneous interventions to families. The multicomponent intervention programs presented here are university-derived and are delivered in clinic, school and/or community settings. We review the procedures for conducting different multicomponent programs and corresponding research evaluation data.

Child- and Parent/Family-Focused Interventions

Combining child with parent/family interventions provides an opportunity to affect the most immediate concerns in a family. This strategy targets child, social/peer, and family factors. Such programs provide social competence training for children and parent and family skills training for their caretakers.

One example of this combination approach is the Webster-Stratton and colleagues combined child and parent training program for 3- to 8-year-old children with ACP (Webster-Stratton, 1996b; Webster-Stratton & Hammond, 1997). The child social competence training program, known as Dinosaur School, provides 22 2-hour group-training sessions to young children with ACP. The parents of children in Dinosaur School also participate in approximately 27–28 2-hour parent group sessions derived from the BASIC and ADVANCE parent training curriculums (see Webster-Stratton, 1996b, for details). The interventions are delivered in a clinical setting.

To evaluate this program, Webster-Stratton and Hammond (1997) compared children with ACP who were assigned to combination child and parent training, child training only, parent training only, and control groups. The combination program produced the strongest gains in enhancing children's social competence and in improving their behavior at home. It also was best at promoting adaptive parent–child interactions. The positive intervention gains were maintained at a 1-year follow-up assessment.

Another example is Kazdin and colleagues' combined child problem-solving skills training and parent behavioral training program for 7- to 13-year-old children with conduct disorder (Kazdin, 1996a; Kazdin et al., 1992). This child and parent program is typically delivered in a clinical setting. Children receive 20 child sessions, each lasting 40–50 minutes, that emphasize problem-solving skills training. Their parents also participate in 16 parent skills training sessions.

In one study evaluating this program, Kazdin and colleagues (1992) assigned children with ACP to combined child and parent training, child only training, parent only training, and control conditions. Kazdin and colleagues found that the combination child and parent training program produced the most significant improvements on child and parent measures of child behavior and adjustment. The initial positive effects were maintained at a 1-year follow-up assessment.

Combining child training with parent training has also been tried in preventive efforts such as the Montreal Prevention Experiment (Tremblay, Masse, Pagani, & Vitaro, 1996). This program is for 7- to 9-year-old boys with ACP. They receive ongoing social skills training in school groups over 2 consecutive years. The child groups include normative peers as comembers. The parent interventions are delivered in-home. Parents receive as much parent training as needed to achieve mastery of content (an average of 17.4 sessions). The parents are also engaged in the intervention program for up to 2 years.

The short- and long-term preventive effects of the Montreal Prevention Experiment have been evaluated. Vitaro and Tremblay (1994) determined that boys in the combined child and parent program did much better than boys in a control group on a variety of child functioning measures, with effects favoring the intervention condition over the control condition by a more significant margin at a 3-year follow-up. Children who received the child and parent program were found to associate less with antisocial peers between immediate posttest and 3-year follow-up, which the authors reasoned may have accounted for the positive benefits at the 3-year follow-up assessment. Tremblay, Pagani-Kurtz, Masse, Vitaro, and Pihl (1995) conducted long-term follow-up evaluation when the boys were 12 to 15 years old. Boys from the child and parent program had less severe teachers' ratings of disruptive behavior and less self-reported delinquency than those in the control condition. In subsequent long-term analysis, Vitaro, Brendgen, Pagani, Tremblay, and McDuff (1999) found that those boys who continued to show long-term positive behavior results were less likely to end up associating with antisocial peers.

The model programs presented in this section combine child and parent training. The accompanying research revealed that this approach is effective in improving the functioning of children with ACP and their families. These child and parent programs have been proven effective in both clinical and prevention efforts.

Child-, Parent/Family-, and School-Focused Interventions

Adding a school-focused intervention to child and parent training could be potent in improving the outcomes of children with ACP. The programs reviewed in this section target child-, parent/family-, and school-related concerns. The school provides an excellent setting in which to implement comprehensive intervention programs because of the accessibility of children and most families. It has the added advantage of being able to intervene with the child's behavior in a natural environment.

The PARTNERS program is intended to augment a Head Start intervention for preschool children (Webster-Stratton, 1996b, 1998a). Children's school and social readiness skills are already targeted in Head Start. The PARTNERS program adds to this by training parents and teachers to improve parent–child and teacher–child interactions and child behavior. Parents meet over eight to nine 2-hour sessions and teachers participate in 2-day workshops totaling 16 hours of training. Both parents and teachers receive an abbreviated version of Webster-Stratton's parent training program (summarized in Webster-Stratton, 1996b). The focus is on managing behavior and promoting social competence in children.

Webster-Stratton (1998a) evaluated the PARTNERS program when employed in a Head Start setting. The children in this study were not selected necessarily on the basis of exhibiting ACP, but many children in the sample had risk factors that placed them at risk for its development (e.g., socioeconomic disadvantage, maternal depression, history of abuse/neglect). Webster-Stratton compared families who received the combined Head Start with PARTNERS program to families who received Head Start only. The results favored the combination condition. Direct observation measures showed that mothers in the combined condition were less aversive and more effective in discipline. Their children had fewer behavior problems and evidenced more social competence. The parents were also more involved in their children's education. These effects were largely maintained at a 1-year follow-up assessment.

Webster-Stratton, Reid, and Hammond (2001) extended the Webster-Stratton (1998) intervention by providing more intensive parent and teacher training and by emphasizing school-related outcomes in the training while working with Head Start families. Parents participated in 12 weekly parent group sessions during their child's Head Start year (approximately 30 hours), and 4 weekly booster parent group sessions during their child's transition year to kindergarten (approximately 8 hours). The Head Start teachers attended 6 day-long training workshops conducted over 6 months of the child's Head Start year (approximately 36 hours). Drawing upon the ADVANCE and School Incredible Years programs (see Webster-Stratton, 1996b), the parents learned about behavior management, facilitating children's social and academic competencies, taking care of self, and working effectively with teachers. The teachers were trained in classroom management and in methods to promote children's social and academic competencies.

The results obtained by Webster-Stratton and colleagues (2001) showed that this intensive parent and teacher intervention was effective. When compared to families whose children attended Head Start centers without parent and teacher training, the families in the experimental group were better off in a variety of domains. Observations revealed more improved parent–child interactions. Children evidenced reductions in problematic behavior, and this was most pronounced for those children who had the highest levels of behavioral problems at baseline. There was more evidence of parent–teacher bonding, and teachers were more adept at managing children's behavior in the classroom. One year after the intervention, many effects were maintained for the families in which the parent had attended six or more of the previously offered parent training groups. The improvements in behavior were also maintained for the children who had shown the highest levels of behavioral difficulties initially.

First Steps to Success is a school-based early intervention program for children displaying ACP in kindergarten (Walker et al., 1998). It involves administration of three intervention components during kindergarten. First, all kindergarten children in the school are involved in a universal screening. Teachers rank children for severity of ACP and then complete ratings on children with significant behavior problems. These children are then observed in their classrooms for academic engagement time (i.e., amount of time on task and involved in school activities). Second, the identified children participate in a classroom intervention. It employs a rigorous point system targeting school-related behaviors, at first administered by a consultant and then gradually transitioned to the classroom teacher. Eventually, the point system is faded out and replaced by social approval and recognition. The third component consists of a six-session in-home parent training program, primarily focusing on improving children's school functioning and parent involvement at school.

Walker and colleagues (1998) evaluated the effects of the First Steps to Success program. They found that children who completed the program did better than children assigned to a wait-list control group on four of five measures of behavior and academic engagement. The results were maintained at first grade for one cohort of children followed to first grade and to second grade for another cohort of children followed to second grade.

Linking the Interests of Families and Teachers (LIFT) is a program for children identified as at risk for ACP in the first or fifth grades (Reid, Eddy, Fetrow, & Stoolmiller, 1999). Boys and girls participate in this program during key transitional years in school (i.e., first or fifth grade). LIFT consists of a 10-week universal program that focuses on the child, parent/family, and school domains. At school, children participate in classroom-based social competence training and school playground behavior interventions. A parent–school communication procedure entails using answering machines in classrooms so that parents and teachers can trade voice mail messages. A parent training group is conducted at school. Parents who do not regularly attend the parent group are given the option of in-home visits or home packets covering the same material. Developmental differences are taken into account to make adjustments for first- or fifth-grade students.

Several studies have been reported regarding the LIFT program. At immediate posttest assessment, Reid and colleagues (1999) determined that children who participated in LIFT exhibited more improvements than children in a no intervention control group. Behavioral observations revealed that children who attended LIFT had less physical aggression on the playground. Mother–child interaction observations showed that mothers who participated in LIFT, and were the most aversive to their children before the intervention, evidenced the most improved interactions with their children. Teachers rated LIFT children as exhibiting improved classroom behavior. During the spring assessment following the program, it was discovered that severely aggressive children exhibited reduced aggressive playground behavior (Stoolmiller, Eddy, & Reid, 2000). At a 3-year follow-up assessment, the original first-grade children had lower levels of impulsive behavior, and the original fifth-grade children had a delayed onset of antisocial peer association and alcohol/marijuana use, as compared to children in the control group (Eddy, Reid, & Fetrow, 2000).

Families and Schools Together (FAST Track) is a large multisite demonstration project being conducted in 54 urban and rural elementary schools at four different sites across the United States (Conduct Problems Prevention Research Group, 1992, 1999b). Children are identified in kindergarten as aggressive at both home and school. The interventions address the child, parent/family, and school domains. During the first grade, a universal intervention is provided to all children in the 54 schools. It consists of a teacher-led classroom-based social skills program. Specific interventions are also provided for at-risk aggressive children. They participate in additional small-group social skills training sessions while their parents go to small-group parent training meetings. Parts of the meetings are devoted to parent–child interaction activities. This part of the program is held on a weekly basis throughout first grade. Families also receive home visits and weekly phone contacts during the first grade on a biweekly basis. School-based interventions include academic and reading tutoring, as well as peer-pairing play sessions to facilitate friendship making at school.

The initial evaluation of FAST Track occurred after the first-grade intervention. Eight hundred ninety-one aggressive children, mostly African American and European American boys, participated in the research project. The Conduct Problem Prevention Research Group (1999b) found that a majority of families participated in most of the programming. Significant results favoring the FAST Track group over a no intervention control group were found on measures related to social, emotional, and academic skills, as well as peer interactions and social status at school. Parents used less aversive discipline strategies and displayed more positive and warm parent–child interactions. Parents also reported high parental satisfaction and involvement in their children's schooling. Although parent and teachers ratings of children's behavior did not change, direct observations of children's behavior revealed that the FAST Track children were less disruptive in the school setting compared to children in the control group.

FAST Track is designed for children to participate in it through 10th grade (Conduct Problems Prevention Research Group, 2000). The planned interventions are designed to unfold and build upon each other over time. The universal classroom intervention will keep going through fifth grade. The child and parent groups will continue to meet on a biweekly basis through second grade, and then on a monthly basis through sixth grade. The children will attend "identity development workshops" during grades seven and eight. Individualized academic-, home-, peer-, and identity development-oriented interventions will be administered to children up to the 10th grade. Further evaluation results will determine the long-term effects of the FAST Track program.

The Metropolitan Area Child Study is a cognitive–ecological prevention program targeting inner-city children with ACP (Guerra, Eron, Huesmann, Tolan, & Van Acker, in press; Huesmann et al. 1996; Metropolitan

Area Child Study Research Group, in press). The children are divided into early (grades two and three) or late (grades five and six) groups. Children in this program receive a universal culturally sensitive classroom intervention designed to enhance teacher–child interaction, teacher's classroom management skills, and children's social competencies. High-risk children also meet in small social skills training groups designed to change the cognitive distortions and deficiencies that are common in aggressive children. The universal classroom and small-group program unfolds over 2 years. A family intervention incorporating parent skills training and family interaction enhancement is also administered for 1 year.

The Metropolitan Area Child Study Research Group (in press) compared the effects of the full program described above to classroom with social skills training only, classroom only, and no intervention control conditions using children with ACP as subjects. They reported that children in the full program condition who attended "high-resource" schools (i.e., those with good financial support, low staff turnovers, etc.) evidenced reduced aggression. Unexpectedly, young children in the full program who attended "low-resource" schools (i.e., those with limited financial support, high staff turnovers, etc.) and older children who received the classroom and social skills only intervention actually got worse. The results for positive and negative findings were similar for boys and girls. The authors hypothesized that children enrolled in low-resource schools were confronted with higher levels of poverty and community violence. In this context, the program may not have been intensive enough and may have actually constituted another burden on families due to the demands of participation. As for the older children who got worse, the authors hypothesized that at this age it may be unwise to put children with ACP together in small groups because they could potentially reinforce each others' problematic behavior (see Dishion et al., 1999). This study showed, however, that early child-, family-, and school-focused preventive programs have the potential to reduce aggression with young children in high-resource schools. The long-term effects of the Metropolitan Area Child Study await further inquiry.

The comprehensive programs reviewed in this section bring together child-, parent/family-, and school-focused interventions. The research cited showed that these programs achieve good results for children with ACP (or children who are at risk for ACP) and their families. More research is needed to fully appreciate the long-term benefits of these comprehensive programs.

Child-, Parent/Family-, and School-Focused
Interventions with Medications

Recently, a comprehensive intervention program, known as the Multimodal Treatment of ADHD (MTA), was developed and implemented. The MTA program provides training for children and families, school-focused interventions, and medications for children with ADHD and comorbid conditions. This comprehensive program provides state-of-the-art interventions focused on multiple domains of functioning with this difficult population of children.

The MTA program combines psychosocial interventions and medications for 7- to 10-year-old children who are carefully diagnosed as ADHD, combined type, with and without comorbid disorders (MTA Cooperative Group, 1999a, 1999b). Children and families in a combination condition participate in an intensive psychosocial intervention that includes behavioral parent training sessions, teacher consultation regarding contingency management, paraprofessional aide in the classroom, and home–school notes, and the children themselves go to an 8-week summer program emphasizing contingency management and social/recreational skills. Children in the combination condition also receive systematic well-managed medication treatment (mostly methylphenidate). Medication treatment includes individualized dosage titration to find each child's optimal dosage and careful monitoring by a physician. The program is delivered to participants over 14 months.

The MTA Cooperative Group (1999a, 1999b) compared the combination treatment approach discussed above to psychosocial intervention alone, medication treatment alone, and "regular community care" groups. At the 14-month evaluation, most psychosocial interventions had been completed, while children assigned to medication conditions continued to use medications. The MTA research team found that the combination and medication alone conditions were both superior to the psychosocial intervention alone and regular community care groups on many child adjustment measures. The combination condition was equally effective to medications alone in reducing children's ADHD symptoms. The positive findings for both the combination and medication alone conditions were largely attributed to the medications that the children received. The combination condition, however, showed an advantage in reducing parent-rated internalizing and oppositional/aggressive symptoms and produced more children rated as exhibiting "excellent response." Interestingly, a majority of children also received medication in the regular community care group, yet they did not fare as well as children who received medication in the MTA program. This likely resulted from children in the MTA program having received higher average daily doses which were administered three times a day (Schachar, 2000). It was also determined that children with ADHD and comorbid anxiety and internalizing problems benefited the most from the psychosocial intervention whether or not they had received medications. Parents voiced greater satisfaction in the conditions employing psychosocial interventions; children in the combined condition achieved good effects with a lower medication dosage than children who received medication alone (Pelham, 2000). Long-term follow-up of children who completed the MTA program is underway.

The MTA multicomponent program brings together comprehensive psychosocial interventions and medications for children diagnosed as ADHD with or without comorbid behavioral disorders. The results of the MTA study provided compelling evidence about the utility of well-managed medication management for this group of children. It also revealed that medications should be combined with empirically validated child-, parent/family-, and school-focused psychosocial interventions to obtain the best outcome for these children.

Child-, Parent/Family-, and School-Focused Interventions Delivered via Community-Based Practitioners

The Early Risers program described below provides child-, parent/family-, and school-focused interventions in an accessible community delivery context. It combines many intervention components to deal with multiple risk and protective factors. The community delivery procedure is designed to engage children and families and strengthen the impact of the intervention.

Early Risers is an intensive multicomponent, multiyear preventive intervention for children with ACP who are at risk for delinquency and substance abuse (August, Realmuto, Bloomquist, & Hektner, 2001; August, Realmuto, Hektner, & Bloomquist, 2001). It is designed for 6-year-old children who exhibit aggressive behavior in the school setting. "Family advocates" deliver Core and Flex intervention components to children and families over 3 years. Core includes child-, parent/family-, and school-focused interventions. Each year children participate in a 6-week summer program where they are exposed to behavioral contingencies, social skills training, recreational enrichment, and tutoring. The Early Risers children and their parents also attend a family program consisting of social skills training for children and parent training/support for parents during the academic year. The family advocates monitor the children's progress in school and consult with school officials regarding educational planning. Flex is a proactive case management strategy in which the family advocates meet with families on an as-needed basis (a minimum of three times per year). The family advocates assess the strengths and needs of each family and assist them in setting goals for their child and family. The family advocates also help families access available community resources to meet family needs not addressed in Core (e.g., financial assistance, referrals for mental health treatments, educational planning, etc.). Importantly, the Early Risers program is integrated into the communities where the children and their families live. The staff is employed in local human service organizations, but they conduct most of the interventions in local schools. They work as intervention providers and coordinate all aspects of the program. University-based prevention specialists designed the program, monitor its implementation, and evaluate its effects.

The Early Risers program was compared to a no intervention control condition for its effects following 2 and 3 years of continuous intervention delivered to children with ACP residing in a semirural community (August, Realmuto, Hektner, & Bloomquist, 2001; August, Hektner, Egan, Realmuto, & Bloomquist, in press). August and colleagues found that severely aggressive Early Risers children exhibited more improved self-regulation (e.g., reduced aggression and hyperactivity/impulsivity) than severely aggressive control children, at both the 2- and 3-year assessments. On a measure of social competence, no statistically significant group differences were found after 2 years, but after 3 years of intervention the Early Risers children exhibited significantly more improvements than the control children. This suggests that it may take up to 3 years of continuous intervention to make improvements in children's social competence. At both the 2- and 3-year assessments, Early Risers children emerged as significantly more improved than controls on a measure of academic achievement; parents who attended 50% or more of parent groups improved on a measure of discipline. Long-term follow-up of this program is underway. Early Risers is also being currently tested on children with ACP residing in a low-income urban community.

Early Risers has been shown to have initial promise as a multicomponent, community-based prevention program. Long-term follow-up evaluation will determine whether or not it is powerful enough to prevent children with early-onset ACP from developing antisocial problems in later years. Additional studies of similar programs are warranted.

Summary

Table 11.1 provides a summary of the selected multicomponent intervention model programs and their general effects. It is important to note that the effects of these model programs are based on the premise of utilizing the standardized procedures described by the program developers. The results of these programs should be viewed as preliminary because many of the multicomponent programs are in the early stages of evaluation. More evaluation and replication will enhance practitioners' confidence in using these types of programs. Nonetheless, we think these multicomponent intervention programs could serve as models for combining interventions for children with ACP and their families.

We realize it may be difficult to replicate these university-derived multicomponent programs in real-life practice settings. We do think, however, that these types of programs can be approximated if practitioners and

TABLE 11.1. Summary of Selected Multicomponent Intervention Program Models

Models	General effects[a]
Child- and parent/family-focused interventions	Child training and parent training with preschool and elementary-age children with ACP is effective in clinical settings.[1, 2] Child training in schools and in-home parent training over 2 years with early elementary-age children with ACP is effective and has preventive effects.[3]
Child-, parent/family-, and school-focused interventions	Teacher and parent behavioral training embedded in child-focused Head Start program or kindergarten is effective with children at risk for ACP.[4, 5] Combining universal child classroom-based skills training and playground interventions, parent training, and school–home communication is effective with early elementary children with ACP or who are at risk.[6] Combining universal child classroom-based training, intensive social skills training, family skills training,[7,8] and academic tutoring[7] is effective with early elementary children with ACP.
Child-, parent/family-, and school-focused interventions with medications	Medication is essential to any treatment involving children with ADHD (with or without comorbid ODD/CD).[9] Medications with intensive child training/contingency management, parent training, and school-focused interventions provide additional benefit for children with ADHD with comorbid disorders.[9]
Child-, parent/family-, and school-focused interventions delivered via community-based practitioners	Intensive multiyear interventions including standardized child social skills training, parent training, and academic interventions, as well as flexible case management utilizing personnel from local human services organizations, is effective with young elementary-age children with ACP.[10]

Note. This table is a brief summary of general effects of these programs. See text and original citations for details. The general effects occur when standardized procedures described by program developers are utilized.

[a]References: 1, Webster-Stratton and Hammond (1997); 2, Kazdin et al. (1992); 3, Vitaro and Tremblay (1994), Tremblay et al. (1995), Vitaro et al. (1999); 4, Webster-Stratton (1998a), Webster-Stratton et al. (2001); 5, Walker et al. (1998); 6, Reid et al. (1999), Stoolmiller et al. (2000), Eddy et al. (2000); 7, Conduct Problems Prevention Research Group (1992, 1999b); 8, Guerra et al. (in press), Huessman et al. (1996), Metropolitan Area Child Study Research Group (in press); 9, MTA Cooperative Group (1999a, 1999b); 10, August, Realmuto, Bloomquist, & Hektner (2001); August, Hektner, et al. (in press).

service agencies collaborate and provide coordinated services. In the next section we provide examples of coordinated services programs that incorporate elements of the multicomponent programs to varying degrees.

COORDINATED SERVICES PROGRAM MODELS

Children with ACP and their families often interface with mental health, education, child welfare, juvenile justice, and community-based family support systems. Each of these systems has a unique mandate and is based in a unique setting. The mental health system provides treatment to children with mental health disorders in clinical settings. The education system educates children in school settings. The child welfare system supports and protects children using interventions delivered in community agencies. The juvenile justice system rehabilitates and diverts offenders who have committed crimes. Finally, the community-based family support system (e.g., neighborhood centers, recreation organizations, churches, etc.) provides practical assistance to address immediate concerns of families. Children with ACP and their families are often involved with several or all of these systems. The dilemma is how to best serve these children within and across these different systems.

Service systems have traditionally operated independently, which means that they are fragmented, uncoordinated, hard to access, and underutilized by the children who need them (Oswald & Singh, 1996; Tuma, 1989b). It is estimated that many children who need mental health treatments, for example, do not receive them (Kazdin, 1996b). The gap between need and utilization is in part attributable to fragmented service systems (Tuma, 1989b; Weist, 1997). In addition, each system only addresses one or several risk factors, which means that ultimately each will be less effective because research tells us that children with ACP are faced with multiple risks and stressors. There is a need for coordinated services to effectively deal with the multitude of problems manifested by children with ACP and their families.

In recent years there has been a move away from unitary delivery of narrow services toward community-based coordinated "systems of care" (Burns & Goldman, 1999; Oswald & Singh, 1996). In fact, the U.S. surgeon general (U.S. Department of Health and Human Services, 1999) has recommended the expansion and development of coordinated services programs to address the significant unmet mental health needs of children in the United States. This model of programming entails coordinating services across practitioners and agencies to address a wide array of child and family problems. In this coordinated service model, practitioners view the family as a partner who assists in directing the interventions provided. There is less focus on remediation and more emphasis on providing family support. Interventions are delivered in a culturally compatible manner. The main goal is to enhance access to existing services so that children and families can receive the benefit of a full continuum of care. The outcomes desired include having the families access needed services easier, utilize less restrictive interventions, avoid duplication of services, and improve functioning. Although coordinated services approaches are not necessarily set up to serve only children with ACP, such children would benefit greatly from such services.

Coordinated services programs use different strategies that involve use of existing or new organizational structures (Oswald & Singh, 1996; Pumariega & Glover, 1998). These different strategies enable families to experience varying levels of coordinated services. One strategy is to colocate services into another setting. This calls for a practitioner or agency to physically move its operations into a new setting (e.g., a mental health clinic moves into a school to provide services). Another strategy is to implement a multisystemic approach. To accomplish this, a practitioner delivers some services and also acts as a case manager to assist families in accessing the services of other practitioners and/or agencies. Still another strategy is to use integrated services. A new organizational structure is created to accomplish service integration. The integrated services model involves many agencies, but is administered by a central coordinating collaborative entity. Various agencies come together, pool their resources, and offer "seamless" access to a wide variety of interventions. Case management is an important part of all the strategies used to provide coordinated services. The common thread across these different strategies of coordinated services is bringing practitioners, agencies, and service systems together for the sake of the families being served.

What follows is a review of selected coordinated services program models. We review coordinated services programs that are focused on mental health, family preservation, and juvenile justice outcomes, as well as comprehensive community-based "wraparound" approaches. We cannot offer an exhaustive review, but the programs we selected reveal different ways of operating coordinated services programs. The programs can serve as models for practitioners. Unfortunately, due to the emphasis on practice, many of these programs have not been subjected to rigorous research evaluation.

Mental Health-Focused Coordinated Services

The programs reviewed here emphasize improving the mental health outcomes of children. They attempt to improve families' access to mental health services and to coordinate with other agencies in the community. We present examples of community- and school-based mental health-focused coordinated services programs.

The Fort Bragg Demonstration Project is a mental health-focused *community-based* model of coordinated services (Bickman, 1996). In this program a mental health clinic coordinates care for an insurance beneficiary associated with the Fort Bragg Army Base in Fayetteville, North Carolina. Children are referred for a variety of mental health problems, including those that are related to ACP. The mental health clinic provides a full range of accessible mental health treatments for children and families ranging from outpatient therapy, to in-home interventions, to day treatment, to crisis management. The families enter the system at their own request and then receive an initial intake review to determine their needs. A treatment team ensures that the families' needs are met. Case managers coordinate mental health treatments and help families obtain other school, social services, and health-related interventions.

Bickman (1996) compared children in the coordinated services model to children who received "traditional services" (mostly fragmented outpatient and institutional interventions). A quasi-experimental design was employed that did not involve random assignment to groups. One positive finding was that children and families receiving coordinated services were able to access greater numbers of interventions and experienced greater continuity of service provision. Families also had higher client satisfaction and used less restrictive treatments. Contrary to expectation, however, children who received coordinated services were no better off than children who received traditional services in terms of clinical outcome, and more money was spent per child. There was also no differences between the coordinated and traditional services groups for clinical outcome at a 5-year follow-up assessment (Bickman, Lambert, Andrade, & Penaloza, 2000). One possible explanation is that the coordinated services program resulted in families obtaining more services, but that the services received within the coordinated services program were ineffective (e.g., the family received services from a mental health clinic but clinic therapy did not work) (Bickman, 1996; Weisz, Han, & Valeri, 1997).

School-based mental health programs are being developed across the United States (Dryfoos, 1997; Hunter, 2001). These programs are often part of a larger school-based health clinic or involve practitioners establishing a satellite office in a school. Children with ACP are often among the clientele serviced in these clinics. The mental health practitioners who work there augment existing school psychology and school social work services already present. Mental health practitioners provide assessment, individual therapy, group therapy, family therapy, consultation with educational staff, and other preventive interventions. Typically, mental health practitioners in schools interface with the other providers who together deliver combined mental health, educational, social, and health-related interventions to children. When this model is employed, more children receive interventions because they are already in the school setting. Another potential benefit is that children are potentially less stigmatized by seeing providers who are in the school rather than going to an outside agency. One drawback to this system is difficulty in getting insurance providers to pay for mental health services rendered in school settings (Weist, 1997).

There is very little data pertaining to the utility of school-based mental health programs. Dryfoos (1997), Hunter (2001), and Weist (1997) reviewed the "spotty" research that does exist. Most of this research does not employ randomized controlled experimental designs. It suggested that school-based mental health interventions are associated with increased services utilization and improved behavioral and emotional adjustment for children and adolescents. Researchers reported that it is hard to involve parents in school-based interventions (Weist, 1997). Apparently, parents will consent to their children being seen, but do not necessarily participate themselves. This model seems potentially very useful, but more research evaluation is needed to ultimately demonstrate its utility, cost-effectiveness, and outcome.

As documented elsewhere in this book, some children with ACP do exhibit mental health problems. Mental health-focused coordinated services models of intervention have the potential to assist these children. The programs reviewed above have improved access to services for children and families, but the results are mixed as to whether or not these models actually improve children's mental health status. It has been argued that the interventions employed within the coordinated services programs need to be empirically supported.

Family-Preservation-Focused Coordinated Services

One model of child welfare–focused coordinated services is family preservation (Illback, 1994; Oswald & Singh, 1996; Schoenwald & Henggeler, 1997). These programs target children who are placed out of home or who are at risk for such placement. Many of the children involved have experienced child maltreatment. Children with ACP are commonly among the clientele served by family preservation. These efforts are primarily led by child welfare systems and typically are funded by federal, state, and local governments. Typically, interventions are delivered in home and/or are community-based. The focus is on providing practical parenting strategies, crisis management, respite care, "concrete" assistance (e.g., transportation), and assisting the family to access available community resources. Case management is an essential component in coordinating services for families. Case managers usually have small caseloads and provide many hours of service per week (with the assistance of an on-call team for around-the-clock coverage).

Few studies evaluating the effects of family preservation are available; those that do exist often have methodological problems. The available research shows mixed results for family preservation. It appears as though family preservation programs are effective in assisting families in accessing services and in reducing out-of-home placements. Unfortunately, these programs do not improve the long-term outcome of a child staying with his or her family any better than traditional child welfare services (see reviews by Illback, 1994; Oswald & Singh, 1996; Schoenwald & Henggeler, 1999).

As with mental health-focused coordinated services programs, we observe that family-preservation-focused coordinated services programs are good at providing a wide array of services to families, but are equivocal as to whether they actually improve important outcomes. Perhaps this is due to the severe level of problems common to families in which maltreatment has been documented. Another explanation could be that empirically supported interventions might not always be employed once services are accessed. In any event, we believe family-preservation-focused coordinated services programs need continued development and evaluation.

Juvenile Justice-Focused Coordinated Services

The emphasis of programs we review in this section is on improving juvenile justice outcomes by providing coordinated services. Police or juvenile courts usually refer children to these programs because they have committed a crime. Community agencies then provide the services.

One example of comprehensive community-based coordinated services is multisystemic therapy (Henggeler et al., 1998). Multisystemic therapy has often been utilized to provide interventions for adolescents involved in the juvenile justice system and their families. Often juvenile courts refer adolescents to multisystemic therapy. Although this book is geared toward younger children, we think it is beneficial to review the basic strategies of multisystemic therapy because of its effectiveness in dealing with severe adolescents' problems. Multisystemic therapy targets multiple influences of adolescent antisocial behavior. As such, interventions are focused on child, family, peer, school, and neighborhood factors. It incorporates empirically validated procedures (typically practical, behavioral, and family approaches) and is delivered mostly via in-home family sessions with additional school, neighborhood, and community interventions employed as needed. The practitioner provides direct services and acts as a case manager to assist families in accessing other community-based services. Practitioners not only refer adolescents and families for additional services, but also make sure that they actually attend them. The practitioners have low caseloads and are able to provide intensive, time-limited services to adolescents and families over 4 to 6 months. The families receive many hours of contact each week with their practitioner. The families can access flexible 24-hour-a-day, 7-day-a-week programming (through an on-call rotation system).

Henggeler and colleagues have conducted many university-based and public-sector studies with juvenile delinquents who have histories of conduct disorder, substance abuse, and sexual offending (see Henggeler et al., 1998, for a review). Multisystemic therapy has consistently proven to be better than a variety of alternative interventions in reducing adolescent symptoms, out-of-home placement, and recidivism, as well as in improving family functioning. Multisystemic therapy has been proven cost-effective and is able to maintain long-term improvements in the adolescents. We think similar programs could be adapted for use with younger children too.

The Earlscourt Under 12 Outreach Project is a coordinated services program for children (mostly boys) under age 12 who are referred by police because they have committed a crime (Day, 1998; Day & Hrynkiw-Augimeri, 1996; Hrynkiw-Augimeri, Pepler, & Goldberg, 1993). It involves the Earlscourt Child and Family Center, the Toronto Police Department, and a variety of child welfare, educational, and community agencies in Toronto, Canada. After referral, children and families are assessed for the presence of risk factors, and then assigned to various intervention components that are delivered at Earlscourt Child and Family Center or other community agencies. The four main intervention components include a 12-week child social competence training group, a 12-week parent training group, individual befriending (mentoring) that links the children to other community services, and academic tutoring (emphasizing reading). Children and families also have access to crisis intervention, individualized family interventions (to address additional family needs), school advocacy, and victim restitution procedures.

Over 15 years, the Earlscourt Under 12 Outreach Project has served approximately 650 families and has conducted three evaluation studies (Day, 1998; Day & Hrynkiw-Augimeri, 1996; Hrynkiw-Augimeri et al., 1993). The Earlscourt Under 12 Outreach Project has been found to reduce children's externalizing behaviors and associations with antisocial peers, as well as to reduce parents' stress and improve their parenting skills. The effects have been maintained at 6- and 12-month follow-up assessments. At a long-term follow-up assessment, it was determined that over 50% of children who attended the intervention did not have court contact as teens and adults.

The Earlscourt Child and Family Center is currently developing and evaluating a gender-specific program for girls under 12 who are referred after committing a crime. This program, known as Girls Connection, includes a 14-week anger management program, a 14-week parent training program, and daughter–mother groups to promote healthy sexuality and bonding. Other interventions such as those used in the original Earlscourt Under 12 Outreach Project are also employed. Initial program evaluation results showed that after 1 year of intervention, parents reported fewer behavior problems in the girls, improved parenting, and improved daughter–

mother relationships (Madsen, Levene, Pepler, & Andreacachi, 1999). Research is underway to assess the long-term effectiveness of this program.

Juvenile justice-focused coordinated services programs have been shown to facilitate coordination of services and to improve child and family functioning. These example programs not only provide coordinated services, but also use empirically supported interventions within the intervention components. This may account for the clearer pattern of effectiveness for these programs, as compared to the mental health- and family-preservation-focused programs that were previously reviewed.

Community-Based Wraparound Delivery of Comprehensive Coordinated Services

Wraparound is a community-based strategy used to provide interventions to a family involved in coordinated service efforts. It is often used with children and families who are already involved in multiple systems (e.g., child welfare and juvenile justice) and exhibit a severe level of functional problems. Theses families may require the coordinated efforts of many agencies and systems to effect change. Community-based wraparound models of coordinated services are intended to provide an intensive level of services to assist these multiproblem families.

Goldman (1999) defined wraparound as "a philosophy of care that includes a definable process involving the child and family that results in a unique set of community services and natural supports individualized for that child and family to achieve a positive set of outcomes" (p. 6). It begins with an evaluation of child and family needs, and then provides tailored services that cut across practitioners and agencies within a community. The family is a partner with the community-based service providers in developing and carrying out the intervention plan. Essential elements of wraparound are that it be community-based, that individualized strengths-based services and supports be provided, that interventions be delivered in a culturally competent manner, that families be full partners working with a team, that flexible formal and informal community and family resources be tapped, that providers make an unconditional commitment to families, that community agencies and community-neighborhood programs collaborate, and that outcomes be measured (Goldman, 1999).

Burns, Goldman, Faw, and Burchard (1999) summarized available research evaluating wraparound interventions. Sixteen evaluation studies were identified, but only two studies employed a randomized controlled research methodology. The focus was on children with emotional/behavior problems and families with multiple problems. The wraparound process was led by different intervention sectors (e.g., mental health, child welfare, etc.), but involved coordination across service systems. Interventions offered through interagency collaboration included crisis management, individual/

group/family therapies, individualized family case management, medication, respite care, mentors, school consultation, in-home visits, and so on. While many studies reviewed were not scientifically rigorous, they did shed light on the potential of wraparound. Most studies found evidence that children and families engaged in wraparound accessed a wide variety of services. The studies differed on whether this actually resulted in improvements in child and family functioning.

Community-based wraparound could potentially have a significant impact on children and families. It apparently is a good strategy to help families access services, but the interventions offered through it may or may not adhere to best practices; this could account for the differential outcome effects. Obviously, more scientifically rigorous research is needed to further evaluate the potential of wraparound.

Summary

Table 11.2 summarizes the general effects of the selected coordinated services program models. The summarized programs are consistently associated with greater service utilization among families who participate in them. There is mixed evidence, however, that these coordinated services programs actually improve the outcome of children and families. It could be that families end up receiving more services, but that the services received are not always effective. Those coordinated services programs that use empirically supported interventions within it tend to derive better out-

TABLE 11.2. Summary of Selected Coordinated Services Program Models

Models	General effects
Mental health-focused coordinated services	Coordinated mental health services delivered in community and/or school-based agencies results in greater services utilization; there is mixed evidence as to whether child and family functioning is improved.
Family-preservation-focused coordinated services	Coordinated in-home and community-based interventions results in greater services utilization; there is mixed evidence as to whether child and family functioning is improved.
Juvenile justice-focused coordinated services	Coordinated home and community-based empirically supported interventions results in greater services utilization and improved child and parent functioning.
Community-based wraparound delivery of comprehensive coordinated services	Coordinated mental health, in-home, and community-based services results in greater service utilization; there is mixed evidence as to whether child and family functioning is improved.

comes for children and families (see "Juvenile Justice-Focused Coordinated Services" section).

BEST PRACTICES FOR COORDINATED SERVICES PROGRAMS

Up to now we have presented model programs that illustrate how multicomponent and coordinated services programs work. In this section we review the essential components that cut across the different models of coordinated services programming and reveal best practices. In our opinion, the procedures reviewed are applicable in implementing coordinated services programs and can be adapted to deploy multicomponent interventions in the real world.

We derived best practices from seven sources that describe procedures of coordinated services programs. These sources include (1) Stroul and Friedman's (1996) review of methods for developing systems of care; (2) Oswald and Singh's (1996) discussion of emerging trends in children's mental health services; (3) Kutash and colleagues' (Kutash & Duchnowski, 1997; Kutash, Duchnowski, Meyers, & King, 1997) articulation of community-based service programming for youth; (4) Hyde, Burchard, and Woodworth's (1996) presentation of wraparound services in urban settings; (5) Goldman's (1999) suggested practice parameters in implementing community-based wraparound services; (6) Henggeler and colleagues' (Henggeler et al., 1998) description of practice parameters for multisystemic therapy; and (7) August and colleagues' (August, Realmuto, Hektner, & Bloomquist, 2001; August et al., in press), Early Risers integrated service model of prevention. The rest of this section will review best practices in providing coordinated services based on these sources.

Interagency and Family Collaboration

Agencies from mental health, education, child welfare, juvenile justice, medical, and the broader community (e.g., churches, neighborhood centers, recreational programs, etc.) collaborate with each other and the family to provide needed services. As we mentioned earlier, this collaboration could involve practitioners colocating services to another setting, practitioners delivering some services and acting as a case manager, or affiliated agencies working together to provide a continuum of integrated services. Each of these collaborative strategies results in the child and family receiving varying levels of coordinated services.

Practitioners must also collaborate with the family. In most coordinated service models, family members participate in assessments of their strengths and needs, formulation of a plan, and implementation of a plan, and are assessed to determine the effects of the plan on the family. Active family involvement empowers the family. This sense of empowerment likely contributes to them achieving a better outcome.

Typically a "team" is formed consisting of the practitioners (across agencies and service systems) and the family. This team could be several practitioners or multiple practitioners working collaboratively with the family. The composition of the team varies depending on the unique strengths and needs of the family.

Developing Individualized Assessments and Service Plans

An assessment needs to be conducted to determine the strengths and needs of the child and family, as well as to consider the effects of other contextual factors on the family (e.g., peer, school, and neighborhood). It is conducted using standardized assessment procedures and by gathering information from practitioners who are already familiar with the family. The child's strengths and needs are evaluated in the areas of behavioral, social, academic, recreational, and mental health functioning. The strengths and needs of the family are also determined in the financial, legal, safety, cultural, spiritual, vocational, parenting, and family mental health areas. In addition, information is gathered pertaining to the child's peer group, school, and neighborhood. All available data is organized to reflect strengths and needs in the child, family, peer, school, and neighborhood domains. See Chapter 3 for more details on assessment.

The family attends a team meeting to discuss assessment information and develop a service plan. The team comes to a consensus regarding the strengths and needs of the family. Interventions are planned accordingly. The interventions selected for the plan are those that can be carried out within the coordinated services delivery network. A plan is drawn up, referrals are made, and team members decide who is ultimately responsible for implementing different parts of the plan.

The team plans how to monitor the progress of the family over the course of the intervention. It is a good idea to designate specific goals and outcomes for a particular family. This could include reducing the number of school suspensions for the child, enhancing the parenting skills of the parents, improving the social competencies of the child, obtaining affordable housing for the family, enrolling the child in a community-based recreational program, finding a mentor for the child, accessing respite care for the family, and so on. A goal attainment scaling procedure can be used to determine if goals are reached. See Chapter 3 for details on goal attainment scaling and the assessment of intervention effects.

The plan should also account for the eventual improvement of the child and family. There needs to be a procedure in place for transitioning the child and family out of the coordinated services program to a single practitioner or agency who can monitor the child and family over time.

Eventually services are terminated all together once the child and family has made sufficient progress.

Conducting Case Management

Someone on the team assumes the coordinating role of case manager. This could be a practitioner already working with the family or a "family care coordinator" whose main job is to conduct case management. To be most effective, case managers need to have small caseloads to allocate sufficient time necessary to engage families and access needed services for them.

The duties of the case manager can range from making informal telephone calls to attending meetings to organizing a continuum of services for a family. The case manager connects the families to practitioners and agencies in the community and coordinates across them to avoid duplication of services. This person also responds to any crises that may come up. The case manager tracks family participation, and determines whether or not the agencies and practitioners involved in the service plan are following through in providing needed services. Finally, the case manager keeps track of whether or not the child and family are improving. See Chapter 10 for further discussion of case management.

Using Family- and Community-Based Services

A full continuum of community-based services needs to be available when providing services to children with ACP and/or multiproblem children and their families. As we mentioned earlier, the exact interventions a family receives is determined by their own unique strengths and needs. Some families will require practical assistance, such as obtaining financial aid, job training for the parents, mentoring for the child, advocating for the child at school, and so on. Other families will benefit from skills training procedures that improve the child's social competencies and parent and family skills. Finally, institutional interventions provided by mental health, education, juvenile justice, and child welfare systems may need to be accessed for some families.

The interventions need to be accessible and relevant to the family. Accessibility can be increased with an in-home outreach approach or by providing interventions in community settings that are close to the family. Interventions need to be culturally relevant and compatible for the child and family. See Chapter 12 for procedures to use in engaging families and making interventions culturally compatible.

Employing Empirically Supported Interventions within the Coordinated Services Program

The models of coordinated services programming focus primarily on assisting families in accessing services. It is not enough, however, just to make it

easier for families to obtain services. As we previously discussed, coordinated services programming is most effective if it incorporates empirically
supported intervention components. Therefore the intervention components that are eventually accessed need to be empirically supported. We advise that the empirically supported best practice procedures discussed
throughout this book be used in each intervention component.

Providing Standardized and Tailored Services

Several models of coordinated services provide both standardized and tailored services to families. Standardized interventions focus on "generic"
risk factors that are usually observed in a certain population of families.
This might include, for example, addressing common parent–child interaction problems by providing parent and family skills training to all families.
Tailored interventions address unique risk factors that are specific to a family. This might entail a practitioner assessing the needs of a family and then
trying to meet those needs through additional interventions. The combination of standardized and tailored interventions could be potent in assisting
families with multiple problems.

Both the Early Risers and Earlscourt Under 12 Outreach programs
(discussed earlier in this chapter) are programs that illustrate the incorporation of standardized and tailored services. All families in these programs
are offered the opportunity to participate in child social competence training and parent and family skills training. These intervention approaches
target important factors that are relevant to most, if not all, of the participants. These same programs also make provisions to individualize the interventions to each family. Early Risers accomplishes this by providing flexible case management and support to families. Each family is assessed for
strengths and needs and is plugged into additional school- and community-
based interventions. The Earlscourt Under 12 Outreach Project tailors
interventions by determining each families' needs and offering crisis intervention, individualized family interventions, school advocacy, and victim
restitution procedures if indicated. It is noteworthy that both of these programs have achieved good outcomes with the families they have served. It is
possible that the combination of standardized and tailored services may
have something to do with those positive results.

Summary

Table 11.3 summarizes the best practices observed across the different
types of coordinated services programs. The implementation of these best
practices is necessary to effectively bring together many needed services for
children and families confronted with multiple problems and challenges. To
ensure the best outcome for families, it is necessary that best practices be

used in each service component that is brought together in a coordinated services program. The combination of both standardized and tailored interventions within a coordinated services program has great potential.

We recommend that practitioners move toward employing university-derived multicomponent interventions in coordinated services programs. Coordinated services programs will be more effective if they use intervention components that are similar to the ones used in the multicomponent program models described earlier.

CONCLUSION

In this chapter we presented models of multicomponent and coordinated services programs for children with ACP and their families. Those children with higher levels of ACP will undoubtedly require, and potentially benefit from, these comprehensive intervention programs. Practitioners need to provide comprehensive programs to families that focus on multiple domains of child and family functioning and target many risk and protective factors. It is our belief that the university-derived multicomponent intervention programs should inform the development of coordinated services pro-

TABLE 11.3. Summary of Best Practices for Coodinated Services Programs

Procedures	Best practices
Interagency and family collaboration	Unite practitioners from mental health, education, child welfare, juvenile justice, and community agencies with families in coordinated service delivery.
Developing individualized assessments and service plans	Assess child and family needs and strengths to determine what services are indicated; design a plan to make sure needed services are provided.
Conducting case management	Provide active coordination and assistance for each family in accessing services and responding to crises.
Using family and community-based services	Provide a full continuum of in-home and/or locally accessible interventions.
Employing empirically supported interventions within the coordinated services program	Empirically supported interventions must be delivered within each component of a coordinated services program.
Providing standardized and tailored services	It may be efficacious to provide a combination of broad services relevant to all families and specific services to meet the unique needs of each family.

grams. Practitioners in mental health, education, child welfare, juvenile justice, and broader community systems should look to research findings regarding multicomponent interventions to determine the components of coordinated services programs.

We recognize that it is difficult for practitioners to provide the multicomponent and coordinated services programs described in this chapter. We encourage individual practitioners to develop collaborative relationships with other agencies and/or to act as case managers. This would move toward providing the comprehensive interventions that are needed to address the complex problems of children with ACP and their families. We are also cognizant of the fact that current organizational structures within service systems provide a formidable barrier to practitioners intent on implementing these types of programs. Chapter 12 provides ideas on how to make the necessary organizational and systems changes to make comprehensive intervention programs more likely to succeed.

CHAPTER 12

Challenges in Implementing Effective Interventions

Engaging Families
and Coordinating Service Systems

*T*hus far we have presented information and procedures for interventions as if they could always be carried out accoring to plan. But those with experience know that when providing services for children with ACP and their families, and attempting to do so by coordinating across service systems, life often does not go according to plan! In fact, we can predict that there will be challenges in engaging families and making the systems work to accommodate their many needs.

In this chapter we review procedures for meeting challenges in providing effective interventions at the family and systems levels. First we discuss factors that commonly impede families from participating in interventions. Then we present suggestions and strategies to engage families and to make interventions culturally compatible. Next we discuss service systems policies that make it difficult to provide coordinated services to families. In the final section we offer suggestions and strategies to adapt current service systems to better accommodate coordinated services programs. Successfully engaging families and making service systems better coordinated should promote the implementation of effective interventions.

THE FAMILY ENGAGEMENT CHALLENGE

Consensus exists among practitioners and researchers alike that it is hard to engage the families of children with ACP in the intervention process. Up

333

to 70% of children and adolescents in need of mental health services do not receive them, and 40–60% of children and families who initially begin intervention drop out prematurely (Kazdin, 1996b). These utilization and dropout statistics are more pronounced for low SES and minority children as compared to middle-class Caucasian children (Hoberman, 1992; Kazdin, Stolar, & Marciano, 1995). In addition, it is sometimes difficult to get the parents of children with special needs involved in their children's education and participate in important school activities (Lynn et al., 2001).

There are many potential explanations as to why it is difficult to engage families in needed services. Some of the reasons have to do with the families themselves, while others are inherent to the way practitioners and service systems operate. First, the very same risk factors that are implicated in the development and acceleration of ACP in children are also risk factors for intervention failure (Kazdin, 1996b). That is, the risk factors and related stressors that confront many of these families may make it hard for them to participate. Second, parents' attributions about the cause of the "problem" and their expectations concerning what the intervention can accomplish relate to their level of engagement (Morrissey-Kane & Prinz, 1999; Prinz & Miller, 1996). If a parent blames the child or the school for the problem, or thinks the intervention will provide a quick "cure," the parent may eventually disengage because the interventions do not conform to his or her way of thinking. Third, the "burden of treatment" predicts poor mental health services utilization and dropout for children with ACP and their families (Kazdin, Holland, & Crowley, 1997). Factors such as transportation problems, scheduling difficulties, child care, and the demands of participation are formidable barriers that could impede a family's participation in an intervention. Fourth, when it comes to schools, many parents feel unwelcome, experience poor communication with school officials, find it hard to access school staff, and lack direct information on how to be involved (Lynn et al., 2001). Whether schools are actually that way or whether they are mistakenly perceived by parents as that way leads to the same end result: poor parental participation. Finally, many available interventions are not culturally compatible with the families who receive them (Brondino et al., 1997; Dumas, Rollock, Prinz, Hops, & Blechman, 1999; Tharp, 1991). Individuals from varying cultural backgrounds may find some interventions irrelevant or even insensitive if they are not culturally contextualized. We assume that all these challenges are evident when trying to engage families in school, community, and clinic settings.

In the next two sections of this chapter we review strategies and procedures that can be utilized to meet the challenges of implementing effective interventions with children with ACP and their families. We present procedures for facilitating family engagement and making interventions culturally relevant. Our focus is primarily on parents (or other guardians who act as parents). This is because parents are primarily responsible for bringing children to interventions. Moreover, research suggests that parent factors are strongly linked to poor participation in child and adolescent services (Armbruster & Kazdin, 1994). We believe these strategies and procedures are applicable to engaging families in school, community, and clinic settings.

BEST PRACTICES FOR ENGAGING FAMILIES IN INTERVENTIONS

In this section we review information from seven research or service delivery programs to derive best practices for engaging families in interventions. Some of these programs pertain to research where specific engagement and retention strategies have been tested, while others are descriptions of procedures used in intervention programs. The seven programs include (1) Kazdin and colleagues' (Kazdin, 1996b; Kazdin, Holland, & Crowley, 1997; Kazdin, Holland, Crowley, & Breton, 1997) research program addressing factors related to dropout in outpatient treatment of children with ACP; (2) McCay and colleagues' (McCay, Nudelman, McCadam, & Gonzales, 1996; McCay, Stoewe, McCadam, & Gonzales, 1998) evaluation of engagement strategies to increase urban children's utilization of outpatient children's mental health services; (3) Cunningham and colleagues' (Cunningham, 1996; Cunningham, Bremner, & Boyle, 1995) evaluation of a community-based parent program for preschool children with ACP; (4) Prinz and colleagues' (Morrissey-Kane & Prinz, 1999; Prinz & Miller, 1996) discussion of engagement procedures for parents of children with ACP; (5) Webster-Stratton's (1998b) description of delivery methods to enhance participation in parent groups for young children with ACP; (6) Lynn and colleagues' (Lynn et al., 2001) ideas to improve parent involvement in schools; and (7) Henggeler and colleagues' (Henggeler et al., 1998; Henggeler, Pickrel, Brondino, & Crouch, 1996) multisystemic therapy model for hard-to-engage delinquent adolescents and families. These seven programs have focused on engagement with low-income urban families. In the rest of this section we review techniques and strategies that are found in these programs. Other sources that elaborate procedures will also be presented.

Preparing the Family for Intervention

Early contacts with the family can be used to increase the probability of its later engagement in an intervention. In traditional practice the first contact with a family involves gathering assessment information through interviews to determine strengths and needs. The First Interview Engagement Procedure can be used to augment the initial assessment procedure and simultaneously prepare families for interventions (McCay et al., 1996, 1998). In addition to asking the traditional intake questions (e.g., presenting problems, history, etc.), the First Interview Engagement Procedure incorporates four engagement strategies:

1. Introduce self and fully discuss methods and procedures of the intervention.
2. Set the stage for collaboration. Allow child and parents to have input into the intervention plan and listen to the family's "stories."
3. Offer practical and concrete assistance early on in managing crises, and assist the family in negotiating systems.
4. Identify barriers—for example, practical problems such as appointment time, transportation, and child care—and provide solutions. Examine the parents' thoughts and feelings regarding possible previous negative experiences with interventions and practitioners. Consider race and gender differences between practitioner and family and make adjustments to accommodate family preferences.

The specific strategies discussed later in this section expand on how to provide practical assistance, reduce barriers, examine parent thoughts, and the like. The First Interview Engagement Procedure highlights the need to attend to these factors during the initial contact with the family.

An in-home visit can also be used to prepare families prior to participating in an intervention (Capaldi, Chamberlain, Fetrow, & Wilson, 1997). This entails a home visitor fully explaining the program to the family and going over an easy-to-read handout or brochure. The home visitor answers the family's questions regarding the program. The home visitor attempts to establish rapport and a relationship with the family.

Researchers have investigated the utility of early family preparation efforts. The engagement interview, especially if combined with a telephone interview addressing similar issues prior to the first appointment, increases the rates of intervention enrollment and completion better than traditional intake procedures with a clinical focus (McCay et al., 1996, 1998). In-home preparation visits are associated with improved enrollment and subsequent attendance in a prevention program (Capaldi et al., 1997).

Enhancing "Bonding" with a Program

One way to connect a family to an intervention or program is to get them to "bond" with it and the agency where it is delivered. Lynn and colleagues (2001) summarized some recent research on procedures to get parents more involved in schools and create an initial working relationship with them. We think these same strategies would be especially useful in school and community intervention settings. Parents can be invited to "welcoming" events, such as informal open houses and dinner parties, or celebrations prior to and throughout an intervention. Special events that showcase parents' children (e.g., musical performances, skits, art project exhibits) are a particularly good way to draw in parents. Agencies could also sponsor practical information events such as job fairs, health fairs, or broader community meetings. Subsequent intervention activities may be better attended once parents have become familiar with the intervention setting and have developed a sense of belonging in the agency.

Making the agency "inviting" will go a long way in engaging families. This can be accomplished by displaying culturally relevant artwork, providing coffee, having comfortable chairs to sit on, allowing people to use the phone in the lobby, and so on. Prospective "clients" will be drawn to these amenities and will be more likely to return after having experienced them.

Identifying Risk Factors and Barriers Related to Dropout

To facilitate engagement, determine the risk factors present in a family (Kazdin, 1996b). This can be accomplished by gathering information through diagnostic interview and testing procedures regarding child, parents, and family functioning, and organizing the information according to risk factors. Each family can be described by a different risk factor profile. Chapter 3 provides a methodology for assessing risk factors in children with ACP and their families. As the number and magnitude of risk factors go up, so too should the amount of effort that the practitioner puts into engaging the family.

Engagement can be enhanced if potential barriers that could impede a family's participation in interventions are identified. Kazdin and colleagues (Kazdin, Holland, & Crowley, 1997; Kazdin, Holland, Crowley, & Breton, 1997) suggested interviewing parents to assess the following four domains of perceived barriers:

1. Determine a parent's perception of stressors and obstacles that compete with the intervention. These include conflicts with others regarding the merits of intervention (e.g., spouse questions the value of the intervention), and other life stressors and problems that may interfere with participation (e.g., financial stress, housing problems, health concerns).
2. Determine a parent's perception of whether or not the intervention is demanding, confusing, difficult, costly, and/or burdensome. The parent may believe that it will be too much work and effort to participate.
3. Determine a parent's perception of whether or not the intervention

is addressing relevant problem areas and meeting the parent's expectations. The parent may believe the family is not getting what is needed.

4. Determine a parent's perception of a potentially poor relationship with the practitioner. The parent may not feel "connected" to the practitioner.

Identify these barriers and try to reduce them to improve participation and outcome in an intervention (Kazdin, Holland, & Crowley, 1997; Kazdin, Holland, Crowley, & Breton, 1997; Kazdin & Wassell, 1999). Obtain information regarding risk factors and perceived barriers as described above so that engagement strategies can be planned accordingly. The next few sections give ideas on how to reduce risk factors and lessen barriers.

Providing Practical Assistance

It may be necessary to provide practical assistance to reduce stressors so the family will be able to participate in interventions. In particular, addressing immediate family needs and/or broader contextual risk factors that relate to basic needs can be critical for success. For example, the family may need help to find affordable housing, to fill out insurance papers, to obtain mental health services, to advocate for a child who requires special education services at school, or to help a single mother obtain occasional weekend respite care for her children. Other interventions might have to be postponed until the family's basic needs are met.

It is also important to reduce barriers related to the burden of participating in the intervention. This can be accomplished by providing transportation, using flexible scheduling (e.g., evenings and weekends), providing child care, serving meals, maintaining frequent contact through telephone calls, and making home visits if a parent or family misses a meeting. Sometimes incentives are provided, such as paying families a small stipend for attending or offering a chance to win prizes through a raffle drawing.

Practitioners can employ these practical assistance strategies to reduce risks and barriers. The exact strategies used should be based on an assessment of unique risks and barriers for each family. The provision of these practical strategies should increase utilization of the interventions and decrease dropout among children with ACP and their families.

Using Interpersonal and Cognitive Strategies to Enhance Motivation in Parents

What transpires between the practitioner and the parent has much to do with the level of subsequent family participation in the intervention. Prinz and colleagues (Morrissey-Kane & Prinz, 1999; Prinz & Miller, 1996) and

Webster-Stratton (1998b) described the importance of the interpersonal process between the practitioner and parent. They recommend that the practitioner should avoid a "hierarchical" or "expert" communication style. Furthermore, it is counterproductive for the practitioner to offer advice, criticize, use sarcasm, interrupt, or be perceived as inattentive. Such communication patterns and behaviors will be interpreted as blaming and condescending, which could lead to premature termination of the intervention. The practitioner will be much more effective if he or she emphasizes collaboration. It is important to elicit parent input, to listen, to ask questions, and to reflect on what parents say. This type of communication will be interpreted as understanding and sincere. Obviously parents will more likely attend future meetings if they feel understood and think of the practitioner as sincere.

As we mentioned earlier, parent attributions and expectations can adversely influence their participation in interventions. Fortunately, these attributions and expectations can be positively modified through the use of cognitive strategies. One technique is education and reframing. For example, a parent could describe his or her child as "the cause of all the family's problems" when explaining the family's difficulties. A parent with such a viewpoint might not understand why a practitioner would suggest a family-focused intervention and might well drop out if one is started. Therefore educating the parent about the multiple causes of ACP in children may assist the parent in seeing the "big picture," and make the parent more willing to focus on areas other than the child. It may be helpful to reframe the child's behavior as "delays in development," and to suggest that the child can "catch up" through intervention. Or suppose the parent has an expectation that the intervention will "cure" the child and "make the problems go away." The parent with that point of view might stop coming in for services if he or she does not see the child's problems dissipate soon. In this case it may be helpful to educate the parent about the "chronic" nature of ACP problems in children and to indicate that a realistic goal would be to make gradual improvements. Further, it can be facilitative to reframe the intervention as "assisting the child in development" and to indicate that "development in children takes time." If a parent receives accurate information and adopts a developmental perspective about his or her child's difficulties, he or she should understand the problems better and be more amenable to intervention.

Cognitive restructuring is another technique that can be used to modify the way parents think. This involves teaching a parent how to identify his or her own "unhelpful" thoughts (attributions and expectations), understand how these thoughts are unhelpful, and counter them with more accurate and constructive ways of thinking. Cognitive restructuring exercises for parents can be used to accomplish this goal. An example of this approach was described in Chapter 5 (see Figure 5.4). If the parent's attributions and expectations are modified accordingly, it should lead to better participation with an intervention.

Collaborating with Parents and Community Members

Many of the best practice programs we cited earlier state that it is essential to collaborate with parents and community members to allow them to shape the goals and focus of an intervention. Such collaboration should enhance engagement and increase the odds of program completion. It is helpful to obtain input from parents and community members both prior to the onset of an intervention and throughout its implementation.

Webster-Stratton (1998b) provided a good example to illustrate collaboration at the parent level when conducting a parent training intervention. In this program, practitioners collaborate with the parents during each session to allow them to shape the content and overall experience. Parents provide weekly evaluations for each session; they rate the relevance of the content covered and recommend new content they wish to see addressed in upcoming parent groups. Webster-Stratton explained that when parent training interventions are delivered in this fashion, it makes the parents feel empowered, increases their "ownership" of the program, and leads to increased levels of engagement.

Another parent collaboration strategy is to survey parents about what they want to see happening in a school- or community-based program. This empowers parents and also makes the programs more responsive to them. For example, when such surveys have been used previously in schools, parents indicated they wanted academic-related help for their children, extracurricular activities, and after-school programming (Lynn et al., 2001). The survey method of collaboration should lead to greater parent participation if practitioners and agencies respond to the surveys by providing what parents want.

At the community level, Webster-Stratton (1998b) advised the use of an "advisory committee." Taking into account the unique needs of children and families within a given community, this committee suggests ways to shape the intervention. It can be helpful to gain the endorsement of a respected community member to give the program credibility.

Conducting Interventions in Accessible Locations

Many practitioners advocate working with parents in school or community settings to increase intervention accessibility and reduce attrition in families. Cunningham and colleagues (1995), for example, took a previously clinically validated parent training program and recast it for use with larger groups of parents in a community setting. Cunningham and colleagues hypothesized that the community setting would increase availability to a larger number of parents and reduce logistical and psychological barriers that might be associated with clinic settings. They compared a 12-week community-based parent training program to a 12-week clinic-based parent training program and a wait-list control group. Families were randomly assigned to one of the above conditions and then invited to attend the program. The community-based parent training program was found to be superior to the clinic-based parent training program in engagement, cost-effectiveness, and outcome for parents and children immediately following the intervention and at a 6-month follow-up. Cunningham and colleagues found that the community-based parent training program was more effective in engaging immigrant families with English as a second language and families whose children had more severe behavior problems. Those families were more likely to enroll in and to complete the community-based parent training program and to derive a better outcome than those families with similar attributes in the clinic-based program.

If it's hard to get families to an intervention, then it may be wise to bring the intervention to them using an outreach approach. In-home multisystemic therapy has been found to be effective in reducing intervention dropout rates in substance-abusing delinquent adolescents (Henggeler et al., 1996). Perhaps most important is the fact that the intervention is delivered using an in-home outreach approach. The intervention staff have low caseloads so that they can devote much time and energy to engaging families. The intervention staff utilizes flexible scheduling to arrange appointments when they are convenient for the families (e.g., evenings and weekends). All potential barriers are identified and creative strategies are employed to reduce them. Henggler et al. found that 98% of adolescents engaged in in-home multisystemic therapy completed a full intervention, which averaged 130 days of intensive services (average 40 hours of total contact). This was compared to approximately 22% of adolescents completing full or partial intervention through the "usual community services." We think similar outreach methods could be used to engage younger children with ACP and their families.

Summary

Table 12.1 provides a summary of best practices for facilitating family engagement in interventions. Practitioners need to use engagement procedures such as those described here to initiate and maintain a family's involvement in an intervention.

BEST PRACTICES FOR MAKING
INTERVENTIONS CULTURALLY COMPATIBLE

Practitioners cannot assume a "one size fits all" mentality when delivering interventions to diverse groups. Rather, interventions need to be tailored to

TABLE 12.1. Summary of Best Practices for Engaging Families in Interventions

Procedures	Best practices
Preparing the family for intervention	Conduct initial interview to fully explain intervention and begin collaboration regarding its focus; use an in-home information-sharing visit prior to the onset of the intervention.
Enhancing "bonding" with a program	Use "welcoming" events to get parents "in the door"; create an inviting atmosphere to keep them there.
Identifying risk factors and barriers related to dropout	Organize assessment information according to known risk factors and barriers to participation and attempt to reduce them.
Providing practical assistance	Offer assistance related to basic family needs and immediate concerns; provide transportation, flexible scheduling of meetings, child care, meals, incentives, and home visits as needed.
Using interpersonal and cognitive strategies to enhance motivation in parents	Use effective communication when interacting with parents and cognitive strategies to modify any attributions and expectations that may reduce the likelihood of their participation.
Collaborating with parents and community members	Obtain input from families and community members about the content and procedures of an intervention.
Conducting interventions in accessible locations	Use community settings and in-home interventions with hard-to-engage families.

account for cultural differences and be delivered in a culturally compatible manner (Tharp, 1989, 1991). In this section we review general guidelines from researchers and practitioners who employ culturally compatible methods and procedures to engage families in a variety of interventions. Our guidelines are derived from six primary sources: (1) Brondino and colleagues' (1997) efforts to make multisystemic therapy culturally sensitive in treating diverse urban delinquent adolescents; (2) Dumas and colleagues' (1999) procedures to make preventive interventions and research culturally sensitive; (3) Tharp's (1989, 1991) review of cultural diversity in the education and treatment of children; (4) Flanagan and Miranda's (1995) discussion of practices for school psychologists working with diverse families; (5) Mason, Benjamin, and Lewis's (1996) description of the Child and Adolescent Service System Program cultural competence model of service delivery; and (6) McGoldrick and Giordano's (1996) family therapy for families from different ethnic backgrounds. Together these sources enable us to present guidelines to make interventions culturally relevant to participants. Other sources that embellish procedures pertaining to specific cultural groups will also be reviewed.

Understanding the Need for Cultural Contextualization

We begin by defining terms that are commonly used in discussions of cultural contextualization of interventions. "Ethnicity" refers to a group of individuals who share a similar heritage and a mutual identification. It interacts with SES, race, religion, and political ideology to inform how an individual views him- or herself. "Culture" is the personal identity and meaning system that guides the behavior of individuals. It is based on the past and current circumstances of a particular group. "Acculturation" is the extent to which an individual is influenced by a culture of origin or a current majority culture. Levels of acculturation can differ within a group or family. A "minority" is someone who belongs to a group that is low in absolute numbers relative to the majority culture. Minorities often live within the context of socioeconomic disadvantage. Issues related to ethnicity, culture, acculturation, and minority status need to be accounted for in interventions. The broader term "culture" is, however, most often used when articulating procedures to make interventions compatible with individuals from diverse backgrounds.

Our presentation focuses on the most common minority cultural groups in the United States: African Americans, Asian Americans, Latino/ Hispanic Americans, and Native Americans. These cultural groups differ from each other and the majority culture in many ways. The family, defined as a sociocultural socialization unit where norms, values, and behaviors are learned, operates in different ways across these cultural groups. Families differ in terms of parenting and marital roles, kinship patterns, and structure. They also differ as far as cultural practices, customs, and traditions are concerned. People of different groups vary in verbal and nonverbal styles of expression and how they interpret others' behavior. The way in which people from different cultural groups process information may be unique to them. Their beliefs and assumptions influence how they interpret and process ongoing events. The amount and types of stressors can also be unique across cultural groups. Minority cultural groups also experience the stressors of prejudice and discrimination. Socioeconomic disadvantage and different levels of acculturalization within families or groups causes stress. Finally, help-seeking behavior may be different across cultural groups. Some groups prefer to take care of their own problems and seek help from family members, while others may be more inclined to seek help from professionals.

Developing Cultural Awareness

Developing cultural awareness involves understanding self and others. The practitioner must first be aware of his or her own cultural influences and potential biases that can influence his or her perception and behavior. It is

INTEGRATION AND CHALLENGES

also necessary for the practitioner to be aware of cultural differences in others to be able to make appropriate adjustments in the delivery and content of interventions. Through education, reading, and experience, practitioners can accumulate a cultural competence for a given cultural group. It may be helpful to consult cultural informants within a particular community to derive a better understanding of a particular cultural group.

What follows is a brief review of cultural variables that are associated with the families of the primary minority cultural groups in the United States. It is beyond our scope in this book to review the minority cultural groups in detail. Interested readers should consult the works we cite below for more information. These cultural descriptions are global and should not be applied in a stereotypic manner. There will be differences among individuals within each cultural group. We offer this cultural information as a starting point for developing cultural awareness.

African American Families

Black (1996), Moore-Hines and Boyd-Franklin (1996), Paniagua (1994), and Tharp (1991) provided information regarding the African American culture. It is important to note that the African American culture has been influenced by many different ethnic groups of African origin. The African American culture has also been shaped by prior experience in Africa and the United States. The history of slavery, racial discrimination, and inequitable allocation of resources within the current economic system have also influenced African American culture. The family is emphasized. Close friends and extended family (including friends and members of the community) are important. The ideas that women can be providers for the family and work outside of the home are widely accepted. Religion or spirituality is important for most African Americans, whether followers of African-based religions or Christianity. African Americans are said to be spiritual even if they are not practicing an organized religion.

Asian American Families

Lee (1996), Tharp (1991), and Paniagua (1994) described the Asian American culture. Numerous ethnic groups with origins in Asia and the Pacific Islands have influenced Asian American culture. In addition, historical experiences, such as war in different Asian countries, and discrimination in the United States upon immigration have influenced Asian American culture. The family unit is valued over the individual. An individual's behavior is said to reflect on the family unit. The husband is viewed as the authority and leader of the family. The wife is typically thought of as the homemaker, as the child bearer, and as the one who provides nurturance to family members. Older siblings are expected to take care of younger children.

Acculturalization across and within specific ethnic groups in the Asian American community causes stress. Conflict can exist between parents who may have traditional beliefs and children who are influenced by contemporary American beliefs and customs. "Culture shock" is said to be high among Asian Americans who have recently immigrated. Self-control and repression of emotions are valued among individuals in the Asian American community. Individuals typically do not publicly acknowledge their problems. They interact with others in a polite and deferential manner. East Asian-based and Christian religious beliefs are common among Asian Americans. Religion is important to Asian Americans' ethnic identity.

Latino/Hispanic American Families

Garcia-Preto (1996), Tharp (1991), and Paniagua (1994) articulated the Latino/Hispanic American culture. Numerous ethnic groups with origins in Spanish-speaking countries have influenced the Latino/Hispanic American culture. Poverty is highly prevalent among Latino/Hispanic American groups. This cultural group has experienced significant discrimination and disrespect in the United States. Many immigrants have been traumatized by war in their countries of origin and experience significant cultural shock when immigrating to the United States. All these experiences shape the Latino/Hispanic American's ethnic identity. The family unit is very important in the Latino/Hispanic American cultural group. Obligation to family is valued over individual pursuits. The extended family (including friends, godparents, etc.) is important in everyday life. Machismo (aggression and authority) is valued among men and marinismo (submission and servitude) is valued among women in the traditional Latino/Hispanic American culture. The Spanish language is very important in transmitting cultural traditions and customs. Many Latino/Hispanic Americans are Roman Catholic in their religious orientation. Spiritual pursuits are valued over material gain.

Native American Families

Paniagua (1994), Tafoya and Del Vecchio (1996), and Sutton and Broken Nose (1996) have reviewed characteristics of the Native American culture. This culture has been influenced by numerous and diverse Native American tribes, each of which have their own distinct characteristics. Historical traumas, such as the dominate culture taking over Native American lands and attempting to "resocialize" them, as well as current discrimination, have shaped the Native American culture. The family is very important and valued over individual pursuits. The extended family (which includes all adults in the family) is involved in the socialization of children. The roles of grandparents and other elders an valued. Grandparents are often deferred to over the parent in socialization practices. Elders are influential within the family system. Individuals who marry into a family are highly regarded. For example, a legal daughter-in-law functions like a daughter within her married family. The communication style of Native Americans is often indirect. They value listening and show respect for others. Their sense of time is flexible and is not bound by artificial constraints (such as a clock). Native Americans tend to live in the present moment. A sense of community is also important. Individuals share their fortunes and assist each other in times of need. The spirituality of Native Americans has much to do with living in harmony with nature. Christianity can also be important for many Native Americans.

All Cultural Groups

All the minority cultural groups discussed above have music, dance, art, food, and customs that originate in their culture of origin. They also celebrate unique holidays and historical events. Practitioners should be aware of the customs and historical events for the cultural group being served.

Delivering Culturally Contextualized Interventions

The interventions described throughout this book will be better received and more effective if they are culturally contextualized. The same authors who were cited in the preceding section on developing cultural awareness also provided suggestions for making interventions culturally compatible for the families being served. The descriptions of culturally contextualized interventions that follow are global and should be viewed only as guidelines. They should not be applied in an absolute or stereotypic manner.

African American Families

Practitioners working with African Americans would do well to present themselves in a "down-to-earth" manner and communicate respect. They should avoid hierarchical relationships and try to be egalitarian in their style. African Americans profit most from time-limited, problem-solving focused, and child-directed interventions with an active and directive practitioner. It is essential that family and community resources be identified and strengthened.

Asian American Families

Practitioners who approach Asian Americans in a polite, formal, and professional manner will be more likely to achieve success. They should avoid direct eye contact and direct solicitation of emotional expression. Practical family and behavioral treatment approaches are preferred. It is important to engage the family, set goals, and utilize practical strategies to build family strengths.

Latino/Hispanic American Families

An instructing and professional practitioner style is said to be constructive in working with Latino/Hispanic Americans. It is important to listen carefully to clients and allow time for their expression and validation of stories. Traditional family structures should be strengthened and solidified. It may be important to discuss spiritual issues. Typically, the extended family can be productively involved in the intervention process. It is important to use family and behavioral approaches to solve immediate concerns and difficulties. Latino/Hispanic Americans can also profit from problem-focused group therapies.

Native American Families

Native Americans work well with practitioners who are genuine and authentic. They are not as impressed with the practitioner's credentials as they are with his or her personal style. It is important to allow Native Americans to express their cultural identity and for the practitioner to make the effort to understand it. Family approaches are preferred. In particular, it is important to support and reinforce traditional family structures. Concrete and practical strategies are effective. It may also be important to discuss how Native Americans can better cope with the dominant culture.

All Cultural Groups

Several other procedures may be helpful across all cultural groups. One strategy is to match the ethnicity of the practitioner to the families being served. Of course, the importance of this may vary across individuals. Other factors, such as the social class, gender, and age of the practitioner may be equally (or more) important to match with some families. As we previously mentioned, all the minority ethnic cultural groups have unique customs originating in their culture of origin. It is therefore a good idea to incorporate culturally specific arts, foods, customs, and celebrations into the intervention. Allow participants to be involved in shaping culturally referenced nuances into the intervention.

It is important to collaborate with the families being served to determine how the intervention should be culturally contextualized. This can be accomplished by asking individual families for suggestions or by forming a "cultural advisory committee" to advise program developers. Practitioners will be more successful if they obtain input about how a planned intervention fits in with the norms, values, customs, and traditions of a given cultural group, and then make appropriate accommodations.

Summary

Table 12.2 summarizes best practices for making interventions culturally compatible. Interventions will be more effective if they are culturally compatible with the families being served. The guidelines presented here may assist in that effort, but due to individual differences within a group they should not be applied in a stereotypic manner.

THE SERVICE SYSTEM COORDINATION CHALLENGE

We have repeatedly made the case throughout this book that many children with ACP require comprehensive and coordinated services. We defined coordinated services and reviewed issues pertaining to providing them at the family level in Chapter 11. Most practitioners agree that coordinated services are needed. They also agree that it is a great challenge to actually deliver coordinated services, in part because of the organizational and policy-related challenges inherent in current delivery systems.

For a number of reasons, it is difficult to incorporate coordinated services programs into current service delivery systems. First, the professionals who work in existing systems often do not understand coordinated services methods, are comfortable with what they were originally trained to do, and may resist changes. Second, the organizations where professionals currently work can be rigid and set up in such a way that their mandate and purpose

TABLE 12.2. Summary of Best Practices for Making Interventions Culturally Compatible

Procedures	Best practices
Understanding the need for cultural contextualization	Understand influence of ethnicity, culture, acculturation, and minority status on family functioning; take into account differences in language, information processing, stressors experienced, and help-seeking behaviors of families from different cultural groups.
Developing cultural awareness	Understand one's own culture and its influence on perceptions, evaluations, and behavior; learn the cultural influences and practices of each cultural group being served; do not apply this information in an absolute or stereotypic manner.
Delivering cultural contextualized interventions	Utilize strategies that are compatible with specific cultural groups; consider matching ethnicity of practitioner with family participants; incorporate culturally specific arts, foods, customs, and celebrations into the intervention; do not apply these strategies in an absolute or stereotypic manner.

is narrowly defined. Issues related to administrative support, "turf," allocation of staff time, leadership, and adjusting the roles of professionals come into play at the organizational level. Third, existing financing practices provide a formidable barrier to implementing coordinated services programs. Most existing public and private funding mechanisms adhere to categorical funding strategies with strict eligibility requirements that are tied to narrow service system mandates. Finally, many programs do not evaluate the services they provide to make sure they are really addressing the concerns of the families they serve. As a result, agencies may not be providing the most needed services to families.

In the next section we provide an overview of effective program- and policy-level procedures for developing coordinated services programs. It is beyond our scope in this chapter to provide an in-depth review of all the organizational and policy matters related to coordinated services programs. Rather, our goal is to present some of the broader strategies to facilitate development in this important area.

BEST PRACTICES FOR CREATING
COORDINATED SERVICES PROGRAMS

Information from six sources pertaining to program development and policy is reviewed to suggest best practices in developing and maintaining coordinated services programs. These sources are (1) Short's (1997) discussion of education and training of professionals; (2) Friedman's (1994) suggestions for restructuring systems to emphasize prevention and family support; (3) Kutash and Duchnowski's (1997) ideas for creating comprehensive and collaborative systems; (4) Orland, Danegger, and Foley's (1997) and Pasters's (1997) reviews of financial strategies for funding coordinated services programs; (5) Illback, Kalafat, and Sanders's (1997) procedures for evaluating programs; and (6) Oswald and Singh's (1996) presentation of trends in children's mental health service delivery. Together these sources give pertinent information regarding program development and policy issues for coordinated services programs.

Training Professionals in the Methods
of Coordinated Services Programs

Several of the cited best practice sources suggested training parameters for professionals. Educators who teach courses and provide training should be experienced in actually developing and implementing coordinated services programs. The content of training should focus on enhancing practitioners' understanding of the broader needs of children and families and on promoting professional collaboration. Training should stress within-discipline and between-discipline knowledge and skills. Specific training about interagency collaboration, organizational procedures, financial strategies, and program evaluation is essential. Professionals need to be trained in the best practices of coordinated services programs and family engagement such as those detailed in Chapters 11 and 12 of this book. It will also be helpful for professionals to have hands-on practicum experiences and to participate in a coordinated services program. The broad desired outcome of this training is that professionals will have a better understanding of families' needs, problems within the existing service delivery systems, and knowledge of practical procedures that pertain to developing and operating coordinated services programs.

Restructuring Organizational Practices

Changes in organizational practices are needed to accommodate coordinated services programs. To begin with, a change of organizational mandate may be necessary. To coordinate services across agencies, the organization mission needs to move away from a narrow mandate that is system-specific to a broader mandate that entails interprofessional collaboration. Administrators within the organization need to champion the cause of coordinated services to facilitate its development and maintenance. The administration needs to allocate resources such as personnel, time, and money to the coordinated services mission. Practical issues between agencies need to be defined and resolved, including procedures for sharing information, determining where services should be located, and defining the specific roles of different agencies within the larger program. Decision making needs to move away from agency-specific procedures to shared decision making involving families, community members, and other agencies involved in service coordination. Finally, allowances need to be made for ongoing professional development of staff who are involved in these efforts.

Using Creative Financing Strategies

A new vision of how money is spent is needed. Governmental and managed care entities need to move away from primarily financing expensive institutional treatments and move toward financing family-friendly community-based services. In the public financial domain, flexible allocation of funds is needed. Money should be freed from categories of spending. Instead, money needs to be blended across agencies with fewer restrictions. Local governments and agencies should be allowed to make decisions as to where money and resources are allocated. For example, federal block grants can be given to states that allow local communities to make decisions regarding how these resources are allocated. Public monies should also be geared toward funding results-based programs that use program evaluation to show how clients have benefited. This means that money is allocated toward trying to achieve demonstrated outcomes (e.g., reductions in special education placements, reductions in recidivism within juvenile justice systems, etc.). In the private domain, citizens, corporations, and foundations are increasingly funding innovative coordinated services programs with fewer procedural requirements.

Administrators need to access funds to develop coordinated services programs. These include government funds and grants, foundation funds and grants, demonstration project grants, Medicaid, private insurance and managed care monies (Paster, 1997). These funding streams often provide money for children's and family services organizations that can be used to develop and maintain coordinated services programs.

Conducting Program Evaluation

Program evaluation should be utilized from the planning stage through the implementation stage in developing and carrying out a coordinated services program (Illback et al., 1997). Evaluation information can be utilized for purposes of accountability and for determining the outcome of a program. This information can assist in designing and maintaining the program.

Program evaluation should be used at all phases of program development and implementation. At the planning stage, the program is developed and evaluation techniques are determined. Initially, it is important to start with a needs assessment to determine the needs of families in the community being served by the coordinated services program. Interviews or surveys of community informants and/or family members in the community can be used for this purpose. Then specifications of the program need to be articulated. This involves clearly defining what the program is and what aspects of it will be evaluated. It is also important to specify program design components in measurable terms and to identify methods that can be used to evaluate them. Next, evaluators should assess implementation of the program. This determines whether or not the program was executed as planned. Information is gathered to see if the program complied with its original intent. Retrospective monitoring, where staff self-report on implementation, and/or naturalistic monitoring, where evaluators observe the program in operation, can be utilized for this purpose. Finally, outcome evaluation is necessary to determine the effects of the program. Data can be collected to see if consumers were satisfied and derived benefit and to determine whether the program was cost-effective. Information collected via the program evaluation process can be used to modify and strengthen an intervention.

Summary

Table 12.3 summarizes the best practices of program development and policies of coordinated services. We argue that coordinated services programs

TABLE 12.3. Summary of Best Practices for Creating Coordinated Services Programs

Procedures	Best practices
Training professionals in methods of coordinated services programs	Train professionals regarding broader child/family needs, enhance interdisciplinary knowledge, and provide education pertaining to coordinated services program practices.
Restructuring organizational practices	Set up organizations so they have a clear mandate for coordinated services, leadership that supports it, resources allocated to it, shared decision making to implement it, and practical procedures to facilitate it; ongoing staff development should also be a priority.
Using creative financing strategies	Change emphasis of financing patterns from institutional treatment approaches to family-centered community-based systems of care; public financing should emphasize flexible decategorization approaches that are locally determined; private financing should promote innovative coordinated services programs.
Conducting program evaluation	Evaluate coordinated services programs from planning through implementation to determine community needs, whether or not the program was implemented as intended, and whether or not the program achieved desired outcomes.

are necessary to address the complex problems of children with ACP and their families. This type of program holds much promise if organizational structures and effective policy are in place to allow it to happen.

CONCLUSION

This book is primarily about describing effective interventions for children with ACP and their families. Throughout the book we have attempted to present best practices for these effective interventions. Many challenges come up, however, that make it difficult to actually implement these interventions. It seems to us that successfully engaging families, and creating co-ordinated service delivery systems to provide comprehensive interventions, are great challenges faced by practitioners and administrators. This chapter reviewed family engagement and coordinated services program development and policy procedures. These procedures can increase the probability of success in delivering effective interventions to children with ACP and their families.

Epilogue
Future Directions

While we were writing this book, it occurred to us many times that there are gaps related to our understanding of ACP, assessment and intervention methods, and related public policy. In our view, these gaps need to be addressed to go to the next level of providing effective services to children with ACP and their families. We will use this epilogue to suggest areas of focus that need to be pursued in the future.

NATURE OF THE PROBLEM

The heterogeneous characteristics and developmental pathways of children with ACP were articulated in Chapters 1 and 2. Most of the information described came from studies of children (mostly boys) who display physical aggression, defiant behavior, and covert antisocial behaviors. Certainly, progress has been made, but more information is needed to adequately describe differing ACP subtypes and developmental pathways, as well as gender and cultural differences that moderate the relationship between problem behaviors and outcomes. In particular, a deeper understanding is required regarding relational aggression, psychopathy, and various comorbid conditions that exist with ACP. The developmental pathways unique to these different subtypes and comorbid conditions need to be better articulated. This information would assist in making assessment and intervention activities more precise and effective.

We need to know more about risk and protective factors associated with different characteristics and long-term outcomes in children with ACP. Presently, most research provides evidence about the broad relationships among different risk and protective factors and outcomes. More research is required to define specific risk and protective factors that are associated with specific outcomes. For example, it could be that certain risk factors are more predictive of some characteristics of ACP than others, and/or that a certain protective factor buffers the effects of a particular risk factor better than another in a certain subtype of ACP. Assessment and intervention strategies would be modified accordingly to account for this specificity.

ASSESSMENT

Assessment is well developed in terms of defining and measuring global dimensions that relate to ACP. We think, however, that there is much work to be done in the area of assessment. To begin with, there are few well-developed assessment measures that assess less common dimensions and/or ACP subtypes. Although several rating scales exist that assess relational aggression, psychopathy, and reactive/proactive forms of aggression (see Chapter 3), they have limited psychometric and normative data. These rating scales, as well as others that measure different dimensions of ACP, need to be further developed. In addition, it would be useful to have well-developed standardized interview procedures to assess various forms of ACP in children.

More effort needs to be put into developing effective and useful screening procedures. Everyone agrees that children with ACP should be identified as early as possible so that interventions can be administered accordingly. Unfortunately, early screening of children is prone to high levels of false positive and false negative identification of ACP, and may also have limited predictive validity (see Chapter 3). Screening procedures that incorporate both identification of specific problems and delineation of risk and protective factors may improve the utility and predictive validity of screening procedures. Further development in this important area is warranted.

Additional work needs to be done in developing a structured methodology with which to assess and organize the presence of risk and protective factors. Currently, delineation of risk and protective factors is somewhat of a "judgment call." We are not aware of many empirically based decision-making strategies that can be used to articulate all of the many possible risk and protective factors for a child. Development of a methodology to match interventions with the presence or absence of specific risk and protective factors is needed. This would certainly aid in effective intervention planning and intervention.

INTERVENTION

Most of the intervention information presented in this book pertains to children exhibiting overt aggression, covert behavior problems, bullying, and delinquency. We were unable to describe with much specificity those interventions that may be useful for children who exhibit specific problems such as relational aggression, psychopathy, and so on. We fault ourselves for not being specific enough and our tendency to rely on general intervention strategies for a wide variety of children with ACP. Our book does, however, reflect what appears to us to be the state of the art in intervention.

One way to improve this situation would be to develop specific interventions that are useful with specific ACP subtypes and pathways. More information regarding which interventions works with which populations under which conditions would be useful. Moreover, there is a need to evaluate already available interventions regarding their effectiveness with different subtypes of ACP. For example, would parent and family skills training work equally effectively with children exhibiting relational aggression as it does with children exhibiting overt aggression?

We need to continue developing a continuum of community-based coordinated services programs. Currently most existing coordinated services programs focus on assisting families in better accessing services. Not enough attention is devoted to providing empirically supported interventions within the components of intervention that are eventually accessed by the families. Coordinated services programs that incorporate standardized and tailored interventions also need to be further developed. The standardized interventions would deal with generic risks that are common to all children with ACP, while the tailored interventions would focus on specific risks that are unique to each individual child and family. The point was also made in Chapter 11 that coordinated services interventions should be available for children over time as needed. In this regard, well-articulated coordinated service strategies for dealing with children over the course of development need to be developed.

There is a need to better develop and evaluate certain promising interventions that presently have been subjected to only preliminary research evaluation. These include school- and community-based interventions such as mentoring, peer mediation, and violence prevention curriculums. We need not only to determine the effects of these types of programs, but also to better articulate how to actually use these methods in real life practice.

A wide gap still exists between research and practice. Many effective standardized interventions have been developed, but these are relatively infrequently utilized in real-life practice settings. We believe it is possible to use validated and standardized intervention procedures in practice settings. Interventions need to be delivered according to best practices and/or by using existing intervention manuals. The effects of such efforts need to be determined through program evaluation. There is a need to make systematic and administrative changes to allow this to happen (see Chapter 12 for additional suggestions).

Everyone who works with children that have ACP and their families knows that it is hard to engage them in the intervention process. Unfortunately, there is limited empirical research evaluating whether or not certain engagement strategies work better than others do. We believe that improving the engagement level of families needs to become a priority in both research and practice efforts. We need to know which engagement strategies work best with different families. Much more effort needs to be put into developing culturally compatible methods that engage families from diverse backgrounds in interventions.

PUBLIC POLICY

Currently, much research and service delivery dollars are allocated to reactive treatment approaches in multiple services sectors. Often children need to cross a certain threshold of severe levels of problems and dysfunction to access these services. By the time children cross this line, they exhibit severe and entrenched problems that are difficult and costly to treat.

Surely everyone agrees that proactive preventive approaches are better than reactive treatments for children with ACP and their families. Information presented in Chapter 11 revealed that many effective and promising early intervention and prevention methodologies already exist. We strongly believe that emphasis must be placed on preventive activities. We need to develop methods to assess children with ACP and related known risk factors early in life and focus research and intervention activities on early and preventive interventions.

Resources need to be allocated more toward community-based coordinated services. Administrators need to provide continuing education to practitioners, as well as incentives to staff in developing these types of programs. Finally, accountability needs to be a hallmark of practice. Program evaluation would lead to the reduction in use of intervention strategies that do not work and promotion of strategies that do. Program evaluation should be more widely used to determine what really works and what can legitimately be referred to as a "best practice" in real-life settings.

References

Abate, C., Brennan, L., & Conrad, B. (1995). New York's family-centered intensive case management program. In B. J. Friesen & J. Poertner (Eds.), *From case management to service coordination for children with emotional, behavioral, or mental disorders: Building on family strengths* (pp. 277–299). Baltimore: Brookes.

Aber, J. L., Jones, S. M., Brown, J. L., Chaudry, N., & Samples, F. (1998). Resolving conflict creatively: Evaluating the developmental effects of a school-based violence prevention program in neighborhood and classroom context. *Development and Psychopathology, 10,* 187–213.

Abidin, R. R. (1995). *Parenting Stress Index—professional manual* (3rd ed.). Odessa, FL: Psychological Assessment Resources.

Abikoff, H. (1991). Cognitive training in ADHD children: Less to it than meets the eye. *Journal of Learning Disabilities, 24,* 205–209.

Abikoff, H. (2001). Tailored psychological treatments for ADHD: The search for a good fit. *Journal of Clinical Child Psychology, 30,* 122–125.

Abikoff, H., & Klein, R. G. (1992). Attention-deficit hyperactivity and conduct disorder: Comorbidity and implications for treatment. *Journal of Consulting and Clinical Psychology, 60,* 881–892.

Achenbach, T. M. (1991). *Manual for the Child Behavior Checklist/4–18 and 1991 Profile.* Burlington: Department of Psychiatry, University of Vermont.

Achenbach, T. M., Bird, H. R., Canino, G., Phares, V., Gould, M. S., & Rubio-Stipec, M. (1990). Epidemiological comparisons of Puerto Rican and U.S. mainland children: Parent, teacher, and self-report. *Journal of the American Academy of Child and Adolescent Psychiatry, 29,* 84–93.

Achenbach, T. M., & Edelbrock, C. (1986). *Manual for the Teachers Report Form and teacher version of the Child Behavior Profile.* Burlington: Department of Psychiatry, University of Vermont.

Achenbach, T. M., & McConaughy, S. H. (1997). *Empirically based assessment of child and adolescent psychopathology: Practical applications* (2nd ed.). London: Sage.

Ackerman, B. P., Kogos, J., Youngstrom, E., Schoff, K., & Izard, C. (1999). Family instability and the problem behaviors of children from economically disadvantaged families. *Developmental Psychology, 35,* 258–268.

Aguilar, B., Sroufe, L. A., Egeland, B., & Carlson, E. (2000). Distinguishing the early-onset/persistent and adolescent-onset antisocial behavior types: From birth to 16 years. *Development and Psychopathology, 12,* 109–132.

Ajibola, O., & Clement, P. W. (1995). Differential effects of methylphenidate and self-reinforcement on attention-deficit hyperactivity disorder. *Behavior Modification, 19,* 211–233.

Alexander, J. F., Barton, C., Schiavo, R. S., & Parsons, B. V. (1976). Systems-behavioral intervention with families of delinquents: Therapist characteristics, family behavior, and outcome. *Journal of Consulting and Clinical Psychology, 44,* 656–664.

Allen, N. B., Lewinsohn, P. M., & Seeley, J. R. (1998). Prenatal and perinatal influences on risk for psychopathology in childhood and adolescence. *Development and Psychopathology, 10,* 513–530.

American Academy of Child and Adolescent Psychiatry. (1997a). Practice parameters for assessment and treatment of children and adolescents with conduct disorder. *Journal of the American Academy of Child and Adolescent Psychiatry, 36,* 122S–139S.

American Academy of Child and Adolescent Psychiatry. (1997b). Practice parameters for assessment and treatment of children, adolescents, and adults with attention-deficit/hyperactivity disorder. *Journal of the American Academy of Child and Adolescent Psychiatry, 36,* 85S–121S.

American Psychiatric Association. (1994). *Diagnostic and statistical manual of mental disorders* (4th ed.). Washington, DC: Author.

Anastasi, A., & Urbina, S. (1997). *Psychological testing.* Upper Saddle River, NJ: Prentice-Hall.

Anastopoulos, A. D., Shelton, T. L., DuPaul, G. J., & Guevremont, D. C. (1993). Parent training for ADHD: Its impact on parent functioning. *Journal of Abnormal Child Psychology, 21,* 581–596.

Anastopoulos, A. D., Smith, J. M., & Wien, E. E. (1998). Counseling and training parents. In R. A. Barkley, *Attention-deficit hyperactivity disorder: A handbook for diagnosis and treatment* (2nd ed., pp. 373–393). New York: Guilford Press.

Anderson, C. A., Hinshaw, S. P., & Simmel, C. (1994). Mother–child interactions in ADHD and comparison boys: Relationships with overt and covert externalizing behavior. *Journal of Abnormal Child Psychology, 22,* 247–265.

Andrade, A. R., Lambert, E. W., & Bickman, L. (2000). Dose effect in child psychotherapy: Outcomes associated with negligible treatment. *Journal of the American Academy of Child and Adolescent Psychiatry, 39,* 161–168.

Antil, L. R., Jenkins, J. R., Wayne, S. K., & Vadasy, P. F. (1998). Cooperative learning: Prevalence, conceptualizations, and the relation between research and practice. *American Educational Research Journal, 35,* 419–454.

Armbruster, P., & Kazdin, A. E. (1994). Attrition in child psychotherapy. In T. H. Ollendick & R. J. Prinz (Eds.), *Advances in clinical child psychology* (Vol. 16, pp. 81–108). New York: Plenum Press.

Arnold, D. H., Lonigan, C. J., Whitehurst, G. J., & Epstein J. N. (1994). Accelerating language development through picture book reading: Replication and extension to a videotape training format. *Journal of Educational Psychology, 86,* 235–243.

Arnold, D. H., Ortiz, C., Curry, J. C., Stowe, R. M., Goldstein, N. E., Fisher, P. H., Zeljo, A., & Yershova, K. (1999). Promoting academic success and preventing disruptive behavior disorders through community partnership. *Journal of Community Psychology, 27,* 589–598.

Arnold, D. S., O'Leary, S. G., Wolff, L. S., & Acker, M. M. (1993). The Parenting Scale: A measure of dysfunctional parenting in discipline situations. *Psychological Assessment, 5,* 137–144.

Asarnow, J. R., Aoki, W., & Elson, S. (1996). Children in residential treatment: A follow-up study. *Journal of Clinical Child Psychology, 25,* 209–214.

Attar, B. K., Guerra, N. G., & Tolan, P. H. (1994). Neighborhood disadvantage, stressful life events, and adjustment in urban elementary-school children. *Journal of Clinical Child Psychology, 23,* 391–400.

Augimeri, L. K., Webster, C. D., Koegl, C. J., & Levene, K. S. (1998). *Early Assessment Risk List for Boys: Version I, consultation edition.* Toronto: Earlscourt Child and Family Centre.

August, G. J., Anderson, D., & Bloomquist, M. L. (1992). Competence enhancement training for children: An integrated child, parent, and school approach. In S. Christenson & J. C. Conoley (Eds.), *Home–school collaboration: Enhancing children's academic and social competence* (pp. 175–213). Silver Springs, MD: National Association of School Psychologists.

August, G. J., Hektner, J. M., Egan, E. A., Realmuto, G. M., & Bloomquist, M. L. (in press). Effects of family participation rates on proximal outcomes in a community-based, longitudinal prevention trial with children at-risk for substance abuse: The Early Risers program. *Psychology of Addictive Behaviors.*

August, G. J., Realmuto, G. M., Bloomquist, M. L., & Hektner, J. M. (2001). *The Early Risers "Skills for Success" program: A high-risk, high-intensity intervention model for preventing substance abuse in aggressive elementary school children.* Manuscript submitted for publication.

August, G. J., Realmuto, G. M., Crosby, R. D., & MacDonald III, A. W. (1995). Community-based multiple-gate screening of children at risk for conduct disorder. *Journal of Abnormal Child Psychology, 23,* 521–543.

August, G. J., Realmuto, G. M., Hektner, J. M., & Bloomquist, M. L. (2001). An integrated components preventive intervention for aggressive elementary school children: The Early Risers program. *Journal of Consulting and Clinical Psychology, 69,* 614–626.

August, G. J., Realmuto, G. M., Joyce, T., & Hektner, J. M. (1999). Persistence and desistance of oppositional defiant disorder in a community sample of children with ADHD. *Journal of the American Academy of Child and Adolescent Psychiatry, 30,* 1262–1270

August, G. J., Realmuto, G. M., MacDonald, A. W., Nugent, S. M., & Crosby, R. D. (1996). Prevalence of ADHD and comorbid disorders among elementary school children screened for disruptive behavior. *Journal of Abnormal Child Psychology, 24,* 571–595.

Axelrod, S. (1997). *Behavior modification for classroom teachers.* New York: McGraw-Hill.

Baden, A. D., & Howe, G. H. (1992). Mothers' attributions and expectancies regarding their conduct-disordered children. *Journal of Abnormal Child Psychology, 20,* 467–485.

Bank, L., Forgatch, M. S., Patterson, G. R., & Fetrow, R. A. (1993). Parenting practices of single mothers: Mediators of negative contextual factors. *Journal of Marriage and the Family, 55*, 371–384.

Barkley, R. A. (1997). *Defiant children: A clinician's manual for assessment and parent training* (2nd ed.). New York: Guilford Press.

Barkley, R. A. (1998). *Attention-deficit hyperactivity disorder: A handbook for diagnosis and treatment* (2nd ed.). New York: Guilford Press.

Barkley, R. A. (2000). *Taking charge of ADHD: The complete, authoritative guide for parents* (rev. ed.). New York: Guilford Press.

Barkley, R. A., & Benton, C. M. (1998). *Your defiant child: 8 steps to better behavior.* New York: Guilford Press.

Barkley, R. A., & Edelbrock, C. S. (1987). Assessing situational variation in children's problem behaviors: The Home and School Situations Questionnaires. In R. J. Prinz (Ed.), *Advances in behavioral assessments of children and families* (Vol. 3, pp. 157–176). New York: JAI Press.

Barkley, R. A., Fischer, M., Edelbrock, C., & Smallish, L. (1991). The adolescent outcome of hyperactive children diagnosed by research criteria: III. Mother–child interactions, family conflicts and maternal psychopathology. *Journal of Child Psychology and Psychiatry, 32*, 233–255.

Barkley, R. A., Shelton, T. L., Crosswait, C., Moorehouse, M., Fletcher, K., Barrett, S., Jenkins, L., & Metevia, L. (2000). Multi-method psycho-educational intervention for preschool children with disruptive behavior: Preliminary results at post-treatment. *Journal of Child Psychology and Psychiatry, 41*, 319–332.

Battistich, V. (2000). *Effects of an elementary school intervention on students' involvement in positive and negative behaviors during middle school: Preliminary findings from a follow-up study of the child development project.* Paper presented at the meeting of the Society for Research on Adolescence, Chicago.

Battistich, V., Watson, M., Solomon, D., Schaps, E., & Solomon, J. (1991). The Child Development Project: A comprehensive program for the development of prosocial character. In W. M. Kurtines & J. L. Gewirtz (Eds.), *Handbook of moral behavior and development* (pp. 1–34). Hillsdale, NJ: Erlbaum.

Bay-Hintz, A. K., Peterson, R. F., & Quilitch, R. (1994). Cooperative games: A way to modify aggressive and cooperative behaviors in young children. *Journal of Applied Behavior Analysis, 27*, 435–446.

Bear, G. G. (1998). School discipline in the United States: Prevention, correction, and long-term social development. *School Psychology Review, 27*, 14–32.

Becker, W. C., & Carnine D. W. (1980). Direct instruction: An effective approach to educational intervention with the disadvantaged and low performers. In B.B. Lahey & A. E. Kazdin (Eds.), *Advances in clinical child psychology* (Vol. 3, pp. 429–473). New York: Plenum Press.

Beelmann, A., Pfingsten, U., & Losel, F. (1994). Effects of training social competence in children: A meta-analysis of recent evaluation studies. *Journal of Clinical Child Psychology, 23*, 260–271.

Bellak, L., & Bellak, S. S. (1966). *CAT-H: Children's Apperception (human figure) manual.* Larchmont, NY: C.P.S.

Bengtson, M. L., & Boll, T. J. (2001). Neuropsychological assessment of the child. In C. E. Walker & M. C. Roberts (Eds.), *Handbook of clinical child psychology* (3rd ed., pp. 151–171). New York: Wiley.

Bennett, K. J., Lipman, E. L., Brown, S., Racine, Y., Boyle, M. N., & Offord, D. R. (1999). Predicting conduct problems: Can high-risk children be identified in kindergarten and grade 1? *Journal of Consulting and Clinical Psychology, 67*, 470–480.

Bennett, K. J., Lipman, E. L., Racine, Y., & Offord, D. R. (1998). Do measures of externalizing behaviour in normal populations predict later outcomes? Implications for targeted interventions to prevent conduct disorder. *Journal of Child Psychology and Psychiatry and Allied Disciplines, 39*, 1059–1070.

Benson, P. L., Scales, P. C., Leffert, N., & Roehlkepartain, E. C. (1999). *Fragile foundation: The state of developmental assets among American youth.* Minneapolis, MN: Search Institute.

Berkowitz, L. (1994). Guns and youth. In L. D. Eron, J. H. Gentry, & P. Schlegel (Eds.), *Reason to hope: A psychological perspective on violence and youth* (pp. 251–280). Washington, DC: American Psychological Association.

Bickett, L. R., Milich, R., & Brown, R. T. (1996). Attributional styles of aggressive boys and their mothers. *Journal of Abnormal Child Psychology, 24*, 457–472.

Bickman, L. (1996). A continuum of care: More is not always better. *American Psychologist, 51*, 698–701.

Bickman, L., Lambert, E. W., Andrade, A. R., & Penaloza, R. V. (2000). The Fort Bragg continuum of care for children and adolescents: Mental health outcomes over 5 years. *Journal of Consulting and Clinical Psychology, 68*, 710–716.

Biederman, J., Faraone, S. V., Chu, M. P., & Wozniak, J. (1999). Further evidence of a bidirectional overlap between juvenile mania and conduct disorder in children. *Journal of American Academy of Child and Adolescent Psychiatry, 38*, 468–476.

Biederman, J., Faraone, S. V., Hatch, M., Mennin, D., Taylor, A., & George, P. (1997). Conduct disorder with and without mania in a referred sample of ADHD children. *Journal of Affective Disorders, 44*, 177–188.

Biederman, J., Faraone, S. V., Mick, E., Wozniak, J., Chen, L., Ouellette, C., Marrs, A., Moore, P., Garcia, J., Mennin, D., & Lelon, E. (1996). Attention-deficit hyperactivity disorder and juvenile mania: An overlooked comorbidity? *Journal of the American Academy of Child and Adolescent Psychiatry, 35*, 997–1008.

Biederman, J., Mick, E., Faraone, S. V., & Burback, M. (2001). Patterns of remission and symptom decline in conduct disorder: A four-year prospective study of an ADHD sample. *Journal of the American Academy of Child and Adolescent Psychiaty, 40*, 290–298.

Biederman, J., Wilens, T., Mick, E., Spencer, T., & Faraone, S. V. (1999). Pharmacotherapy of attention-deficit/hyperactivity disorder reduces risk for substance use disorder. *Pediatrics, 104*, 1–5.

Bierman, K. L. (1983). Cognitive development and clinical interview with children. In B. B. Lahey & A. E. Kazdin (Eds.), *Advances in clinical child psychology* (Vol. 6, pp. 217–250). New York: Plenum Press.

Bierman, K. L., & Furman, W. (1984). The effects of social skills training and peer involvement on social adjustment of preadolescents. *Child Development, 55*, 151–162.

Bierman, K. L., Greenberg, M. T., & Conduct Problems Prevention Research Group (1996). Social skills training in the Fast Track program. In R. D. Peters & R. J. McMahon (Eds.), *Preventing childhood disorders, substance abuse, and delinquency* (pp. 65–89). Thousand Oaks, CA: Sage.

Bierman, K. L., Miller, C. M., & Stabb, S. P. (1987). Improving the social behavior and peer acceptance of rejected boys: Effects of social skill training. *Journal of Consulting and Clinical Psychology, 55,* 194–200.

Bierman, K. L., Smoot, D. L., & Aumiller, K. (1993). Characteristics of aggressive-rejected, aggressive (nonrejected), and rejected (nonaggressive) boys. *Child Development, 64,* 139–151.

Bihm, E. M., Poindexter, A. R., & Warren, E. R. (1998). Aggression and psychopathology in persons with severe or profound mental retardation. *Research in Developmental Disabilities, 19,* 423–438.

Bird, H. R. (1999). The assessment of functional impairment. In D. Shaffer, C. P. Lucas, & J. E. Richters (Eds.), *Diagnostic assessment in child and adolescent psychopathology* (pp. 209–229). New York: Guilford Press.

Bird, H. R., & Gould, M. (1995). The use of diagnostic instruments and global measures of functioning in child psychiatry epidemiological studies. In F. C. Verhulst & H. M. Koot (Eds.), *The epidemiology of child and adolescent psychopathology* (pp. 86–103). New York: Oxford University Press.

Black, L. (1996). Families of African origin: An overview. In M. McGoldrick, J. Giordano, & J. K. Pearce (Eds.), *Ethnicity and family therapy* (2nd ed., pp. 57–65). New York: Guilford Press.

Blanz, B., & Schmidt, M. H. (2000). Practitioner review: Preconditions and outcomes of inpatient treatment in child and adolescent psychiatry. *Journal of Child Psychology and Psychiatry, 41,* 703–712.

Bloomquist, M. L. (1996). *Skills training for children with behavior disorders: A parent and therapist guidebook.* New York: Guilford Press.

Bloomquist, M. L., August, G. J., Brombach, A. M., Anderson, D., & Skare, S. S. (1996). Maternal facilitation of children's problem solving: Relationship to disruptive child behavior and maternal characteristics. *Journal of Clinical Child Psychology, 25,* 308–316.

Bloomquist, M. L., August, G. J., Cohen, C., Doyle, A., & Everhart, K. (1997). Social problem-solving in hyperactive-aggressive children: How and what they think in conditions of automatic and controlled processing. *Journal of Clinical Child Psychology, 26,* 172–180.

Bolger, K. E., Patterson, C. J., Thompson, W. W., & Kupersmidt, J. B. (1995). Psychosocial adjustment among children experiencing persistent and intermittent family economic hardship. *Child Development, 66,* 1107–1129.

Botting, N., Powls, A., Cooke, R., & Marlow, N. (1997). Attention deficit hyperactivity disorder and other psychiatric outcomes in very low birth weight children at 12 years. *Journal of Child Psychology and Psychiatry, 38,* 931–941.

Boyle, M. H., & Pickles, A. R. (1997). Influence of maternal depressive symptoms on ratings of childhood behavior. *Journal of Abnormal Child Psychology, 25,* 399–412.

Braswell, L. (1998). Self-regulation training for children with ADHD: Response to Harris and Schmidt. *ADHD Report, 6,* 1–3.

Braswell, L. (1995). Cognitive-behavioral approaches in the classroom. In S. Goldstein, *Understanding and managing children's classroom behavior* (pp. 319–355). New York: Wiley.

Braswell, L., & Bloomquist, M. L. (1991). *Cognitive-behavioral therapy with ADHD children: Child, family, and school interventions.* New York: Guilford Press.

Brestan, E. V., & Eyberg, S. M. (1998). Effective psychosocial treatments of conduct-disordered children and adolescents: 29 years, 82 studies, and 5272 kids. *Journal of Clinical Child Psychology, 27,* 180–189.

Brigham, T. A. (1992). A brief commentary on the future of self-management interventions in education. *School Psychology Review, 21,* 264–268.

Brody, G. H., & Flor, D. L. (1997). Maternal psychological functioning, family processes, and child adjustment in rural, single-parent, African-American families. *Developmental Psychology, 33,* 1000–1011.

Brondino, M. D., Henggeler, S., Rowland, M. D., Pickrel, S. G., Cunningham, P. B., & Schoenwald, S. K. (1997). Multisystemic therapy and the minority client: Culturally responsive and clinically effective. In D. K. Wilson, J. R. Rodrigue, & W. C. Taylor (Eds.), *Adolescent health promotion in minority populations* (pp. 92–117). Washington, DC: American Psychiatric Association Books.

Bronfenbrenner, U. (1979). *The ecology of human development.* Cambridge, MA: Harvard University Press.

Brook, J. S., Balka, E. B., Brook, D. W., Win, P. T., & Gursen, M. D. (1998a). Drug use among African-Americans: Ethnic identity as a protective factor. *Psychological Reports, 83,* 1427–1446.

Brook, J. S., Whiteman, M., Balka, E. B., Win, P. T., & Gursen, M. D. (1998b). Drug use among Puerto Ricans: Ethnic identity as a protective factor. *Hispanic Journal of Behavioral Sciences, 20,* 241–254.

Brook, J. S., Whiteman, M., Finch, S. J., & Cohen, P. (1996). Young adult drug use and delinquency: Childhood antecedents and adolescent mediators. *Journal of the American Academy of Child and Adolescent Psychiatry, 35,* 1584–1592.

Brophy, J., & Good, T. L. (1986). Teacher behavior and student achievement. In M. C. Wittrock (Ed.), *Handbook of research on teaching* (3rd ed., pp. 328–375). New York: Macmillan.

Brown, K., Atkins, M. S., Osborne, M. L., & Milnamow, M. (1996). A revised teacher rating scale for reactive and proactive aggression. *Journal of Abnormal Child Psychology, 24,* 473–480.

Buck, J. N. (1948). The House–Tree–Person technique: A qualitative and quantitative scoring manual. *Journal of Clinical Psychology, 4,* 317–396.

Buckner, J. C., Bassuk, E. L., Weinreb, L. F., & Brooks, M. G. (1999). Homelessness and its relation to the mental health and behavior of low-income school-age children. *Developmental Psychology, 35,* 246–257.

Burns, B. J., Farmer, E. M. Z., Angold, A., Costello, E. J., & Behar, L. (1996). A randomized trial of case management for youths with serious emotional disturbance. *Journal of Clinical Child Psychology, 25,* 476–486.

Burns, B. J., & Goldman, S. K. (Eds.). (1999). *Systems of care: Promising practices in children's mental health, 1998 Series: Vol. IV: Promising practices in wraparound for children with serious emotional disturbance and their families* [Online]. Washington, DC: Center for Effective Collaboration and Practice, American Institute for Research. Available: www.air-dc.org/cecp/promisingpractices/1998monographs/documents.htm#4

Burns, B. J., Goldman, S. K., Faw, L., & Burchard, J. (1999). The wraparound evidence base. In B. J. Burns & S. K. Goldman (Eds.), *Systems of care: Promising practices in children's mental health, 1998 series: Vol. IV. Promising practices in wraparound for children with serious emotional disturbance and their families* [Online]. Washington, DC: Center for Effective Collaboration and Practice, American Institute for Research. Available: www.air-dc.org/cecp/promisingpractices/1998monographs/documents.htm#4

Burns, B. J., Gwaltney, E. A., & Bishop, G. K. (1995). Case management research: Issues and directions. In B. J. Friesen & J. Poertner (Eds.), *From case management to service coordination for children with emotional, behavioral, or mental disorders: Building on family strengths* (pp. 353–372). Baltimore: Brookes.

Burton, D. L., Nesmith, A. A., & Badten, L. (1997). Clinicians' views on sexually aggressive children and their families: A theoretical exploration. *Child Abuse and Neglect, 21,* 157–170.

Cadoret, R. J., Leve, L. D., & Devor, E. (1997). Genetics of aggressive and violent behavior. *Psychiatric Clinics of North America, 20,* 301–322.

Cadoret, R. J., Yates, W. R., Troughton, E., Woodsworth, G., & Stewart, M. A. (1995). Genetic–environmental interaction in the genesis of aggressivity and conduct disorders. *Archives of General Psychiatry, 52,* 916–924.

Cameron, J., & Pierce W. D. (1994). Reinforcement, reward, and intrinsic motivation: A meta-analysis. *Review of Educational Research, 64,* 363–423.

Campbell, S. B. (1995). Behavior problems in preschool children: A review of recent research. *Journal of Child Psychology and Psychiatry, 36,* 113–149.

Campis, L. K., Lynam, R. D., & Prentice-Dunn, S. (1986). The parental locus of control scale: Development and validation. *Journal of Clinical Child Psychology, 15,* 260–267.

Canter, A. S. (1997). The future of intelligence testing in the schools. *School Psychology Review, 26,* 255–261.

Capaldi, D. M., Chamberlain, P., Fetrow, R. A., & Wilson, J. E. (1997). Conducting ecologically valid prevention research: Recruiting and retaining a "whole village" in multimethod, multiagent studies. *American Journal of Community Psychology, 25,* 471–492.

Capaldi, D. M., & Patterson, G. R. (1991). Relation of parental transitions to boys' adjustment problems: I. A linear hypothesis. II. Mothers at risk for transitions and unskilled parenting. *Developmental Psychology, 27,* 489–504.

Carlson, C. L., Lahey, B. B., Frame, C. L., Walker, J., & Hynd, G. W. (1987). Sociometric status of clinic-referred children with attention deficit disorders with and without hyperactivity. *Journal of Abnormal Child Psychology, 15,* 537–547.

Carlson, G. A. (1998). Mania and ADHD: Comorbidity or confusion? *Journal of Affective Disorders, 51,* 177–187.

Carr, S. C., & Punzo, R. P. (1993). The effects of self-monitoring of academic accuracy and productivity on the performance of students with behavioral disorders. *Behavioral Disorders, 19,* 241–250.

Carter, J. F. (1993, Spring). Self-management: Education's ultimate goal. *Teaching Exceptional Children,* pp. 28–32.

Catalano, R. F., Arthur, M. W., Hawkins, D. J., Berglund, L., & Olson, J. J. (1998). Comprehensive community- and school-based interventions to prevent antisocial behavior. In R. Loeber & D. P. Farrington (Eds.), *Serious and violent juvenile offenders: Risk factors and successful interventions* (pp. 248–283). Thousand Oaks, CA: Sage.

Center for Effective Collaboration and Practice. (1998). *Addressing student problem behavior: An IEP team's introduction to functional behavioral assessment and behavior intervention plans* [Online]. Available: www.air-dc.org/cecp/cecp.html

Chamberlain, P. (1996). Intensified foster care: Multi-level treatment for adolescents with conduct disorders in out-of-home care. In E. D. Hibbs & P. S. Jensen (Eds.), *Psychosocial treatments for child and adolescent disorders: Empirically based strategies for clinical practice* (pp. 475–495). Washington, DC: American Psychological Association.

Chamberlain, P., & Mihalic, S. F. (1998). *Multidimensional treatment foster care.* Boulder: Institute of Behavioral Science, University of Colorado.

Chamberlain, P., & Reid, J. B. (1998). Comparison of two community alternatives to incarceration for chronic juvenile offenders. *Journal of Consulting and Clinical Psychology, 66,* 624–633.

Chandler, M. (1973). Egocentrism and antisocial behavior: The assessment and training of social perspective-taking skills. *Developmental Psychology, 9,* 326–332.

Charlebois, P., Leblanc, M., Gagnon, C., & Larivee, S. (1994). Methodological issues in multiple-gating screening procedures for antisocial behaviors in elementary students. *Remedial and Special Education, 15,* 44–54.

Chilcoat, H. D., & Anthony, J. C. (1996). Impact of parent monitoring on initiation of drug use through late childhood. *Journal of the American Academy of Child and Adolescent Psychiatry, 35,* 91–100.

Christenson, S. L. (1995). Best practices in supporting home–school collaboration. In A. Thomas & J. Grimes (Eds.), *Best practices in school psychology–III* (pp. 253–267). Washington, DC: National Association of School Psychologists.

Christenson, S. L., & Buerkle, K. (1999). Families as educational partners for children's school success: Suggestions for school psychologists. In C. R. Reynolds & T. B. Gutkin (Eds.), *The handbook of school psychology* (3rd ed., pp. 709–744). New York: Wiley.

Christenson, S. L., Hurley, C. M., Sheridan, S. M., & Fenstermacher, K. (1997). Parents' and school psychologists' perspectives on parent involvement activities. *School Psychology Review, 26,* 111–130.

Christenson, S. L., Rounds, T., & Franklin, M. J. (1992). Home–school collaboration: Effects, issues, and opportunities. In S. L. Christenson & J. C. Conoley (Eds.), *Home–school collaboration: Enhancing children's academic and social competence* (pp. 67–83). Silver Spring, MD: National Association of School Psychologists.

Christenson, S. L., Ysseldyke, J. E., & Thurlow, M. L. (1989). Critical instructional factors for students with mild handicaps: An integrative review. *Remedial and Special Education, 10,* 21–31.

Christian, R. E., Frick, P. J., Hill, N. L., Tyler, L., & Frazer, D. R. (1997). Psychopathy and conduct problems in children: II. Implications for subtyping children with conduct problems. *Journal of the American Academy of Child and Adolescent Psychiatry, 36,* 233–241.

Cicchetti, D. (1994). Integrating developmental risk factors: Perspectives from developmental psychopathology. In C. Nelson (Ed.), *Minnesota Symposia on Child Psychology: Vol. 27. Threats to optimal development: Integrating biological, psychological, and social risk factors* (pp. 229–272). Hillsdale, NJ: Erlbaum.

Clark, R. M. (1983). *Family life and school achievement.* Chicago: University of Chicago Press.

Coie, J. D., & Dodge, K. A. (1998). Aggression and antisocial behavior. In W. Damon (Ed.), *Handbook of child psychology: Vol. 3. Social emotional, and personality development* (5th ed., pp. 779–862). New York: Wiley.

Coie, J. D., Dodge, K. A., & Kupersmidt, J. B. (1990). Peer group behavior and social status. In S. R. Asher & J. D. Coie (Eds.), *Peer rejection in childhood* (pp. 17–59). New York: Cambridge University Press.

Coie, J. D., Dodge, K. A., Terry, R., & Wright, R. (1991). The role of aggression in peer relations: An analysis of aggression episodes in boys' play group. *Child Development, 62,* 812–826.

Coie, J., Terry, R., Lenox, K., Lochman, J., & Hyman, C. (1995). Childhood peer rejection and aggression as predictors of stable patterns of adolescent disorder. *Development and Psychopathology, 7,* 697–713.

Cole, C. L., & Bambara, L. M. (1992). Issues surrounding the use of self-management interventions in the schools. *School Psychology Review, 21,* 193–201.

Coleman, M., & Vaughn, S. (2000). Reading interventions for students with emotional/behavioral disorders. *Behavioral Disorders, 25,* 93–104.

Coltoff, P. (1998). *Community schools: Educational reform and partnership with our nation's social service agencies.* Washington, DC: Child Welfare League of America Press.

Colvin, G., Kameenui, E. J., & Sugai, G. (1993). Reconceptualizing behavior management and school-wide discipline in general education. *Education and Treatment of Children, 16,* 361–381.

Colvin, G., Sugai, G., Good III, R. H., & Lee, Y.-Y. (1997). Using active supervision and precorrection to improve transition behaviors in an elementary school. *School Psychology Quarterly, 12,* 344–363.

Comer, J. P. (1980). *School power: Implications of an intervention project.* New York: Free Press.

Comer, J. P., Haynes, N. M., Joyner, E. T., & Ben-Avie, M. (1996). *Rallying the whole village: The Comer process for reforming education.* New York: Teachers College Press.

Conduct Problems Prevention Research Group. (1992). A developmental and clinical model for the prevention of conduct disorders: The Fast Track program. *Development and Psychopathology, 4,* 509–527.

Conduct Problems Prevention Research Group. (1999a). Initial impact of the Fast Track prevention trial for conduct problems: II. Classroom effects. *Journal of Consulting and Clinical Psychology, 67,* 648–657.

Conduct Problems Prevention Research Group. (1999b). Initial impact of the Fast Track prevention trial for conduct problems: I. The high-risk sample. *Journal of Consulting and Clinical Psychology, 67,* 631–647.

Conduct Problems Prevention Research Group. (2000). Merging universal and indicated prevention programs: The Fast Track model. *Addictive Behaviors, 25,* 913–927.

Connor, D. F., Melloni, R. H., & Harrison, R. J. (1998). Overt categorical aggression in referred children and adolescents. *Journal of the American Academy of Child and Adolescent Psychiatry, 37,* 66–73.

Connors, C. K. (2000). *Conners' Rating Scales—Revised: Technical manual.* North Tonawanda, NY: Multi-Health Systems.

Conrad, M., & Hammen, C. (1989). Role of maternal depression in perceptions of child maladjustment. *Journal of Consulting and Clinical Psychology, 57,* 663–667.

Cook, E. T., Greenberg, M. T., & Kusche, C. A. (1994). The relations between emotional understanding, intellectual functioning, and disruptive behavior problems in elementary-school aged children. *Journal of Abnormal Child Psychology, 22,* 205–219.

Cook, T. D., Hunt, H. D., & Murphy, R. F. (1998). *Comer's School Development Program in Chicago: A theory-based evaluation.* Evanston, IL: Institute for Policy Research, Northwestern University.

Cook, S. B., Scruggs, T. E., Mastropieri, M. A., & Casto, G. C. (1985–1986). Handicapped students as tutors. *Journal of Special Education, 19,* 483–491.

Craig, W. M. (1998). The relationship among bullying, victimization, depression, anxiety, and aggression in elementary school children. *Personality and Individual Differences, 24,* 123–130.

Crawford, D., & Bodine, R. (1996). *Conflict resolution education: A guide to implementing programs in schools, youth-serving organizations, and community and juvenile justice settings: Program report.* Washington, DC: Office of Juvenile Justice and Delinquency Prevention, U.S. Department of Justice and Office of Elementary and Secondary Education, U.S. Department of Education.

Crick, N. R. (1995). Relational aggression: The role of intent attributions, feelings of distress, and provocation type. *Development and Psychopathology, 7,* 313–322.

Crick, N. R. (1996). The role of relational aggression, overt aggression, and prosocial behavior in the prediction of children's future social adjustment. *Child Development, 67,* 2317–2327.

Crick, N. R. (1997). Engagement in gender normative versus gender non-normative forms of aggression: Links to social-psychological adjustment. *Developmental Psychology, 33,* 610–617.

Crick, N., Bigbee, M. A., & Howes, C. (1996). Gender differences in children's normative beliefs about aggression: How do I hurt thee? Let me count the ways. *Child Development, 67,* 1003–1014.

Crick, N., Casas, J. F., & Mosher, M. (1997). Relational and overt aggression in preschool. *Developmental Psychology, 33,* 579–588.

Crick, N. R., & Dodge, K. A. (1994). A review and reformulation of social information-processing mechanisms in children's social adjustment. *Psychological Bulletin, 115,* 74–101.

Crick, N. R., & Dodge, K. A. (1996). Social information-processing mechanisms in reactive and proactive aggression. *Child Development, 67,* 993–1002.

Crick, N. R., & Grotpeter, J. K. (1995). Relational aggression, gender, and social-psychological adjustment. *Child Development, 66,* 710–722.

Crick, N. R., & Werner, N. E. (1998). Response decision processes in relational and overt aggression. *Child Development, 69,* 1630–1639.

Crockenberg, S., & Covey, S. L. (1991). Marital conflict and externalizing behavior in children. In D. Cicchetti & S. L. Toth (Eds.), *Rochester Symposium on Developmental Psychopathology* (pp. 235–260). Rochester, NY: University of Rochester Press.

Cummings, E. M., Davies, P. T., & Campbell, S. B. (2000). *Developmental psychopathology and family process: Theory, research, and clinical implications.* New York: Guilford Press.

Cummings, E. M., Iannotti, R. J., & Zahn-Waxler, C. (1989). Aggression between peers in early childhood: Individual continuity and developmental change. *Child Development, 60,* 887–895.

Cunningham, C. E. (1996). Improving availability, utilization and cost efficacy of parent training programs for children with disruptive behavior disorders. In R. D. Peters & R. J. McMahon (Eds.), *Preventing childhood disorders, substance abuse, and delinquency* (pp. 144–160). Thousand Oaks, CA: Sage.

Cunningham, C. E., Bremner, R., & Boyle, M. (1995). Large group community-based parenting programs for families of preschoolers at risk for disruptive behavior disorders: Utilization, cost effectiveness, and outcome. *Journal of Child Psychology and Psychiatry, 36,* 1141–1159.

Cunningham, C. E., & Cunningham, L. J. (1998). Student-mediated conflict resolution programs. In R. A. Barkley, *Attention-deficit/hyperactivity disorder: A handbook for diagnosis and treatment* (2nd ed., pp. 491–509). New York: Guilford Press.

Cunningham, C. E., Cunningham, L. J., Martorelli, V., Tran, A., Young, J., & Zacharias, R. (1998). The effects of primary division, student-mediated conflict resolution programs on playground aggression. *Journal of Child Psychology and Psychiatry, 39,* 653–662.

Dana, R. H. (1993). *Multicultural assessment perspectives for professional psychology.* Boston: Allyn & Bacon.

Dana, R. H. (1998). Cultural identity assessment of culturally diverse groups. *Journal of Personality Assessment, 70,* 1–16.

Dansforth, J. S., Barkley, R. A., & Stokes, T. F. (1991). Observations of parent–child interactions with hyperactive children: Research and clinical implications. *Clinical Psychology Review, 11,* 703–727.

David, C. F., & Kistner, J. A. (2000). Do positive self-perceptions have a "dark side"? Examination of the link between perceptual bias and aggression. *Journal of Abnormal Child Psychology, 28,* 327–337.

Davidson, P. W., Jacobson, J., Cain, N. N., Palumbo, D., Sloane-Reeves, J., Quijano, L., Van Heyningon, J., Giesow, V., Erhart, J., & Williams, T. (1996). Characteristics of children and adolescents with mental retardation and frequent outwardly directed aggressive behavior. *American Journal on Mental Retardation, 101,* 244–255.

Day, D. M. (1998). Risk for court contact and predictors of an early age for a first court contact among a sample of high risk youths: A survival analysis approach. *Canadian Journal of Criminology, 40,* 421–443.

Day, D. M., Bream, L. A., & Pal, A. (1992). Proactive and reactive aggression: An analysis of subtypes based on teacher perceptions. *Journal of Clinical Child Psychology, 21,* 210–217.

Day, D. M., & Hrynkiw-Augimeri, L. (1996). *Serving children at risk for juvenile delinquency: An evaluation of the Earlscourt Under 12 Outreach Project (ORP).* Report submitted to the Department of Justice, Ottawa, Canada.

Deater-Deckard, K., Dodge, K. A., Bates, J. E., & Pettit, G. S. (1996). Physical discipline among African-American and European American mothers: Links to children's externalizing behaviors. *Developmental Psychology, 32,* 1065–1072.

Deater-Deckard, K., Dodge, K. A., Bates, J. E., & Pettit, G. S. (1998). Multiple risk factors in the development of externalizing behavior problems: Group and individual differences. *Development and Psychopathology, 10,* 469–493.

Deater-Deckard, K., & Plomin, R. (1999). An adoption study of the etiology of teacher and parent reports of externalizing behavior problems in middle childhood. *Child Development, 70,* 144–154.

Deci, E. L., Koestner, R., & Ryan, R. M. (1999). A meta-analytic review of experiments examining the effects of extrinsic rewards on intrinsic motivation. *Psychological Bulletin, 125,* 627–668.

Deklyen, M. (1996). Disruptive behavior disorder and intergenerational attachment patterns: A comparison of clinic-referred and normally functioning preschoolers and their mothers. *Journal of Consulting and Clinical Psychology, 64,* 357–365.

Deklyen, M., Speltz, M. L., & Greenberg, M. T. (1998). Fathering and early onset conduct problems: Positive and negative parenting, father–son attachment, and marital context. *Clinical Child and Family Psychology Review, 1,* 3–22.

Demaray, M. K., Ruffalo, S. L., Carlson, J., Busse, R. T., Olsen, A. E., McManus, S. M., & Leventhal, A. (1995). Social skills assessment: A comparative evaluation of six published rating scales. *School Psychology Review, 24,* 648–671.

Derzon, J. H. (2001). Antisocial behavior and the prediction of violence: A meta-analysis. *Psychology in the Schools, 38,* 93–106.

Dimmock, C. A. J., O'Donoghue, T. A., & Robb, A. S. (1996). Parental involvement in schooling: An emerging research agenda. *Compare, 26,* 5–19.

Dishion, T. J., Andrews, D. W., & Crosby, L. (1995). Antisocial boys and their friends in early adolescence. *Child Development, 66,* 139–151.

Dishion, T. J., Duncan, T. E., Eddy, J. M., Fagot, B. I., & Fetrow, R. (1994). The world of parents and peers: Coercive exchanges and children's social adaptation. *Social Development, 3,* 255–268.

Dishion, T. J., McCord, J., & Poulin, F. (1999). When interventions harm: Peer groups and problem behavior. *American Psychologist, 54,* 755–764.

Dishion, T. J., & McMahon, R. J. (1998). Parental monitoring and the prevention of child and adolescent problem behavior: A conceptual and empirical formulation. *Clinical Child and Family Psychology Review, 1,* 61–75.

Dix, T., & Lochman, J. E. (1990). Social cognition and negative reactions to children: A comparison of mothers of aggressive and non-aggressive boys. *Journal of Social and Clinical Psychology, 9,* 418–438.

Dobkin, P. L., Tremblay, R. E., Masse, L. C., & Vitaro, F. (1995). Individual and peer characteristics predicting boys early onset of substance abuse: A seven-year longitudinal study. *Child Development, 66,* 1198–1214.

Dodge, K. A. (1991). The structure and function of reactive and proactive aggression. In D. J. Pepler & K. H. Rubin (Eds.), *The development and treatment of childhood aggression* (pp. 201–218). Hillsdale, NJ: Erlbaum.

Dodge, K. A. (1993). Social-cognitive mechanisms in the development of conduct disorder and depression in children. *Annual Review of Psychology, 44,* 559–584.

Dodge, K. A., & Coie, J. D. (1987). Social-information processing factors in reactive and proactive aggression in children's peer groups. *Journal of Personality and Social Psychology, 53,* 1146–1158.

Dodge, K. A., Lochman, J. E., Harnish, J. D., Bates, J. E., & Pettit, G. S. (1997). Reactive and proactive aggression in school children and psychiatrically impaired chronically assaultive youth. *Journal of Abnormal Psychology, 106,* 37–51.

Dodge, K. A., Pettit, G. S., & Bates, J. E. (1994a). Effects of physical maltreatment on the development of peer relations. *Development and Psychopathology, 6,* 43–56.

Dodge, K. A., Pettit, G. S., & Bates, J. E. (1994b). Socialization mediators of the relation between socioeconomic status and child conduct problems. *Child Development, 65,* 649–665.

Dodge, K. A., Pettit, G. S., Bates, J. E., & Valente, E. (1995). Social information-processing patterns partially mediate the effects of early physical abuse on later conduct problems. *Journal of Abnormal Psychology, 104,* 632–643.

Donnerstein, E., Slaby, R. G., & Eron, E. D. (1994). The mass media and youth aggression. In L. D. Eron, J. H. Gentry, & P. Schlegel (Eds.), *Reason to hope: A psychological perspective on violence and youth* (pp. 219–250). Washington, DC: American Psychological Association.

Doyle, A., Biederman, J., Seidman, L., Weber, W., & Faraone, S. (2000). Diagnostic efficiency of neuropsychological test scores for discriminating boys with and without attention deficit-hyperactivity disorder. *Journal of Consulting and Clinical Psychology, 68,* 477–488.

Dryfoos, J. G. (1997). School-based youth programs: Exemplary models and emerging opportunities. In R. J. Illback, C. T. Cobb, & H. M. Joseph (Eds.), *Integrated services for children and families: Opportunities for psychological practice* (pp. 23–52). Washington, DC: American Psychological Association.

Dryfoos, J. G. (1999). The role of the school in children's out-of-school time. *The Future of Children: When School is Out, 9,* 117–134.

Dubow, E. F., Edwards, S., & Ippolito, M. F. (1997). Life stressors, neighborhood disadvantage, and resources: A focus on inner-city children's adjustment. *Journal of Clinical Child Psychology, 26,* 130–144.

Dubow, E. F., & Ippolito, M. F. (1994). Effects of poverty and quality of the home environment on changes in the academic and behavioral adjustment of elementary school-age children. *Journal of Clinical Child Psychology, 23,* 401–412.

Dumas, J. E., Blechman, E. A., & Prinz, R. J. (1994). Aggressive children and effective communication. *Aggressive Behavior, 20,* 347–358.

Dumas, J. E., Lafreniere, P. J., & Serketich, W. J. (1995). "Balance of power": A transactional analysis of control in mother–child dyads involving socially competent, aggressive, and anxious children. *Journal of Abnormal Psychology, 104,* 104–113.

Dumas, J. E., Rollock, D., Prinz, R. J., Hops, H., & Blechman, E. A. (1999). Cultural sensitivity: Problems and solutions in applied and preventive intervention. *Applied and Preventive Psychology, 8,* 175–196.

Dumas, J. E., & Serketich, W. J. (1994). Maternal depressive symptomatology and child maladjustment: A comparison of three process models. *Behavior Therapy, 25,* 161–181.

Dumas, J. E., & Wekerle, C. (1995). Maternal reports of child behavior problems and personal distress as predictors of dysfunctional parenting. *Development and Psychopathology, 7,* 465–479.

Dunlap, G., Kern, L., dePerczel, M., Clarke, S., Wilson, D., Childs, K., White, R., & Falk, G. D. (1993). Functional analysis of classroom variables for students with emotional and behavioral disorders. *Behavioral Disorders, 18,* 275–291.

Dunlap, G., White, R., Vera, A., Wilson, D., & Panacek, L. (1996). The effects of multicomponent, assessment-based curricular modifications on the classroom behavior of children with emotional and behavioral disorders. *Journal of Behavioral Education, 6,* 481–500.

DuPaul, G. J. (1998). Peer tutoring for children with ADHD: Effects on classroom behavior and academic performance. *Journal of Applied Behavior Analysis, 31,* 579–592.

DuPaul, G. J., & Barkley, R. A. (1992). Social interactions of children with attention-deficit-hyperactivity disorder: Effects of methylphenidate. In J. McCord & R.E. Tremblay (Eds.), *Preventing antisocial behavior: Interventions from birth through adolescence* (pp. 89–116). New York: Guilford Press.

DuPaul, G. J., & Eckert, T. L. (1997). The effects of school-based interventions for attention-deficit/hyperactivity disorder: A meta-analysis. *School Psychology Review, 26,* 5–27.

DuPaul, G. J., & Eckert, T. L. (1998). Academic interventions for students with attention-deficit/hyperactivity disorder: A review of the literature. *Reading and Writing Quarterly, 14,* 59–82.

DuPaul, G. J., Eckert, T. L., & McGoey, K. E. (1997). Interventions for students with attention-deficit/hyperactivity disorder: One size does not fit all. *School Psychology Review, 26,* 369–381.

DuPaul, G. J., & Ervin, R. A. (1996). Functional assessment of behaviors related to attention-deficit/hyperactivity disorder: Linking assessment to intervention design. *Behavior Therapy, 27,* 601–622.

DuPaul, G. J., McGoey, K. E., & Yugar, J. M. (1997). Mainstreaming students with behavior disorders: The use of classroom peers as facilitators of generalization. *School Psychology Review, 26,* 634–650.

DuPaul, G. J., Power, T. J., & Anastopoulos, A. D. (1998). *ADHD Rating Scale–IV: Checklists, norms, and clinical interpretation.* New York: Guilford Press.

Durlak, J. L. (1995). *School-based prevention programs for children and adolescence.* Newbury Park, CA: Sage.

Dwyer, K., & Osher, D. (2000). *Safeguarding our children: An action guide.* Washington, DC: U.S. Departments of Education and Justice, American Institute for Research.

Early, T. J., & Poertner, J. (1995). Examining current approaches to case management for families with children who have serious emotional disorders. In B. J. Friesen & J. Poertner (Eds.), *From case management to service coordination for children with emotional, behavioral, or mental disorders: Building on family strengths* (pp. 37–59). Baltimore: Brookes.

Eddy, J. M., Reid, J. B., & Fetrow, R. A. (2000). An elementary school-based prevention program targeting modifiable antecedents of youth delinquency and violence: Linking the Interests of Families and Teachers (LIFT). *Journal of Emotional and Behavioral Disorders, 8,* 165–176.

Edens, J. F., Cavell, T. A., & Hughes, J. N. (1999). The self-systems of aggressive children: A cluster-analytic investigation. *Journal of Child Psychology and Psychiatry, 40,* 441–453.

Eiraldi, R. B., Power, T. J., & Nezu, C. M. (1997). Patterns of comorbidity associated with subtypes of attention-deficit hyperactivity among 6- to 12-year-old children. *Journal of the American Academy of Child and Adolescent Psychiatry, 36,* 503–514.

Eisenstadt, T. H., Eyberg, S., McNeil, C. B., Newcomb, K., & Funderburk, B. (1993). Parent–child interaction therapy with behavior problem children: Relative effectiveness of two stages and overall treatment outcome. *Journal of Clinical Child Psychology, 22,* 42–51.

Elliott, S. N., Busse, R. T., & Shapiro, E. S. (1999). Intervention techniques for academic performance problems. In C. R. Reynolds & T. B. Gutkin (Eds.), *The handbook of school psychology* (3rd ed., pp. 664–685). New York: Wiley.

Elliott, D. S., Dunford, F. W., & Huizinga, D. (1987). The identification and prediction of career offenders utilizing self-report and official data. In J. D. Burchard & S. N. Burchard (Eds.), *Preventing delinquent behavior* (pp. 90–121). Newbury Park, CA: Sage.

Epstein, J. L. (1992). School and family partnerships: Leadership roles for school psychologists. In S. L. Christenson & J. C. Conoley (Eds.), *Home–school collaboration: Enhancing children's academic and social competence* (pp. 499–515). Silver Spring, MD: National Association of School Psychologists.

Epstein, N. J., March, J. S., Conners, C. K., & Jackson, D. L. (1998). Using the Conners Teacher Rating Scale with African-American children. *Journal of Abnormal Child Psychology, 26,* 109–118.

Erdley, C. A., & Asher, S. R. (1998). Linkages between children's beliefs about the legitimacy of aggression and their behavior. *Social Development, 7,* 321–339.

Erhardt, D., & Hinshaw, S. P. (1994). Initial sociometric impressions of attention-deficit hyperactivity disorder and comparison boys: Predictions from social behaviors and from nonbehavioral variables. *Journal of Consulting and Clinical Psychology, 62,* 833–842.

Ervin, R. A. (1996). Functional assessment of behaviors related to attention-deficit/hyperactivity disorder: Linking assessment to intervention design. *Behavior Therapy, 27,* 601–622.

Ervin, R. A., Kern, L., Clarke, S., DuPaul, G. J., Dunlap, G., & Friman, P. C. (2000). Evaluating assessment-based intervention strategies for students with ADHD and comorbid disorders within the natural classroom context. *Behavioral Disorder, 25,* 344–358.

Esposito, C. (1999). Learning in urban blight: School climate and its effect on the school performance of urban, minority, low-income children. *School Psychology Review, 28,* 365–377.

Esters, I., Ittenbach, R., & Han, K. (1997). Today's IQ tests: Are they really better than their historical predecessors? *School Psychology Review, 26,* 211–224.

Evans, H. L., & Sullivan, M. A. (1993). Children and the use of self-monitoring, self-evaluation, and self-reinforcement. In A. J. Finch, W. M. Nelson, & E. S. Ott (Eds.), *Cognitive-behavioral procedures with children and adolescents: A practical guide* (pp. 67–89). Boston: Allyn & Bacon.

Evans, M. E., Armstrong, M. I., Dollard, N., Kuppinger, A. D., Huz, S., & Wood, V. M. (1994). Development and evaluation of treatment foster care and family-centered intensive case management in New York. *Journal of Emotional and Behavioral Disorders, 2,* 228–239.

Evans, M. E., Armstrong, M. I., & Kuppinger, A. D. (1996). Family-centered intensive case management: A step toward understanding individualized care. *Journal of Child and Family Studies, 5,* 55–65.

Exner, J. E. (1993). *The Rorschach* (3rd ed., Vol. 1). New York: Wiley.

Eyberg, S. M. (1992). Parent and teacher behavior inventories for the assessment of conduct problems in children. In L. VandeCreek, S. Knapp, & T. L. Jackson

(Eds.), *Innovations in clinical practice: A source book* (Vol. 11, pp. 261–270). Sarasota, FL: Professional Resource Exchange.

Eyberg, S. M., & Boggs, S. R. (1998). Parent–child interaction therapy: A psychosocial intervention for treatment of young conduct-disorders children. In J. M. Briermeister & C. E. Schaefer (Eds.), *Handbook parent training: Parents as cotherapists for children's behavior problems* (2nd ed., pp. 61–97). New York: Wiley.

Eyberg, S. M., Boggs, S. R., & Algina, J. (1995). Parent–child interaction therapy: A psychosocial model for the treatment of young children with conduct problem behavior and their families. *Psychopharmacology Bulletin, 31,* 83–91.

Fagot, B. I., & Pears, K. C. (1996). Changes in attachment during the third year: Consequences and predictions. *Development and Psychopathology, 8,* 325–344.

Fantuzzo, J. W., DePaola, L. M., Lambert, L., Martino, T., Anderson, G., & Sutton, S. (1991). Effects of interpersonal violence on the psychological adjustment and competencies of young children. *Journal of Consulting and Clinical Psychology, 59,* 258–265.

Fantuzzo, J. W., King, J. A., & Heller, L. R. (1992). Effects of reciprocal peer tutoring on mathematics and school adjustment: A component analysis. *Journal of Educational Psychology, 84,* 331–339.

Fantuzzo, J. W., & Polite, K. (1990). School-based behavioral self-management: A review and analysis. *School Psychology Quarterly, 5,* 180–198.

Farrington, D. P. (1993). Understanding and preventing bullying. In M. Tonry (Ed.), *Crime and justice: A review of research* (Vol. 17, pp. 381–458). Chicago: University of Chicago Press.

Farver, J. M. (1996). Aggressive behavior in preschoolers' social networks: Do birds of a feather block together? *Early Childhood Research Quarterly, 11,* 333–350.

Fashola, O. S. (1998). *Report no. 24: Review of extended-day and after-school programs and their effectiveness.* Baltimore: Center for Social Organization of Schools, Johns Hopkins University.

Feil, E., Walker, H., Severson, H., & Ball, A. (2000). Proactive screening for emotional/behavioral concerns in Head Start preschools: Promising practices and challenges in applied research. *Behavioral Disorders, 26,* 13–25.

Felner, R. D., Brand, S., DuBois, D. L., Adan, A. M., Mulhall, P. F., & Evans, E. G. (1995). Socioeconomic disadvantage, proximal environmental experiences, and socioemotional and academic adjustment in early adolescence: Investigation of a mediated effects model. *Child Development, 66,* 774–792.

Fergusson, D. M., & Lynskey, M. T. (1997). Early reading difficulties and later conduct problems. *Journal of Child Psychology and Psychiatry, 38,* 899–907.

Fergusson, D. M., Woodward, L. J., & Horwood, L. J. (1999). Childhood peer relationship problems and young people's involvement with deviant peers in adolescence. *Journal of Abnormal Child Psychology, 27,* 357–370.

Feuerstein, A. (2000). School characteristics and parent involvement: Influences on participation in children's schools. *Journal of Education Research, 94,* 29–38.

Fisher, L., & Blair, R. J. R. (1998). Cognitive impairment and its relationship to psychopathic tendencies in children with emotional and behavioral difficulties. *Journal of Abnormal Child Psychology, 26,* 511–519.

Fisher, P. A., & Chamberlain, P. (2000). Multidimensional treatment foster care: A program for intensive parenting, family support, and skill building. *Journal of Emotional and Behavioral Disorders, 8,* 155–164.

Fitzpatrick, K. M. (1997a). Aggression and environmental risk among low-income African-American Youth. *Journal of Adolescent Health, 21,* 172–178.

Fitzpatrick, K. M. (1997b). Fighting among America's youths: A risk and protective factors approach. *Journal of Health and Social Behavior, 38,* 131–148.

Flanagan, D. P., & Miranda, A. H. (1995). Best practices in working with culturally different families. In A. Thomas, & J. Grimes (Eds.), *Best practices in school psychology–III* (pp. 1049–1060). Washington, DC: National Association of School Psychologists.

Fletcher, K. E., Fischer, M., Barkley, R. A., & Smallish, L. (1996). A sequential analysis of mother–adolescent interactions of ADHD, ADHD/ODD, and normal teenagers during neutral and conflict discussions. *Journal of Abnormal Child Psychology, 24,* 272–297.

Foote, R., Eyberg, S. M., & Schuhmann, E. (1996). Parent–child interaction approaches to the treatment of child behavior problems. In T. H. Ollendick & R. J. Prinz (Eds.), *Advances in clinical child psychology* (Vol. 20, pp. 125–151). New York: Plenum Press.

Forehand, R. L., & McMahon, R. J. (1981). *Helping the noncompliant child: A clinician's guide to parent training.* New York: Guilford Press.

Forgatch, M. S. (1991). The clinical science vortex: Developing a theory for antisocial behavior. In D. Pepler & K. H. Rubin (Eds.), *The development and treatment of childhood aggression* (pp. 291–315). Hillsdale, NJ: Erlbaum.

Forness, S. R., Kavale, K. A., Blum, I. M., & Lloyd, J. W. (1997, July/August). Mega-analysis of meta-analyses: What works in special education and related services. *Teaching Exceptional Children,* pp. 4–9.

Fox, J., Conroy, M., & Heckaman, K. (1998). Research issues in functional assessment of the challenging behaviors of students with emotional and behavioral disorders. *Behavioral Disorders, 24,* 26–33.

Frauenglass, S., & Routh, D. K. (1999). Assessment of the disruptive disorders: Dimensional and categorical approaches. In H. C. Quay & A. E. Hogan (Eds.), *Handbook of disruptive behavior disorders* (pp. 49–71). New York: Kluwer Academic/Plenum Press.

French, D. C. (1988). Heterogeneity of peer-rejected boys: Aggressive and non-aggressive subtypes. *Child Development, 59,* 976–985.

Frey, K. S., Hirschstein, M. K., & Guzzo, B. A. (2000). Second Step: Preventing aggression by promoting social competence. *Journal of Emotional and Behavioral Disorders, 8,* 102–112.

Frick, P. J. (1994). Family dysfunction and the disruptive behavior disorders: A review of recent empirical findings. In T. H. Ollendick & R. J. Prinz (Eds.), *Advances in clinical child psychology* (Vol. 16, pp. 203–226). New York: Plenum Press.

Frick, P.J. (1998a). Callous-unemotional traits and conduct problems: Applying the two-factor model of psychopathy to children. In D. J. Cooke, A. E. Forth, & R. D. Hare (Eds.), *Psychopathy: Theory, research and implication for society* (pp. 161–187). Dordrecht, Netherlands: Kluwer Academic.

Frick, P. J. (1998b). *Conduct disorders and severe antisocial behavior.* New York: Plenum Press.

Frick, P. J., Barry, C. T., & Bodin, S. D. (2000). Applying the concept of psychopathy to children: Implications for the assessment of antisocial youth. In C. B. Gacono (Ed.), *The clinical and forensic assessment of psychopathy: A practitioners guide* (pp. 3–24). Mahwah, NJ: Erlbaum.

Frick, P. J., & Hare, R. D. (in press). *The Psychopathy Screening Device*. Toronto: Multi-Health Systems.

Frick, P. J., Kamphaus, R. W., Lahey, B. B., Loeber, R., Christ, M. G., Hart, E. L., & Tannenbaum, L. E. (1991). Academic underachievement and the disruptive behavior disorders. *Journal of Consulting and Clinical Psychology, 59,* 289–294.

Frick, P. J., Lahey, B. B., Loeber, R., Stouthamer-Loeber, M., Christ, M. G., & Hanson, K. (1992). Familial risk factors to oppositional defiant disorder and conduct behavior: Parental psychopathology and maternal parenting. *Journal of Consulting and Clinical Psychology, 60,* 49–55.

Frick, P. J., Lilienfeld, S. O., Ellis, M., Loney, B., & Silverthorn, P. (1999). The association between anxiety and psychopathy dimensions in children. *Journal of Abnormal Child Psychology, 27,* 383–392.

Frick, P. J., & Loney, B. R. (1999). Outcomes of children and adolescents with oppositional defiant disorder and conduct disorder. In H. C. Quay & A. E. Hogan (Eds.), *Handbook of disruptive behavior disorders* (pp. 507–524). New York: Kluwer Academic/Plenum Press.

Frick, P. J., O'Brien, B. S., Wooton, J. M., & McBurnett, K. (1994). Psychopathy and conduct problems in children. *Journal of Abnormal Psychology, 103,* 700–707.

Frick, P. J., Van Horn, Y., Lahey, B. B., Christ, M. A. G., Loeber, R., Hart, E. A., Tannenbaum, L., & Hanson, K. (1993). Oppositional defiant disorder and conduct disorder: A meta-analytic review of factor analyses and cross-validation in a clinic sample. *Clinical Psychology Review, 13,* 319–340.

Friedman, R. M. (1994). Restructuring of systems to emphasize prevention and family support. *Journal of Clinical Child Psychology, 23,* 40–47.

Frisby, C. L. (1999). Straight talk about cognitive assessment and diversity. *School Psychology Quarterly, 14,* 195–207.

Fuchs, L. S., Fuchs, D., Phillips, N. B., Hamlett, C. L., & Karns, K. (1995). Acquisition and transfer effects of classwide peer-assisted learning strategies in mathematics for students with varying learning histories. *School Psychology Review, 24,* 604–620.

Gagnon, W. A., & Conoley, J. C. (1997). Academic and curriculum interventions with aggressive youths. In A. P. Goldstein & J. C. Conoley (Eds.), *School violence intervention: A practical handbook* (pp. 217–235). New York: Guilford Press.

Galloway, J., & Sheridan S. M. (1994). Implementing scientific practices through case studies: Examples using home–school interventions and consultation. *Journal of School Psychology, 32,* 385–413.

Garcia, M. M., Shaw, D. S., Winslow, E. B., & Yaggi, K. E. (2000). Destructive sibling conflict and the development of conduct problems in young boys. *Developmental Psychology, 36,* 44–53.

Garcia-Preto, N. (1996). Latino families: An overview. In M. McGoldrick, J. Giordano, & J. K. Pearce (Eds.), *Ethnicity and family therapy* (2nd ed., pp. 141–154). New York: Guilford Press.

Garcia-Vázquez, E., & Ehly, S. (1995). Best practices in facilitating peer tutoring programs. In A. Thomas & J. Grimes (Eds.), *Best practices in school psychology–III* (pp. 403–411). Washington, DC: National Association of School Psychologists.

Gaub, M., & Carlson, C. L. (1997). Gender differences in ADHD: A meta-analysis and critical review. *Journal of the American Academy of Child and Adolescent Psychiatry, 36,* 1036–1045.

Gelfand, D. M., & Teti, D. M. (1990). The effects of maternal depression on children. *Clinical Psychology Review, 10,* 329–353.

Geller, B., & Luby, J. (1997). Child and adolescent bipolar disorder: A review of the past 10 years. *Journal of the American Academy of Child and Adolescent Psychiatry, 36,* 1168–1176.

Geller, J., & Johnston, C. (1995). Depressed mood and child conduct problems: Relationships to mother's attributions for their own and their children's experiences. *Child and Family Behavior Therapy, 17,* 19–34.

Gersten, R. (1998). Recent advances in instructional research for students with learning disabilities: An overview. *Learning Disabilities Research and Practices, 13,* 162–170.

Gersten, R., Carnine, D., & Woodward, J. (1987). Direct instruction research: The third decade. *Remedial and Special Education, 8,* 48–56.

Gersten, R., Woodward, J., & Darch, C. (1986). Direct instruction: A research-based approach to curriculum design and teaching. *Exceptional Children, 53,* 17–31.

Gettinger, M. (1988). Methods of proactive classroom management. *School Psychology Review, 17,* 227–242.

Gettinger, M. (1995). Best practices for increasing academic learning time. In A. Thomas & J. Grimes (Eds.), *Best practices in school psychology–III* (pp. 943–954). Washington, DC: National Association of School Psychologists.

Gettinger, M., & Stoiber, K. C. (1999). Excellence in teaching: Review of instructional and environmental variables. In C. R. Reynolds & T. B. Gutkin (Eds.), *The handbook of school psychology* (3rd ed., pp. 933–958). New York: Wiley.

Giancola, P. R., Martin, C. S., Tarter, R., Pelham, W. E., & Moss, H. B. (1996). Executive cognitive functioning and aggressive behavior in preadolescent boys at high risk for substance abuse/dependence. *Journal of Studies on Alcohol, 57,* 352–359.

Giancola, P. R., Moss, H. B., Martin, C. S., Kirisci, L., & Tarter, R. E. (1996). Executive cognitive functioning predicts reactive aggression in boys at high risk for substance abuse: A prospective study. *Alcoholism: Clinical and Experimental Research, 20,* 740–744.

Gillies, R. M., & Ashman, A. F. (1997). The effects of training in cooperative learning on differential student behavior and achievement. *Journal of Classroom Interaction, 32,* 1–9.

Girouard, P. C., Baillargeon, R. H., Tremblay, R. E., Glorieux, J., Lefebvre, F., & Robaey, P. (1998). Developmental pathways leading to externalizing behaviors in 5 year olds born before 29 weeks gestation. *Developmental and Behavior Pediatrics, 19,* 244–253.

Goldman, S. K. (1999). The conceptual framework for wraparound. In B. J. Burns & S. K. Goldman (Eds.), *Systems of care: Promising practices in children's mental health, 1998 series: Vol. IV. Promising practices in wraparound for children with serious emotional disturbance and their families* [Online]. Washington, DC: Center for Effective Collaboration and Practice, American Institute for Research. Available: www.air-dc.org/cecp/promisingpractices/1998monographs/documents.htm#4

Gomez, R., & Sanson, A. V. (1994). Mother–child interactions and noncompliance in hyperactive boys with and without conduct problems. *Journal of Child Psychology and Psychiatry 35*, 477–490.

Goodman, R. F., & Stevenson, J. (1989). A twin study of hyperactivity: II. The etiological role of genes, family relationships and perinatal adversity. *Journal of Child Psychology and Psychiatry, 30*, 691–709.

Gordon, M., & Barkley, R. A. (1998). Tests and observational measures. In R. A. Barkley, *Attention-deficit/hyperactivity disorder: A handbook for diagnosis and treatment* (2nd ed., pp. 294–311). New York: Guilford Press.

Gorman-Smith, D., & Tolan, P. H. (1998). The role of exposure to community violence and developmental problems among inner-city youth. *Development and Psychopathology, 10*, 101–116.

Gray, J. A. (1985). A whole and its part: Behavior, the brain, cognition, and emotion. *Bulletin of the British Psychological Society, 38*, 99–112.

Green, W. H. (1996). Principles of psychopharmacotherapy and specific drug treatments. In M. Lewis (Ed.), *Child and adolescent psychiatry: A comprehensive textbook* (pp. 772–801). Baltimore: Williams & Wilkins.

Greenberg, M. T., Kusche, C. A., Cook, E. T., & Quamma, J. P. (1995). Promoting emotional competence in school-aged children: The effects of the PATHS curriculum. *Development and Psychopathology, 7*, 117–136.

Greenberg, M. T., Lengua, L. J., Coie, J. D., Pinderhughes, E. E., & Conduct Problems Prevention Research Group. (1999). Predicting developmental outcomes at school entry using a multiple-risk model: Four American communities. *Developmental Psychology, 35*, 403–417.

Greenberg, M. T., Speltz, M. L., & Deklyen, M. (1993). The role of attachment in the early development of disruptive behavior problems. *Development and Psychopathology, 5*, 191–213.

Greene, R. W. (1996). Students with attention-deficit hyperactivity disorder and their teachers: Implications of a goodness-of-fit perspective. In T. H. Ollendick & R. J. Prinz (Eds.), *Advances in clinical child psychology* (Vol. 18, pp. 205–230). New York: Plenum Press.

Greenhill, L. L., Abikoff, H. B., Arnold, L. E., Cantwell, D. P., Connors, C. K., Elliot, G., Hechtman, L., Hinshaw, S. P., Hoza, B., Jensen, P. S., March, J. S., Newcorn, J., Pelham, W. E., Severe, J. B., Swanson, J. M., Vitiello, B., & Wells, K. (1996). Medication treatment strategies in the MTA study: Relevance to clinicians and researchers. *Journal of the American Academy of Child and Adolescent Psychiatry, 35*, 1304–1313.

Greenhill, L. L., Halperin, J. M., & Abikoff, H. (1999). Stimulant medications. *Journal of the American Academy of Child and Adolescent Psychiatry, 38*, 503–512.

Greenwood, C. R. (1996). The case for performance-based instructional models. *School Psychology Quarterly, 11*, 283–296.

Greenwood, C. R., Delquadri, J. C., & Hall, R. V. (1989). Longitudinal effects of classwide peer tutoring. *Journal of Educational Psychology, 81*, 371–383.

Greenwood, C. R., Terry, B., Utley, C. A., Montagna, D., & Walker, D. (1993).

Achievement, placement, and services: Middle school benefits of classwide peer tutoring used at the elementary school. *School Psychology Review, 22,* 497–516.

Greenwood, P. W., Model, K. E., Rydell, C. P., & Chiesa, J. (1996). *Diverting children from a life of crime: Measuring costs and benefits.* Santa Monica, CA: Rand.

Greist, D. L., Forehand, R., Wells, K. C., & McMahon, R. J. (1980). An examination of differences between nonclinic and behavior-problem clinic-referred children and their mothers. *Journal of Abnormal Psychology, 89,* 497–500.

Greist, D. L., Wells, K. C., & Forehand, R. (1979). Examinations of predictors of maternal perceptions of maladjustment in clinic-referred children. *Journal of Abnormal Psychology, 88,* 277–281.

Grenell, M. M., Glass, C. R., & Katz, K. S. (1987). Hyperactive children and peer interaction: Knowledge and performance of social skills. *Journal of Abnormal Child Psychology, 15,* 1–13.

Gresham, F. M., & Elliott, S. N. (1990). *The social skills rating system.* Circle Pines, MN: American Guidance Services.

Gresham, F. M., MacMillan, D. L., Bocian, K. M., Ward, S. L., & Forness, S. R. (1998). Comorbidity of hyperactivity–impulsivity–inattention and conduct problems: Risk factors in social, affective, and academic domains. *Journal of Abnormal Child Psychology, 26,* 393–406

Grizenko, N. (1997). Outcome of multimodal day treatment for children with severe behavior problems: A five-year follow up. *Journal of the American Academy of Child and Adolescent Psychiatry, 36,* 989–997.

Grossman, D. C., Neckerman, H. J., Koepsell, T. D., Liu, P.-Y., Asher, K. N., Beland, K., Frey, K., & Rivara, F. P. (1997). Effectiveness of a violence prevention curriculum among children in elementary school: A randomized controlled trial. *Journal of the American Medical Association, 277,* 1605–1611.

Grossman, J. B., & Tierney, J. P. (1998). Does mentoring work? An impact study of the Big Brothers Big Sisters Program. *Evaluation Review, 22,* 403–426.

Groth-Marnat, G. (1998). *Handbook of psychological assessment.* New York: Wiley.

Grych, J. H., Jouriles, E. N., Swank, P. R., McDonald, R., & Norwood, W. D. (2000). Patterns of adjustment among children of battered women. *Journal of Consulting and Clinical Psychology, 68,* 84–94.

Guerra, N. G., Eron, L. D., Huesmann, L. R., Tolan, P. H., & Van Acker, R. (In press). A cognitive–ecological approach to the prevention and mitigation of violence and aggression in inner-city youths. In K. Bijorkquist & D. P. Fry (Eds.), *Styles and conflict resolution: Models and applications from around the world.* Orlando, FL: Academic Press.

Guerra, N. G., Huesmann, L. R., Tolan, P. H., Van Acker, R., & Eron, L. D. (1995). Stressful events and individual beliefs as correlates of economic disadvantage and aggression among urban children. *Journal of Consulting and Clinical Psychology, 63,* 518–528.

Guevremont, D. C. (1990). Social skills and peer relationship training. In R. A. Barkley, *Attention-deficit/hyperactivity disorder: A handbook for diagnosis and treatment* (pp. 540–572). New York: Guilford Press.

Guevremont, D. C., & Foster, S. L. (1993). Impact of social problem-solving training on aggressive boys: Skill acquisition, behavior change, and generalization. *Journal of Abnormal Child Psychology, 21,* 13–27.

Gunter, P. L., & Denny, R. K. (1998). Trends and issues in research regarding academic instruction of students with emotional and behavioral disorders. *Behavioral Disorders, 24,* 44–50.

Guskey, T. (1986). Staff development and the process of teacher change. *Educational Researcher, 15,* 5–12.

Haapasalo, J., & Tremblay, R. E. (1994). Physically aggressive boys from ages 6 to 12: Family background, parenting behavior, and prediction to delinquency. *Journal of Consulting and Clinical Psychology, 62,* 1044–1052.

Halperin, J. M., Newcorn, J. H., Kopstein, I., McKay, K. E., Schwartz, S. T., Siever, L. J., & Vanshdeep, S. (1997) Serotonin, aggression, and parental psychopathology in children with attention-deficit hyperactivity disorder. *Journal of the American Academy of Child and Adolescent Psychiatry, 36,* 1391–1398.

Halperin, J. M., Newcorn, J. H., Matier, K., Bedi, G., Hall, S., & Vanshdeep, S. (1995). Impulsivity and initiation of fights in children with disruptive behavior disorders. *Journal of Child Psychology and Psychiatry, 36,* 1199–1211.

Halperin, J. M., Newcorn, J. H., Schwartz, S. T., Vanshdeep, S., Siever, L. J., Koda, V. H., & Gabriel, S. (1997). Age-related changes in the association between serotonergic function and aggression in boys with ADHD. *Biological Psychiatry, 41,* 682–689.

Halpern, R. (1999). After-school programs for low-income children: Promise and challenges. *The Future of Children: When School Is Out, 9,* 81–95.

Hamilton, S. B., & MacQuiddy, S. L. (1984). Self-administered behavioral parent training: Enhancement of treatment efficacy using a time-out signal seat. *Journal Clinical Child Psychology, 13,* 61–69.

Hammill, D. D., Pearson, N. A., & Wiederholt, J. S. (1996). *Comprehensive Test of Nonverbal Intelligence (C-TONI).* Austin, TX: PRO-ED.

Harnish, J.D., Dodge, K. A., & Valente, J. (1995). Mother–child interaction quality as a partial mediator of the roles of maternal depressive symptoms and SES in development of child behavior problems. *Child Development, 66,* 739–553.

Hartung, C., & Widiger, T. (1998). Gender differences in the diagnosis of mental disorders: Conclusions and controversies of the DSM-IV. *Psychological Bulletin, 123,* 260–278.

Hastings, P. D., Zahn-Waxler, C., Robinson, J., Usher, B., & Bridges, D. (2000). The development of concern for others in children with behavior problems. *Developmental Psychology, 36,* 531–546.

Hausman, A., Pierce, G., & Briggs, L. (1996). Evaluation of comprehensive violence prevention education: Effects on student behavior. *Journal of Adolescent Health, 19,* 104–110.

Haynes, N. M., Emmons, C., & Ben-Avie, M. (1997). School climate as a factor in student adjustment and achievement. *Journal of Educational and Psychological Consultation, 8,* 321–329.

Heckaman, K., Conroy, M., Fox, J., & Chait, A. (2000). Functional assessment-based intervention research on students with or at risk for emotional and behavioral disorders in school settings. *Behavioral Disorders, 25,* 196–210.

Hektner, J. M., August, G. J., & Realmuto, G. M. (2000). Patterns and temporal changes in peer affiliation among aggressive and non-aggressive children participating in a summer school program. *Journal of Clinical Child Psychology, 29,* 603–614.

Henggeler, S. W., Pickrel, S. G., Brondino, M. J., & Crouch, J. L. (1996). Eliminating (almost) treatment dropout of substance abusing or dependent delinquents through home-based multisystemic therapy. *American Journal of Psychiatry, 153,* 427–428.

Henggeler, S. W., Schoenwald, S. K., Borduin, C. M., Rowland, M. D., & Cunningham, P. B. (1998). *Multisystemic treatment of antisocial behavior in children and adolescents.* New York: Guilford Press.

Henrich, C. C., Brown, J. L., & Aber, J. L. (1999). Evaluating the effectiveness of school-based violence prevention: Developmental approaches. *Social Policy Report: Society for Research in Child Development, 13,* 1–17.

Henry, B., Feehan, M., McGee, R., Stanton, W., Moffitt, T. E., & Silva, P. (1993). The importance of conduct problems and depressive symptoms in predicting adolescent substance abuse. *Journal of Abnormal Child Psychology, 21,* 469–480.

Heston, J. D., Kiser, L. J., & Pruitt, D. B. (1996). Child and adolescent partial hospitalization. In M. Lewis (Ed.), *Child and adolescent psychiatry: A comprehensive textbook* (pp. 883–890). Baltimore: Williams & Wilkins.

Hinshaw, S. P. (1992a). Externalizing behavior problems and academic underachievement in childhood and adolescence: Causal relationships and underlying mechanisms. *Psychological Bulletin, 111,* 127–155.

Hinshaw, S. P. (1992b). Academic underachievement, attention deficits, and aggression: Comorbidity and implications for intervention. *Journal of Consulting and Clinical Psychology, 60,* 893–903.

Hinshaw, S. P. (2000). Attention-deficit/hyperactivity disorder: The search for viable treatments. In P. C. Kendall (Ed.), *Child and adolescent therapy: Cognitive-behavioral procedures* (2nd ed., pp. 88–128). New York: Guilford Press.

Hinshaw, S. P., & Anderson, C. A. (1996). Conduct and oppositional defiant disorders. In E. J. Mash & R. A. Barkley (Eds.), *Child psychopathology* (pp. 113–149). New York: Guilford Press.

Hinshaw, S. P., Henker, B., & Whalen, C. K. (1984a). Cognitive-behavioral and pharmacologic interventions for hyperactive boys: Comparative and combined effects. *Journal of Consulting and Clinical Psychology, 52,* 739–749.

Hinshaw, S. P., Henker, B., & Whalen, C. K. (1984b). Self-control in hyperactive boys in anger-inducing situations: Effects of cognitive-behavioral training and of methylphenidate. *Journal of Abnormal Child Psychology, 12,* 55–77.

Hinshaw, S. P., Lahey, B. B., & Hart, E. L. (1993). Issues of taxonomy and comorbidity in the development of conduct disorder. *Development and Psychopathology, 5,* 31–49.

Hinshaw, S. P., & Nigg, J. T. (1999). Behavior rating scales in the assessment of disruptive behavior problems in childhood. In D. Shaffer, C. P. Lucas, & J. E. Richters (Eds.), *Diagnostic assessment in child and adolescent psychopathology* (pp. 91–126). New York: Guilford Press.

Hinshaw, S. P., & Park, T. (1999). Research problems and issues: Toward a more definitive science of disruptive behavior disorders. In H. C. Quay & A. E. Hogan (Eds.), *Handbook of disruptive behavior disorders* (pp. 593–620). New York: Kluwer Academic/Plenum Press.

Hinshaw, S. P., & Zupan, B. A. (1997). Assessment of antisocial behavior in children and adolescents. In D. M. Stoff, J. Breiling, & J. D. Maser (Eds.), *Handbook of antisocial behavior* (pp. 36–50). New York: Wiley.

Hoagwood, K., Hibbs, E., Brent, D., & Jenson, P. (1995). Introduction to the special section: Efficacy and effectiveness in studies of child and adolescent psychotherapy. *Journal of Consulting and Clinical Psychology, 63*, 683–687.

Hoberman, H. M. (1992). Ethnic minority status and adolescent mental health services utilization. *Journal of Mental Health Administration, 19*, 247–267.

Hodges, K. (1993). Structured interviews for assessing children. *Journal of Child Psychology and Psychiatry, 34*, 49–68.

Hogan, A. E. (1999). Cognitive functioning in children with oppositional defiant disorder and conduct disorder. In H. C. Quay & A. E. Hogan (Eds.), *Handbook of disruptive behavior disorders* (pp. 317–335). New York: Kluwer Academic/Plenum Press.

Holleran, P. A., Littman, D. C., Freund, R. D., & Schmaling, K. B. (1982). A signal detection approach to social perception: Identification of negative and positive behaviors by parents of normal and problem children. *Journal of Abnormal Child Psychology, 10*, 547–558.

Horn, W. F., Wagner, A. E., & Ialongo, N. (1989). Sex differences in school-aged children with pervasive attention deficit hyperactivity disorder. *Journal of Abnormal Child Psychology, 17*, 109–125.

Howard, K. A., Flora, J., & Griffin, M. (1999). Violence-prevention programs in schools: State of the science and implications for future research. *Applied and Preventive Psychology, 8*, 197–215.

Hrynkiw-Augimeri, L., Pepler, D., & Goldberg, K. (1993). An outreach project for children having early police contact. *Canada's Mental Health, 41*, 7–12.

Huberty, T. J., & Eaken, G. J. (1994). Personality assessment of anger and hostility in children and adolescents. In M. Furlong & D. Smith (Eds.), *Anger, hostility, and aggression: Assessment, prevention and intervention strategies for youth* (pp. 285–309). Brandon, VT: Clinical Psychology Publishing.

Hudley, C. A. (1994). The reduction of childhood aggression using the Brain Power program. In M. Furlong & D. Smith (Eds.), *Anger, hostility and aggression: Assessment, prevention and intervention strategies for youth* (pp. 97–116). Brandon, VT: Clinical Psychology Publishing.

Hudley, C. A., Britsch, B., Wakefield, W. D., Smith, T., Demorat, M., & Cho, S. (1998). An attribution retraining program to reduce aggression in elementary school students. *Psychology in the Schools, 35*, 271–282.

Hudley, C. A., & Graham, S. (1993). An attributional intervention to reduce peer-directed aggression among African-American boys. *Child Development, 64*, 124–138.

Hudziak, J. J., Rudiger, L. P., Neale, M. C., Heath, A. C., & Todd, R. D. (2000). A twin study of inattentive, aggressive, and anxious/depressed behaviors. *Journal of the American Academy of Child and Adolescent Psychiatry, 39*, 469–476.

Huesmann, L. R., & Guerra, N. G. (1997). Children's normative beliefs about aggression and aggressive behavior. *Journal of Personality and Social Psychology, 72*, 408–419.

Huesmann, L. R., Maxwell, C. D., Eron, L., Dahlberg, L. L., Guerra, N. G., Tolan, P. H., VanAcker, R., & Henry, D. (1996). Evaluating a cognitive/ecological program for the prevention of aggression among urban children. *American Journal of Preventive Medicine, 12*(Suppl. 2), 120–128.

Hughes, C., White, A., Sharpen, J., & Dunn, J. (2000). Antisocial, angry, and unsympathetic: "Hard to manage" preschoolers, peer problems and possible cognitive influences. *Journal of Child Psychology and Psychiatry, 41*, 169–179.

Hughes, J. N. (1988). *Cognitive behavior therapy with children in schools.* New York: Pergamon Press.

Hughes, J. N, Cavell, T. A., & Grossman, P. B. (1997). A positive view of self: Risk or protection for aggressive children? *Development and Psychopathology, 9*, 75–94.

Hughes, J. N., Cavell, T. A., & Jackson, T. (1999). Influence of the teacher–student relationship on childhood conduct problems: A prospective study. *Journal of Clinical Child Psychology, 28*, 173–184.

Hughes, J. N., & Hasbrouck, J. E. (1996). Television violence: Implications for violence prevention. *School Psychology Review, 25*, 134–151.

Hunter, L. (2001). The value of school-based mental health programs. *Report on Emotional and Behavioral Disorders in Youth, 1*, 27–44.

Hyde, K. L., Burchard, J. D., & Woodworth, K. (1996). Wrapping services in an urban setting. *Journal of Child and Family Services, 5*, 67–82.

Illback, R. J. (1994). Poverty and the crisis in children's services: The need for services integration. *Journal of Clinical Child Psychology, 23*, 413–424.

Illback, R. J., Kalafat, J., & Sanders, D. (1997). Evaluating integrated service programs. In R. J. Illback, C. T. Cobb, & H. M. Joseph (Eds.), *Integrated services for children and families: Opportunities for psychological practice* (pp. 323–346). Washington, DC: American Psychological Association.

Jackson, Y., & Frick, P. J. (1998). Negative life events and the adjustment of school-age children: Testing protective models. *Journal of Clinical Child Psychology, 27*, 370–380.

Jenkins, J. M., & Smith, M. A. (1991). Marital disharmony and children's behavior problems: Aspects of a poor marriage that affect children adversely. *Journal of Child Psychology and Psychiatry, 32*, 793–810.

Johnson, D. W., & Johnson, R. T. (1996). Conflict resolution and peer mediation programs in elementary and secondary schools: A review of the research. *Review of Educational Research, 66*, 459–506.

Johnson, D. W., & Johnson, R. T. (1999). Making cooperative learning work. *Theory into Practice, 38*, 67–73.

Johnson, D. W., Johnson, R. T., & Stanne, M. A. (2000). *Cooperative learning methods: A meta-analysis* [Online]. Available: www.clcrc.com

Johnston, C. (1996). Parent characteristics and parent–child interactions in families of non-problem children and ADHD children with higher and lower levels of oppositional-defiant behavior. *Journal of Abnormal Child Psychology, 24*, 85–104.

Johnston, C., & Freeman, W. (1997). Attributions for child behavior in parents of children without behavior disorders and children with attention-deficit hyperactivity disorder. *Journal of Consulting and Clinical Psychology, 65*, 636–645.

Johnstone, B., Frame, C., & Bouman, D. (1992). Physical attractiveness and athletic ability in controversial-aggressive and rejected-aggressive children. *Journal of Social and Clinical Psychology, 11*, 71–79.

Jolivette, K., Wehby, J. H., & Hirsch, L. (1999). Academic strategy identification for students exhibiting inappropriate classroom behavior. *Behavioral Disorders, 24*, 210–221.

Jones, C. B. (1999). Strategies for middle school and high school teachers of ADHD students. *ADHD Report, 7*, 9–11.

Jones, V. F., & Jones, L. S. (1995). *Comprehensive classroom management: Creating positive learning environments for all students* (4th ed.). Boston: Allyn & Bacon.

Jouriles, E. N., Bourg, W. J., & Farris, A. M. (1991). Marital adjustment and child conduct problems: A comparison of the correlation across subsamples. *Journal of Consulting and Clinical Psychology, 59*, 354–357.

Jouriles, E. N., Murphy, C. M., & O'Leary, K. D. (1989). Effects of maternal mood on mother–son interaction patterns. *Journal of Abnormal Child Psychology, 17*, 513–525.

Jouriles, E. N., Pfiffner, L. J., & O'Leary, S. G. (1988). Marital conflict, parenting, and toddler conduct problems. *Journal of Abnormal Child Psychology, 16*, 197–206.

Kamphaus, R. W., & Frick, P. J. (1996). *Clinical assessment of child and adolescent personality and behavior*. Boston: Allyn & Bacon.

Kamps, D., Kravits, T., Rauch, J., Kamps, J. L., & Chung, N. (2000). A prevention program for students with or at-risk for ED: Moderating effects of variation in treatment and classroom structure. *Journal of Emotional and Behavioral Disorders, 8*, 141–154.

Kaslow, N. J., & Thompson, M. P. (1998). Applying the criteria for empirically supported treatments to studies of psychosocial interventions for child and adolescent depression. *Journal of Clinical Child Psychology, 27*, 146–155.

Kaufman, A., & Kaufman, N. (1983). *Kaufman Assessment Battery for Children: Administration and scoring manual*. Circle Pines, MN: American Guidance Services.

Kauffman, J. M., & Wong, K. L. H. (1991). Effective teachers of students with behavioral disorders: Are generic teaching skills enough? *Behavioral Disorders, 16*, 225–237.

Kavale, K. A., & Forness, S. R. (1999). Effectiveness of special education. In C. R. Reynolds & T. B. Gutkin (Eds.), *The handbook of school psychology* (3rd ed., pp. 984–1024). New York: Wiley.

Kazdin, A. E. (1995). *Conduct disorders in childhood and adolescence* (2nd ed.). Thousand Oaks, CA: Sage.

Kazdin, A. E. (1996a). Problem solving and parent management in treating aggressive and antisocial behavior. In E. S. Hibbs & P. S. Jensen (Eds.), *Psychosocial treatments for child and adolescent disorders: Empirically based strategies for clinical practice* (pp. 377–408). Washington, DC: American Psychological Association.

Kazdin, A. E. (1996b). Dropping out of child psychotherapy: Issues for research and implications for practice. *Clinical Child Psychology and Psychiatry, 1*, 133–156.

Kazdin, A. E. (1997a). Practitioner review: Psychosocial treatments for conduct disorder in children. *Journal of Child Psychology and Psychiatry, 38*, 161–178.

Kazdin, A. E. (1997b). A model for developing effective treatments: Progression and interplay of theory, research, and practice. *Journal of Clinical Child Psychology, 26*, 114–129.

Kazdin, A. E., & Crowley, M. J. (1997). Moderators of treatment outcome in cognitively based treatment of antisocial children. *Cognitive Therapy and Research, 21,* 185–207.

Kazdin, A. E., & Esveldt-Dawson, K. (1986). The Interview for Antisocial Behavior: Psychometric characteristics and concurrent validity with child psychiatric inpatients. *Journal of Psychopathology and Behavioral Assessment, 8,* 289–303.

Kazdin, A. E., Esveldt-Dawson, K., French, N. H., & Unis, A. S. (1987a). Effects of parent management training and problem-solving skills training combined in the treatment of antisocial child behavior. *Journal of the American Academy of Child and Adolescent Psychiatry, 26,* 416–424.

Kazdin, A. E., Esveldt-Dawson, K., French, N. H., & Unis, A. S. (1987b). Problem-solving skills training and relationship therapy in the treatment of antisocial child behavior. *Journal of Consulting and Clinical Psychology, 55,* 76–85.

Kazdin, A. E., Holland, L., & Crowley, M. (1997). Family experience of barriers to treatment and premature termination of child therapy. *Journal of Consulting and Clinical Psychology, 65,* 453–463.

Kazdin, A. E., Holland, L., Crowley, M., & Breton, S. (1997). Barriers to Participation in Treatment Scale: Evaluation and validation in the context of child outpatient treatment. *Journal of Child Psychology and Psychiatry, 38,* 1051–1062.

Kazdin, A. E., & Kagan, J. (1994). Models of dysfunction in developmental psychopathology. *Clinical Psychology: Science and Practice, 1,* 35–52.

Kazdin, A. E., Mazurick, J. L., & Bass, D. (1993). Risk for attrition in treatment of antisocial children and families. *Journal of Clinical Child Psychology, 22,* 2–16.

Kazdin, A. E., Siegel, T., & Bass, D. (1992). Cognitive problem-solving skills training and parent management training in the treatment of antisocial behavior in children. *Journal of Consulting and Clinical Psychology, 60,* 733–747.

Kazdin, A. E., Stolar, M. J., & Marciano, P. L. (1995). Risk factors for dropping out of treatment among white and black families. *Journal of Family Psychology, 9,* 402–417.

Kazdin, A. E., & Wassell, G. (1999). Barriers to treatment participation and therapeutic change among children referred for conduct disorder. *Journal of Clinical Child Psychology, 28,* 160–172.

Keenan, K., Loeber, R., & Green, S. (1999). Conduct disorder in girls: A review of the literature. *Clinical Child and Family Psychology Review, 2,* 3–19.

Keenan, K., & Shaw, D. (1994). The development of aggression in toddlers: A study of low-income families. *Journal of Abnormal Child Psychology, 22,* 53–77.

Keenan, K., Shaw, D., Dellilquadri, E., Giovannelli, J., & Walsh, B. (1998). Evidence for the continuity of early problem behaviors: Application of a developmental model. *Journal of Abnormal Child Psychology, 26,* 441–454.

Keenan, K., & Wakschlag, L. S. (2000). More than the terrible twos: The nature and severity of behavior problems in clinic-referred preschool children. *Journal of Abnormal Child Psychology, 28,* 33–46.

Keller, H. R., & Tapasak, R. C. (1997). Classroom management. In A. P. Goldstein & J. C. Conoley (Eds.), *School violence intervention: A practical handbook* (pp. 107–126). New York: Guilford Press.

Kelley, M. L., & McCain, A. P. (1995). Promoting academic performance in inattentive children: The relative efficacy of school–home notes with and without response cost. *Behavior Modification, 19,* 357–375.

Kendall, P. C., & Braswell, L. (1993). *Cognitive-behavioral therapy for impulsive children* (2nd ed.). New York: Guilford Press.

Kendall, P. C., Chu, B. C., Pimentel, S. S., & Choudhury, M. (2000). Treating anxiety disorders in youth. In P. C. Kendall (Ed.), *Child and adolescent therapy: Cognitive-behavioral procedures* (2nd ed., pp. 235–287). New York: Guilford Press.

Kendall, P. C., & MacDonald, J. P. (1993). Cognition in the psychopathology of youth and its implications for treatment. In K. S. Dobson & P. C. Kendall (Eds.), *Psychopathology and cognition* (pp. 387–430). San Diego: Academic Press.

Kendall, P. C., Reber, M., McLeer, S., Epps, J., & Ronan, K. R. (1990). Cognitive-behavioral treatment of conduct-disordered children. *Cognitive Therapy and Research, 14,* 279–297.

Kendziora, K. T., & O'Leary, S. G. (1998). Appraisals of child behavior by mothers of problem and nonproblem toddlers. *Journal of Abnormal Child Psychology, 26,* 247–255.

Kilgore, K., Snyder, J., & Lentz, C. (2000). The contribution of parental discipline, parental monitoring, and school risk to early-onset conduct problems in African-American boys and girls. *Developmental Psychology, 36,* 835–845.

Kingston, L., & Prior, M. (1995). The development of patterns of stable, transient, and school-age onset aggressive behavior in young children. *Journal of the American Academy of Child and Adolescent Psychiatry, 34,* 348–358.

Kliewer, W., & Kung, E. (1998). Family moderators of the relation between hassles and behavior problems in inner-city youth. *Journal of Clinical Child Psychology, 27,* 278–292.

Knoff, H. M. (2000). Organizational development and strategic planning for the millennium: A blueprint toward effective school discipline, safety, and crisis prevention. *Psychology in the Schools, 37,* 17–32.

Kohler, F. W., & Strain, P. S. (1990). Peer-assisted interventions: Early promises, notable achievements, and future aspiration. *Clinical Psychology Review, 10,* 441–452.

Kokko, K., & Pulkkinen, L. (2000). Aggression in childhood and long-term unemployment in adulthood: A cycle of maladaptation and some protective factors. *Developmental Psychology, 36,* 463–472.

Kolko, D. J. (1996). Education and counseling for child fire setters: A comparison of skills training programs with standard practice. In E. D. Hibbs & P. S. Jensen (Eds.), *Psychosocial treatments for child and adolescent disorders* (pp. 409–433). Washington, DC: American Psychological Association.

Koppitz, E. (1968). *Psychological evaluation of children's human figure drawings.* New York: Grune & Stratton.

Kovacs, M. (1992). *Children's Depression Inventory.* North Tonawanda, NY: Multi-Health Systems.

Kratochwill, T. R., Elliott, S. N., & Rotto, P.C. (1995). Best practices in school-based behavioral consultation. In A. Thomas & J. Grimes (Eds.), *Best practices in school psychology–III* (pp. 519–537). Washington, DC: National Association of School Psychologists.

Kumpulainen, K., Rasanen, E., Henttonen, I., Almquist, F., Kresanor, K., Lina, S., Moilanen, I., Piha, J., Puura, K., & Tamminen, T. (1998). Bullying and psychiatric symptoms among elementary school-age children. *Child Abuse and Neglect, 22,* 705–717.

Kupersmidt, J. B., Griesler, P. C., DeRosier, M. E., Patterson, C. J., & Davis, P. W. (1995). Childhood aggression and peer relations in context of family and neighborhood factors. *Child Development, 66,* 360–375.

Kutash, K., & Duchnowski, A. J. (1997). Create comprehensive and collaborative systems. *Journal of Emotional and Behavioral Disorders, 5,* 66–75.

Kutash, K., Duchnowski, A. J., Meyers, J., & King, B. (1997). Community- and neighborhood-based services for youth. In S. W. Henggeler & A. B. Santos (Eds.), *Innovative approaches for difficult-to-treat populations* (pp. 47–63). Washington, DC: American Psychiatric Press.

Lahey, B. B., Loeber, R., Quay, H. C., Applegate, B., Shaffer, D., Waldman, I., Hart, E. L., McBurnett, K., Frick, P. J., Jensen, P. S., Dulcan, M. K., Canino, G., & Bird, H. (1998). Validity of DSM-IV subtypes of conduct disorder based on age of onset. *Journal of the American Academy of Child and Adolescent Psychiatry, 37,* 435–442.

Lahey, B. B., Miller, T. L., Gordon, R. A., & Riley, A. W. (1999). Developmental epidemiology of the disruptive behavior disorders. In H. C. Quay & A. E. Hogan (Eds.), *Handbook of disruptive behavior disorders* (pp. 23–48). New York: Kluwer Academic/Plenum Press.

Lahey, B. B., Pelham, W. E., Stein, M. A., Loney, J., Trapani, C., Nugent, K., Kipp, H., Schmidt, E., Lee, S., Cale, M., Gold, E., Hartung, C.M., Willcutt, B., & Baumann, B. (1998). Validity of DSM-IV attention-deficit/hyperactivity disorder for younger children. *Journal of the American Academy of Child and Adolescent Psychiatry, 37,* 695–702.

Lahey, B. B., Piacentini, J. C., McBurnett, K., Stone, P., Hartdagen, S., & Hynd, G. (1988). Psychopathology in the parents of children with conduct disorder and hyperactivity. *Journal of the American Academy of Child and Adolescent Psychiatry, 27,* 163–170.

Lahey, B. B., Schaughency, E. A., Hynd, G. W., Carlson, C. L., & Nieves, N. (1987). Attention deficit disorder with and without hyperactivity: Comparison of behavioral characteristics of clinic-referred children. *Journal of the American Academy of Child and Adolescent Psychiatry, 26,* 718–723.

Lahey, B. B., Schaughency, E. A., Strauss, C. C., & Frame, C. L. (1984). Are attention deficit disorders with and without hyperactivity similar or dissimilar disorders? *Journal of the American Academy of Child and Adolescent Psychiatry, 23,* 302–309.

Lambert, E. W., Wahler, R. G., Andrade, A. R., & Bickman, L. (2001). Looking for the disorder in conduct disorder. *Journal of Abnormal Psychology, 110,* 110–123.

Larzelere, R. E. (2000). Child outcomes of nonabusive and customary physical punishment by parents: An updated literature review. *Clinical Child and Family Psychology Review, 3,* 199–221.

Larzelere, R. E., & Patterson, G. R. (1990). Parental management: Mediator of the effects of socioeconomic status on early delinquency. *Criminology, 28,* 301–324.

Ledingham, J. E. (1999). Children and adolescents with oppositional defiant disorder and conduct disorder in the community: Experiences with school and with peers. In H. C. Quay & A. E. Hogan (Eds.), *Handbook of disruptive behavior disorders* (pp. 353–370). New York: Kluwer Academic/Plenum Press.

Lee, E. (1996). Asian American families: An overview. In M. McGoldrick, J. Giordano, & J. K. Pearce (Eds.), *Ethnicity and family therapy* (pp. 227–248). New York: Guilford Press.

Lemerise, E. A., & Arsenio, W. F. (2000). An integrated model of emotion processes and cognition in social information processing. *Child Development, 71,* 107–118.

Levendoski, L. S., & Cartledge, G. (2000). Self-monitoring for elementary school children with serious emotional disturbances: Classroom applications for increased academic responding. *Behavioral Disorders, 25,* 211–224.

Leventhal, T., & Brooks-Gunn, J. (2000). The neighborhoods they live in: The effects of neighborhood residence on child and adolescent outcomes. *Psychological Bulletin, 126,* 309–337.

Levy, F., Hay, D. A., McStephen, M., Wood, C., Hons, B. B. S., & Waldman, I. (1997). Attention-deficit hyperactivity disorder: A category or a continuum? Genetic analysis of a large-scale twin study. *Journal of the American Academy of Child and Adolescent Psychiatry, 36,* 737–744.

Lewis, M., Summerville, J. W., & Graffagnino, P. N. (1996). Residential treatment. In M. Lewis (Ed.), *Child and adolescent psychiatry: A comprehensive textbook* (pp. 894–902). Baltimore: Williams & Wilkins.

Lindsey, M. L. (1998). Culturally competent assessment of African American clients. *Journal of Personality Assessment, 70,* 43–53.

Lochman, J. E., Burch, P. R., Curry, J. F., & Lampron, L. B. (1984). Treatment and generalization effects of cognitive-behavioral and goal setting interventions with aggressive boys. *Journal of Consulting and Clinical Psychology, 52,* 915–916.

Lochman, J. E., & Conduct Problems Research Group. (1995). Screening of child behavior problems from prevention programs at school entry. *Journal of Consulting and Clinical Psychology, 63,* 549–559.

Lochman, J. E., & Dodge, K. A. (1994). Social-cognitive processes of severely violent, moderately aggressive and nonaggressive boys. *Journal of Consulting and Clinical Psychology, 62,* 366–374.

Lochman, J. E., Lampron, L. B., Gemmer, T. C., & Harris, S. R. (1987). Anger coping intervention with aggressive children: A guide to implementation in school settings. In P. A. Keller & S. R. Heyman (Eds.), *Innovations in clinical practice: A source book* (Vol. 6, pp. 339–356). Sarasota, FL: Professional Resource Exchange.

Lochman, J. E., Lampron, L. B., Gemmer, T. C., & Harris, S. R. (1989). Teacher consultation and cognitive-behavioral interventions with aggressive boys. *Psychology in the Schools, 26,* 179–188.

Lochman, J. E., & Lenhart, L. A. (1993). Anger coping intervention for aggressive children: Conceptual models and outcome effects. *Clinical Psychology Review, 13,* 785–805.

Lochman, J. E., & Wells, K. C. (1996). A social-cognitive intervention with aggressive children: Prevention effects and contextual implementation issues. In R. D. Peters & R. J. McMahon (Eds.), *Preventing childhood disorders, substance abuse, and delinquency* (pp. 111–143). Thousand Oaks, CA: Sage.

Lochman, J. E., Whidby, J. M., & FitzGerald, D. P. (2000). Cognitive-behavioral assessment and treatment with aggressive children. In P. C. Kendall (Ed.), *Child and adolescent therapy: Cognitive-behavioral procedures* (2nd ed., pp. 31–87). New York: Guilford Press.

Loeber, R., Burke, J. D., Lahey, B. B., Winters, A., & Zera, M. (2000). Oppositional defiant and conduct disorder: A review of the past 10 years, Part I. *Journal of the American Academy of Child and Adolescent Psychiatry, 39,* 1468–1484.

Loeber, R., & Dishion, T. J. (1984). Boys who fight at home and in school: Family conditions influencing cross-setting consistency and discontinuity. *Journal of Consulting and Clinical Psychology, 52,* 759–768.

Loeber, R., & Farrington, D. P. (2000). Young children who commit crime: Epidemiology, developmental origins, risk factors, early interventions, and policy implications. *Development and Psychopathology, 12,* 737–762.

Loeber, R., Farrington, D. P., Stouthamer-Loeber, M., Moffitt, T. E., & Caspi, A. (1998). The development of male offending: Key findings from the first decade of the Pittsburgh Youth Study. *Studies on Crime and Crime Prevention, 7,* 141–171.

Loeber, R., Green, S. M., Lahey, B. B., & Kalb, L. (2000). Physical fighting in childhood as a risk factor for later mental health problems. *Journal of the American Academy of Child and Adolescent Psychiatry, 39,* 421–428.

Loeber, R., & Hay, D. F. (1994). Developmental approaches to aggression and conduct problems. In M. Rutter & D. F. Hay (Eds.), *Development through life: A handbook for clinicians* (pp. 488–516). Malden, MA: Blackwell Scientific.

Loeber, R., & Hay, D. F. (1997). Key issues in the development of aggression and violence from childhood to early adulthood. *Annual Review of Psychology, 48,* 371–410.

Loeber, R., & Schmaling, K. B. (1985). Empirical evidence for overt and covert patterns of antisocial conduct problems: A meta-analysis. *Journal of Abnormal Child Psychology, 13,* 337–352.

Loeber, R., & Stouthamer-Loeber, M. (1998). Development of juvenile aggression and violence: Some common misconceptions and controversies. *American Psychologist, 53,* 242–259.

Loeber, R., Stouthamer-Loeber, M., & White, H. R. (1999). Developmental aspects of delinquency and internalizing problems and their association with persistent juvenile substance use between ages 7 and 18. *Journal of Clinical Child Psychology, 28,* 322–332.

Loeber, R., Wung, P., Keenan, K., Giroux, B., Stouthamer-Loeber, M., Van Kammen, W. B., & Maughan, B. (1993). Developmental pathways in disruptive child behavior. *Development and Psychopathology, 5,* 101–131.

Lonigan, C. J., Elbert, J. C., & Johnson, S. B. (1998). Empirically supported psychosocial interventions for children: An overview. *Journal of Clinical Child Psychology, 27,* 138–145.

Lovejoy, M. C., Graczyk, P. A., O'Hare, E., & Neuman, G. (2000). Maternal depression and parenting behavior: A meta-analytic review. *Clinical Psychology Review, 20,* 561–592.

Lovell, R., & Pope, C. E. (1993). Recreational interventions. In A. P. Goldstein & C. R. Huff (Eds.), *The gang intervention handbook* (pp. 319–332). Champaign, IL: Research Press.

Luthar, S. S., Cicchetti, D., & Becker, B. (2000). The construct of resilience: A critical evaluation and guidelines for future work. *Child Development, 71,* 543–562.

Lynam, D. R. (1996). Early identification of chronic offenders: Who is the fledgling psychopath? *Psychological Bulletin, 120,* 209–234.

Lynam, D. R. (1997). Pursuing the psychopath: Capturing the fledgling psychopath in the nomological net. *Journal of Abnormal Psychology, 106,* 425–438.

Lynam, D. R. (1998). Early identification of the fledgling psychopath: Locating the psychopathic child in the current nomenclature. *Journal of Abnormal Psychology, 107,* 566–575.

Lynch, M., & Cicchetti, D. (1998). An ecological–transactional analysis of children and contexts: The longitudinal interplay among child maltreatment, community violence, and children's symptomatology. *Development and Psychopathology, 10*, 235–257.

Lynn, C. J., McKay, M. M., Hibbert, R., Carrera, S., Lawrence, R., Miranda, A., Jarvis, A., Gamble, D., & Palacios, J. (2001). Developing collaborations with parents and schools to promote urban-child mental health. *Report on Emotional and Behavioral Disorders in Youth. 1*, 31–45.

Lyons-Ruth, K. (1996). Attachment relationships among children with aggressive behavior problems: The role of disorganized early attachment patterns. *Journal of Consulting and Clinical Psychology, 64*, 64–73.

Maag, J. W., & Reid, R. (1994). Attention-deficit hyperactivity disorder: A functional approach to assessment and treatment. *Behavioral Disorders, 20*, 5–23.

Madan-Swain, A., & Zentall, S. S. (1990). Behavioral comparisons of liked and disliked hyperactive children in play contexts and the behavioral accommodations by their classmates. *Journal of Consulting and Clinical Psychology, 58*, 197–209.

Madsen, K., Levene, K., Pepler, D., & Andreacachi, M. (1999). *The Earlscourt Girls Connection: An outcome study.* Unpublished manuscript, Earlscourt Child and Family Center, Toronto, Canada.

Magnus, K. B., Cowen, E. L., Wyman, P. A., Fagen, D. B., & Work, W. C. (1999a). Correlates of resilient outcomes among highly stressed African-American and white urban children. *Journal of Community Psychology, 27*, 473–488.

Magnus, K. B., Cowen, E. L., Wyman, P. A., Fagen, D. B., & Work, W. C. (1999b). Parent–child relationship qualities and child adjustment in highly stressed urban black and white families. *Journal of Community Psychology, 27*, 55–71.

Maguin, E., & Loeber, R. (1996). Academic performance and delinquency. In M. Tonry (Ed.), *Crime and justice* (Vol. 20, pp. 102–123). Chicago: University of Chicago Press.

Mahoney, A., Jouriles, E. N., & Scavone, J. (1997). Marital adjustment, marital discord over child rearing, and child behavior problems: Moderating effects of child age. *Journal of Clinical Child Psychology, 26*, 415–423.

Mahoney, J. L. (2000). School extracurricular activity participation as a moderator in the development of antisocial patterns. *Child Development, 71*, 502–516.

Malo, J., & Tremblay, R. E. (1997). The impact of paternal alcoholism and maternal social position on boys' school adjustment, pubertal maturation and sexual behavior: A test of two competing hypotheses. *Journal of Child Psychology and Psychiatry, 38*, 187–197.

Manly, J. T., Cicchetti, D., & Barnett, D. (1994). The impacting subtype, frequency, chronicity and severity of child maltreatment on social competence and behavior problems. *Development and Psychopathology, 6*, 121–144.

Mann, B. J., & Mackenzie, E. P. (1996). Pathways among marital function, parental behaviors, and child behavior problems in school-age boys. *Journal of Clinical Child Psychology, 25*, 183–191.

Maquin, E., & Loeber, R. (1996). Academic performance and delinquency. In M. Tonry (Ed.), *Crime and justice: A review of research* (Vol. 20, pp. 145–246). Chicago: University of Chicago Press.

Marcon, R. A. (1999). Positive relationships between parent school involvement and public school inner-city preschoolers' development and academic performance. *School Psychology Review, 28*, 395–412.

Martens, B. K., & Kelly, S. Q. (1993). A behavioral analysis of effective teaching. *School Psychology Quarterly, 8,*10–26.

Martens, B. K., Witt, J. C., Daly III, E. J., & Vollmer, T. R. (1999). Behavior analysis: Theory and practice in educational settings. In C. R. Reynolds & T. B. Gutkin (Eds.), *The handbook of school psychology* (3rd ed., pp. 638–663). New York: Wiley.

Mash, E. J., & Johnston, C. (1990). Determinants of parenting stress: Illustrations from families of hyperactive children and families of physically abused children. *Journal of Clinical Child Psychology, 19,* 313–328.

Mash, E. J., & Terdal, L. G. (1997). Assessment of child and family disturbance: A behavioral–systems approach. In E. J. Mash & L. G. Terdal (Eds.), *Assessment of childhood disorders* (3rd ed., pp.3–68). New York: Guilford Press.

Mason, J. L., Benjamin, M. P., & Lewis, S. A. (1996). The cultural competence model: Implications for child and family mental health services. In C. A. Heflinger & C. T. Nixon (Eds.), *Families and the mental health system for children and adolescents: Policy, services, and research* (pp. 63–74). Thousand Oaks, CA: Sage.

Masten, A. S., & Coatsworth, J. D. (1998). The development of competence in favorable and unfavorable environments: Lessons from research on successful children. *American Psychologist, 53,* 205–220.

Masten, A. S., & Garmezy, N. (1986). Risk, vulnerability and protective factors in developmental psychopathology. In B. B. Lahey & A. E. Kazdin (Eds.), *Advances in clinical child psychology* (Vol. 8, pp. 1–52). New York: Plenum Press.

Masten, A. S., Hubbard, J. J., Gest, S. D., Tellegen, A., Garmezy, N., & Ramirez, M.-L. (1999). Competence in the context of adversity: Pathways to resilience and maladaptation from childhood to late adolescence. *Development and Psychopathology, 11,* 143–169.

Matthys, W., Cuperus, J. M., & Van Engeland, H. (1999). Deficient social problem-solving in boys with ODD/CD, with ADHD, and with both disorders. *Journal of the American Academy of Child and Adolescent Psychiatry, 38,* 311–321.

Mayer, G. R. (1995). Preventing antisocial behavior in the schools. *Journal of Applied Behavior Analysis, 28,* 467–478.

McArthur, D. S., & Roberts, G. E. (1982). *Roberts Apperception Test for Children: Manual.* Los Angeles: Western Psychological Services.

McBurnett, K., Lahey, B. B., Rathouz, P. J., & Loeber, R. (2000). Low salivary cortisol and persistent aggression in boys referred for disruptive behavior. *Archives of General Psychiatry, 57,* 38–43.

McCay, M., Nudelman, R., McCadam, K., & Gonzales, J. (1996). Evaluating a social work engagement approach to involving inner-city children and their families in mental health care. *Research on Social Work Practice, 6,* 462–472.

McCay, M., Stoewe, J., McCadam, K., & Gonzales, J. (1998). Increasing access to child mental health services for urban children and their caregivers. *Health and Social Work, 23,* 9–15.

McCloskey, L. A., Figueredo, A. J., & Koss, M. P. (1995). The effects of systematic family violence on children's mental health. *Child Development, 68,* 1239–1261.

McConaughy, S. H., & Achenbach, T. M. (1994). *Manual for the Semistructured Clinical Interview for Children and Adolescents.* Burlington: Department of Psychiatry, University of Vermont.

McEvoy, A., & Welker, R. (2000). Antisocial behavior, academic failure, and school climate: A critical review. *Journal of Emotional and Behavioral Disorders, 8,* 130–140.

McFadyen-Ketchum, S. A., Bates, J. E., Dodge, K. A., & Pettit, G. S. (1996). Patterns of change in early childhood aggressive-disruptive behaviors: Gender differences in predictions from early coercive and affectionate mother–child interactions. *Child Development, 67,* 2417–2433.

McFadyen-Ketchum, S. A., & Dodge, K. A. (1998). Problems in social relationships. In E. J. Mash & R. A. Barkley (Eds.), *Treatment of childhood disorders* (2nd ed., pp. 338–365). New York: Guilford Press.

McGee, R., Share, D., Moffitt, T. E., Williams, S., & Silva, P. A. (1988). Reading disability, behaviour problems, and juvenile delinquency. In D. H. Sadlofske & S. B. G. Eysenck (Eds.), *Individual differences in children and adolescents: International perspectives* (pp. 158–172). London: Hodder & Stoughton.

McGill, D. E., Mihalic, S. F., & Grotpeter, J. K. (1997). *Big Brothers Big Sisters of America.* Boulder: Institute of Behavioral Science, University of Colorado.

McGoldrick, M., & Giordano, J. (1996). Overview: Ethnicity and family therapy. In M. McGoldrick, J. Giordano, & J. K. Pearce (Eds.), *Ethnicity and family therapy* (pp. 1–27). New York: Guilford Press.

McLoyd, V. C. (1990). The impact of economic hardship on black families and children: Psychological distress, parenting, and socioemotional development. *Child Development, 61,* 311–346.

McLoyd, V. C. (1998). Socioeconomic disadvantage and child development. *American Psychologist, 53,* 185–204.

McMahon, R. J. (1994). Diagnosis, assessment, and treatment of externalizing problems in children: The role of longitudinal data. *Journal of Consulting and Clinical Psychology, 62,* 901–917.

McMahon, R. J., & Estes, A. M. (1997). Conduct problems. In E. J. Mash & L. G. Terdal (Eds.), *Assessment of childhood disorders* (3rd ed., pp. 130–193). New York: Guilford Press.

McMahon, R. J., & Forehand, R. (1984). Parent training for the noncompliant child: Treatment outcome, generalization, and adjunctive therapy procedures. In R. F. Dangel & R. A. Polster (Eds.), *Parent training: Foundations of research and practice* (pp. 298–328). New York: Guilford Press.

McMahon, R. J., Slough, N. M., & Conduct Problems Prevention Research Group (1996). Family-based intervention in the Fast Track program. In R. D. Peters & R. J. McMahon (Eds.), *Preventing childhood disorders, substance abuse and delinquency* (pp. 90–110). Thousand Oaks, CA: Sage.

McNeil, C. B., Eyberg, S., Eisenstadt, T. H., Newcomb, K., & Funderburk, B. (1991). Parent–child interaction therapy with behavior problem children: Generalization of treatment effects to the school setting. *Journal of Clinical Child Psychology, 20,* 140–151.

McPartland, J. M., & Nettles, S. M. (1991, August). Using community adults as advocates or mentors for at-risk middle school students: A two-year evaluation of project RAISE. *American Journal of Education,* pp. 568–586.

McQuillan, K., DuPaul, G. J., Shapiro, E. S., & Cole, C. L. (1996). Classroom performance of students with serious emotional disturbance: A comparative study of evaluation methods for behavior management. *Journal of Emotional and Behavioral Disorders, 4,* 162–170.

Melnick, S. M., & Hinshaw, S. P. (2000). Emotion regulation and parenting in AD/HD and comparison boys: Linkages with social behaviors and peer preference. *Journal of Abnormal Child Psychology, 28,* 73–86.

Metropolitan Area Child Study Research Group. (in press). A cognitive–ecological approach to preventing aggression in urban settings: Initial outcomes for high-risk children. *Journal of Consulting and Clinical Psychology.*

Middlebrook, J. L., & Forehand, R. (1985). Maternal perceptions of deviance in child behavior as a function of stress and clinic versus nonclinic status of the child: An analogue study. *Behavior Therapy, 16,* 494–502.

Miles, D. R., & Carey, G. (1997). Genetic and environmental architecture of human aggression. *Journal of Personality and Social Psychology, 72,* 207–217.

Milich, R., & Nietzel, M. T. (1993). Introduction. *Clinical Psychology Review, 13,* 695–697.

Miller, G. E., & Prinz, R. J. (1990). Enhancement of social learning family interventions for childhood conduct disorder. *Psychological Bulletin, 108,* 291–307.

Miller, L. S., Wasserman, G. A., Neugebauer, R., Gorman-Smith, D., & Kamboukos, D. (1999). Witnessed community violence and antisocial behavior in high-risk, urban boys. *Journal of Clinical Child Psychology, 28,* 2–11.

Miller, S. A. (1995). Parents' attributions for their children's behavior. *Child Development, 66,* 1557–1584.

Miller-Johnson, S., Coie, J. D., Maumary-Gremaud, A., Lochman, J. E., & Terry, R. (1999). Relationship between childhood peer rejection and aggression and adolescent delinquency severity and type among African-American youth. *Journal of Emotional and Behavioral Disorders, 7,* 137–146.

Miller-Johnson, S., Lochman, J. E., Coie, J. D., Terry, R., & Hyman, C. (1998). Comorbidity of conduct and depressive problems at sixth grade: Substance use outcomes across adolescence. *Journal of Abnormal Child Psychology, 26,* 221–232.

Moffitt, T. E. (1993). Adolescent-limited and life-course persistent antisocial behavior: A developmental taxonomy. *Psychological Review, 100,* 674–701.

Moffitt, T. E., & Caspi, A. (2001). Childhood predictors differentiate life-course persistent and adolescent-limited antisocial pathways among males and females. *Development and Psychopathology, 13,* 355–375.

Moffitt, T. E., Caspi, A., Dickson, N., Silva, P., & Stanton, W. (1996). Childhood-onset versus adolescent-onset antisocial conduct problems in males: Natural history from ages 3 to 18 years. *Development and Psychopathology, 8,* 399–424.

Molina, B. S. G., Smith, B. H., & Pelham, W. E. (1999). Interactive effects of ADHD and CD on early adolescent substance use. *Psychology of Addictive Behaviors, 113,* 344–358.

Moore Hines, P., & Boyd-Franklin, N. (1996). African American families. In M. McGoldrick, J. Giordano, & J. K. Pearce (Eds.), *Ethnicity and family therapy* (2nd ed., pp. 66–84). New York: Guilford Press.

Moos, R., & Moos, B. (1983). Clinical applications of the Family Environment Scale. In E. Filsinger (Ed.), *Marriage and family assessment: A sourcebook for family therapy* (pp. 253–273). Beverly Hills, CA: Sage.

Morgan, A. B., & Lilienfeld, S. O. (2000). A meta-analytic review of the relation between antisocial behavior and neuropsychological measures of executive function. *Clinical Psychology Review, 20,* 113–136.

Morrison, G. M., Robertson, L., & Harding, M. (1998). Resilience factors that support the classroom functioning of acting out and aggressive students. *Psychology in the Schools, 35,* 217–227.

Morrissey-Kane, E., & Prinz, R. J. (1999). Engagement in child and adolescent treatment: The role of parental cognitions and attributions. *Clinical Child and Family Psychology Review, 2,* 183–198.

Morrow, K. V., & Styles, M. B. (1995). *Building relationships with youth in program settings: A study of Big Brothers Big Sisters.* Philadelphia: Public/Private Ventures.

Moss, H. B., Mezzich, A., Yao, J. K., Gavaler, J., & Martin, C. S. (1995). Aggressivity among sons of substance-abusing fathers: Association with psychiatric disorder in father and son, paternal personality, pubertal development, and sociometric status. *American Journal of Drug and Alcohol Abuse, 21,* 195–208.

Moss, H. B., Vanyukov, M. M., & Martini, C. S. (1995). Salivary cortisol responses and the risk for substance abuse in prepubertal boys. *Biological Psychiatry, 38,* 547–555.

Moss, H. B., & Yao, J. K. (1996). Platelet dense granule secretion in adolescents with conduct disorders and substance abuse: Preliminary evidence for variation in signal transduction. *Biological Psychiatry, 40,* 892–898.

MTA Cooperative Group. (1999a). Fourteen-month randomized clinical trial of treatment strategies for attention-deficit/hyperactivity disorder. *Archives of General Psychiatry, 56,* 1073–1086.

MTA Cooperative Group. (1999b). Effects of comorbid anxiety, poverty, session attendance, and community medication in treatment outcome in children with attention-deficit/hyperactivity disorder. *Archives of General Psychiatry, 56,* 1088–1096.

Mulvey, E. P., Arthur, M. W., & Reppucci, N. D. (1993). The prevention and treatment of juvenile delinquency. *Clinical Psychology Review, 13,* 133–168.

Mulvey, E. P., & Woolard, J. L. (1997). Themes for consideration in future research on prevention and intervention with antisocial behaviors. In D. M. Stoff, J. Breiling, & J. D. Maser (Eds.), *Handbook of antisocial behavior* (pp. 454–460). New York: Wiley.

Munk, D. D., & Repp, A. C. (1994). The relationship between instructional variables and problem behavior: A review. *Exceptional Children, 60,* 390–401.

Nagin, D., & Tremblay, R. E. (1999). Trajectories of boys' physical aggression, opposition and hyperactivity on the path to physically violent and nonviolent juvenile delinquency. *Child Development, 70,* 1181–1196.

Nastasi, B. K., & Clements, D. H. (1991). Research on cooperative learning: Implications for practice. *School Psychology Review, 20,* 110–131.

Neisser, U., Boodoo, G., Bouchard Jr., T., Boykin, A. W., Brody, N., Ceci, S., Halpern, D., Loehlin, J., Perloff, R., Sternberg, R., & Urbina, S. (1996). Intelligence: Knowns and unknowns. *American Psychologist, 51,* 77–101.

Nelson, J. R. (1996). Designing schools to meet the needs of students who exhibit disruptive behavior. *Journal of Emotional and Behavioral Disorders, 4,* 147–161.

Nelson, J. R., Roberts, M. L., Mathur, S. R., & Rutherford Jr., R. B. (1999). Has public policy exceeded our knowledge base? A review of the functional behavioral assessment literature. *Behavioral Disorders, 24,* 169–179.

Nelson, J. R., Smith, D. J., Young, R. K., & Dodd, J. M. (1991). A review of self-management outcome research conducted with students who exhibit behavioral disorders. *Behavioral Disorders, 16,* 168–179.

Nicolosi, E. M., & Stavrou, E. (2000). IQ tests and their fairness for Native American students. *School Psychologist, 54*, 58–79

Nigg, J. T., & Hinshaw, S. P. (1998). Parent personality traits and psychopathology associated with antisocial behaviors in childhood attention-deficit hyperactivity disorder. *Journal of Child Psychology and Psychiatry, 39*, 145–159.

Nix, R. L., Pinderhughes, E. E., Dodge, K. A., Bates, J. E., Pettit, G. S., & McFadyen-Ketchum, S. A. (1999). The relation between mothers' hostile attribution tendencies and children's externalizing behavior problems: The mediating role of mothers' harsh discipline practices. *Child Development, 70*, 896–909.

Novaco, R. W. (1978). Anger and coping with stress: Cognitive-behavioral intervention. In J. P. Foreyet & D. P. Rathjen (Eds.), *Cognitive behavioral therapy: Research and application* (pp. 135–173). New York: Plenum Press.

Office of Juvenile Justice and Delinquency Prevention. (1998). *1998 report to Congress: Juvenile Mentoring Program (JUMP)*. Washington, DC: Author.

Ollendick, T. H., & King, N. J. (1998). Empirically supported treatments for children with phobic and anxiety disorders: Current status. *Journal of Clinical Child Psychology, 27*, 156–167.

Ollendick, T. H., & King, H. J. (2000). Empirically supported treatments for children and adolescents. In P. C. Kendall (Ed.), *Child and adolescent therapy: Cognitive-behavioral procedures* (pp. 386–426). New York: Guilford Press.

Olson, D. H., & Killorin, E (1985). *Clinical rating scale for the Circumplex Model of Marital and Family Systems*. St. Paul: University of Minnesota.

Olson, H. C., Streissguth, A. P., Sampson, P. D., Barr, H. M., Bookstein, F. L., & Thiede, K. (1997). Association of prenatal alcohol exposure with behavioral and learning problems in early adolescence. *Journal of the American Academy of Child and Adolescent Psychiatry, 36*, 1187–1194.

Olweus, D. (1979). Stability of aggressive patterns in males: A review. *Psychological Bulletin, 86*, 852–875.

Olweus, D. (1991). Bully–victim problems among schoolchildren: Basic facts and effects of a school-based intervention program. In D. J. Pepler & K. E. Rubin (Eds.), *The development and treatment of childhood aggression* (pp. 411–448). Hillsdale, NJ: Erlbaum.

Olweus, D. (1994). Bullying at school: Long-term outcomes for the victims and an effective school-based intervention program. In L. R. Huesmann (Ed.), *Aggressive behavior: Current perspectives* (pp. 97–130). New York: Plenum Press.

Olweus, D. (1996). *The revised Olweus Bully/Victim Questionnaire*. Unpublished manuscript, Research Center for Health Promotion (HEMIL), Bergen, Norway.

Olweus, D., Limber, S., & Mihalic, S. (2000). *Blueprints for violence prevention: Bullying prevention program*. Boulder, CO: Center for the Study and Prevention of Violence.

O'Neill, R. E., Horner, R. H., Albin, R. W., Sprague, J. R., Storey, K., & Newton, J. S. (1997). *Functional assessment and program development for problem behavior: A practical handbook*. Pacific Grove, CA: Brooks/Cole.

Oosterlaan, J., Logan, G. D., & Sergeant, J. A. (1998). Response inhibition in AD/HD, CD, AD/HD + CD, anxious, and control children: A meta-analysis of studies with the Stop Task. *Journal of Child Psychology and Psychiatry, 39*, 411–425.

Oosterlaan, J., & Sergeant, J. A. (1996). Inhibition in ADHD, aggressive, and anxious children: A biologically based model of child psychopathology. *Journal of Abnormal Child Psychology, 24*, 19–36.

Orland, M. E., Danegger, A. E., & Foley, E. (1997). The critical role of finance in creating comprehensive support systems. In R. J. Illback, C. T. Cobb, & H. M. Joseph Jr. (Eds.), *Integrated services for children and families: Opportunities for psychological practice* (pp. 93–118). Washington, DC: American Psychological Association.

Osofsky, J. D. (1995). The effects of exposure to violence on young children. *American Psychologist, 50*, 782–788.

Oswald, D. P., & Singh, N. N. (1996). Emerging trends in child and adolescent mental health. In T. H. Ollendick & R. J. Prinz (Eds.), *Advances in clinical child psychology* (Vol. 18, pp. 331–366). New York: Plenum Press.

Paniagua, F. A. (1994). *Assessing and treating culturally diverse clients: A practical guide*. Thousand Oaks, CA: Sage.

Paster, V. S. (1997). Emerging perspectives in child mental health services. In R. J. Illback, C. T. Cobb, & H. M. Joseph Jr. (Eds.), *Integrated services for children and families: Opportunities for psychological practice* (pp. 259–279). Washington, DC: American Psychological Association.

Paschall, M. J., & Hubbard, M. L. (1998). Effects of neighborhood and family stressors on African-American male adolescents' self-worth and propensity for violent behavior. *Journal of Consulting and Clinical Psychology, 66*, 825–831.

Patterson, C. J., Kupersmidt, J. B., & Vaden, N. A. (1990). Income level, gender, ethnicity, and household composition as predictors of children's school-based competence. *Child Development, 61*, 485–494.

Patterson, C. J., Vaden, N. A., & Kupersmidt, J. B. (1991). Family background, recent life events and peer rejection during childhood. *Journal of Social and Personal Relationships, 8*, 347–361.

Patterson, G. R. (1975a). *Families: Applications of social learning to family life* (rev. ed.). Champaign, IL: Research Press.

Patterson, G. R. (1975b). *Professional guide for "Families" and "Living with children."* Champaign, IL: Research Press.

Patterson, G. R. (1976). *Living with children: New methods for parents and teachers* (rev. ed.). Champaign, IL: Research Press.

Patterson, G. R. (1982). *Coercive family process*. Eugene, OR: Castalia.

Patterson, G. R. (1984). Siblings: Fellow travelers in coercive family processes. In R. J. Blanchard (Ed.), *Advances in the study of aggression* (pp. 174–213). New York: Academic Press.

Patterson, G. R., Capaldi, D., & Bank, L. (1991). An early starter model of predicting delinquency. In D. J. Pepler & K. H. Rubin (Eds.), *The development and treatment of childhood aggression* (pp. 139–168). New York: Erlbaum.

Patterson, G. R., & Chamberlain, P. (1988). Treatment process: A problem at three levels. In L. C. Wynne (Ed.), *The state of the art in family therapy research: Controversies and recommendations* (pp. 189–223). New York: Family Process Press.

Patterson, G. R., & Chamberlain, P. (1994). A functional analysis of resistance during parent training therapy. *Clinical Psychology: Science and Practice, 1*, 53–70.

Patterson, G. R., Cobb, J. A., & Ray, R. S. (1973). A social engineering technology for retraining the families of aggressive boys. In H. E. Adams & I. P. Unikel (Eds.), *Issues and trends in behavior therapy* (pp. 139–210). Springfield, IL: Thomas.

Patterson, G. R., DeGarmo, D. S., & Knutson, N. (2000). Hyperactive and antisocial behaviors: Comorbid or two points in the same process. *Development and Psychopathology, 12,* 91–106.

Patterson, G. R., Dishion, T. J., & Yoerger, K. (2000). Adolescent growth in new forms of problem behavior: Macro- and micro-peer dynamics. *Prevention Science, 1,* 3–13.

Patterson, G. R., & Fleischman, M. J. (1979). Maintenance of treatment effects: Some considerations concerning family systems and follow-up data. *Behavioral Therapy, 10,* 168–185.

Patterson, G. R., & Forgatch, M. S. (1985). Therapist behavior as a determinant for client noncompliance: A paradox for the behavior modifier. *Journal of Consulting and Clinical Psychology, 53,* 846–851.

Patterson, G. R., & Forgatch, M. S. (1987). *Parents and adolescents living together: Part 1. The basics.* Eugene, OR: Castalia.

Patterson, G. R., Forgatch, M. S., Yoerger, K. L., & Stoolmiller, M. (1998). Variables that initiate and maintain early-onset trajectories of juvenile offending. *Development and Psychopathology, 10,* 531–547.

Patterson, G. R., & Gullion, M. E. (1968). *Living with children: New methods for parents and teachers.* Champaign, IL: Research Press.

Patterson, G. R., Reid, J. B., Jones, R. R., & Conger R. E. (1975). *A social learning approach to family intervention: Vol. 1. Families with aggressive children.* Eugene, OR: Castalia.

Pearson, J. L., Ialongo, N. S., Hunter, A. G., & Kellam, S. G. (1994). Family structure and aggressive behavior in a population of urban elementary school children. *Journal of the American Academy of Child and Adolescent Psychiatry, 33,* 540–548.

Peed, S., Roberts, M., & Forehand, R. (1977). Evaluation of the effectiveness of a standardized parent training program in altering the interaction of mothers and their noncompliant children. *Behavior Modification, 1,* 323–350.

Peeples, F., & Loeber, R. (1994). Do individual factors and neighborhood context explain ethnic differences in juvenile delinquency? *Journal of Quantitative Criminology, 10,* 141–157.

Pelham, W. E. (2000). Implications of the MTA study for behavioral and combined treatments. *ADHD Report, 8,* 9–16.

Pelham, W., & Hoza, B. (1996). Intensive treatment: Summer treatment program for children with ADHD. In E. D. Hibbs & P. S. Jenson (Eds.), *Psychosocial treatment for child and adolescent disorders: Empirically based strategies for clinical practice* (pp. 311–340). Washington, DC: American Psychological Association.

Pelham, W. E., & Waschbusch, D. A. (1999). Behavioral intervention in attention-deficit/hyperactivity disorder. In H. C. Quay & A. E. Hogan (Eds.), *Handbook of disruptive behavior disorders* (pp. 255–278). New York: Kluwer Academic/Plenum Press.

Pelham Jr., W. E., Wheeler, T., & Chronis, A. (1998). Empirically supported psychosocial treatments for attention deficit hyperactivity disorder. *Journal of Clinical Child Psychology, 27,* 190–205.

Pennington, B. F., & Ozonoff, S. (1996). Executive functions and developmental psychopathology. *Journal of Child Psychology and Psychiatry, 37,* 51–87.

Penno, D. A., Frank, A. R., & Wacker, D. P. (2000). Instructional accommodations for adolescent students with severe emotional or behavioral disorders. *Behavioral Disorders, 25*, 325–343.

Pepler, D. J., Byrd, W., & King, G. (1991). A social-cognitively based social skills training program for aggressive children. In D. J. Pepler & K. H. Rubin (Eds.), *The development and treatment of childhood aggression* (pp. 361–379). Hillsdale, NJ: Erlbaum

Pepler, D. J., Craig, W. M., & Roberts, W. L. (1998). Observations of aggressive and nonaggressive children on the school playground. *Merrill-Palmer Quarterly, 44*, 55–76.

Pettit, G. S. (2000). Mechanisms in the cycle of maladaption: The life-course perspective. *Prevention and Treatment, 3*, 1–6.

Pettit, G. S., Bates, J. E., & Dodge, K. A. (1997). Supportive parenting, ecological context, and children's adjustment: A seven-year longitudinal study. *Child Development, 68*, 908–923.

Pfiffner, L. J., & Barkley, R. A. (1998). Treatment of ADHD in school settings. In R. A. Barkley, *Attention-deficit hyperactivity disorder: A handbook for diagnosis and treatment* (2nd ed., pp. 458–490). New York: Guilford Press.

Piacentini, J. C., Cohen, P., & Cohen, J. (1992). Combining discrepant information from multiple sources: Are complex algorithms better than simple ones? *Journal of Abnormal Child Psychology, 20*, 51–63.

Pianta, R. C., & Egeland, B. (1994). Relation between depressive symptoms and stressful life events in a sample of disadvantaged mothers. *Journal of Consulting and Clinical Psychology, 62*, 1229–1234.

Pierce, C. (1994). Importance of classroom climate for at-risk learners. *Journal of Educational Research, 88*, 37–42.

Pierce, E. W., Ewing, L. J., & Campbell, S. B. (1999). Diagnostic status and symptomatic behavior of hard-to-manage preschool children in middle childhood and early adolescence. *Journal of Clinical Child Psychology, 28*, 44–57.

Pincus, J. H. (1991). A neurological view of violence. In D. H. Crowell, I. M. Evans, & C. R. O'Donnell (Eds.), *Childhood aggression and violence* (pp. 53–73). New York: Plenum Press.

Plomin, R., Owen, M. J., & McGuffin, P. (1994). The genetic bases of complex human behavior. *Science, 264*, 1733–1739.

Pomplun, M. (1997). When students with disabilities participate in cooperative groups. *Exceptional Children, 64*, 49–58.

Pope, A. W., Bierman, K. L., & Mumma, G. H. (1989). Relations between hyperactive and aggressive behavior and peer relations at three elementary grade levels. *Journal of Abnormal Child Psychology, 17*, 253–267.

Pope, A. W., Bierman, K. L., & Mumma, G. H. (1991). Aggression, hyperactivity, and inattention-immaturity: Behavior dimensions associated with peer rejection in elementary school boys. *Developmental Psychology, 27*, 663–671.

Porter, B., & O'Leary, K. D. (1980). Marital discord and child behavior problems. *Journal of Abnormal Child Psychology, 8*, 287–295.

Posner, J. K., & Vandell, D. L. (1999). After-school activities and the development of low-income urban children: A longitudinal study. *Developmental Psychology, 35*, 868–879.

Poulin, F., & Boivin, M. (1999). Proactive and reactive aggression and boys' friendship quality in mainstream classrooms. *Journal of Emotional and Behavioral Disorders, 7,* 168–177.

Poulin, F., & Boivin, M. (2000). The role of proactive and reactive aggression in the formation and development of boys' friendships. *Developmental Psychology, 36,* 233–240.

Powell-Smith, K. A., Shinn, M. R., Stoner, G., & Good, III, R. H. (2000). Parent tutoring in reading using literature and curriculum materials: Impact on student reading achievement. *School Psychology Review, 29,* 5–27.

Price, J. M., & Dodge, K. A. (1989). Reactive and proactive aggression in childhood: Relations to peer status and social context dimensions. *Journal of Abnormal Child Psychology, 17,* 455–471.

Prinz, R. J., Blechman, E. A., & Dumas, J. E. (1994). An evaluation of peer-coping skills training for childhood aggression. *Journal of Clinical Child Psychology, 23,* 193–203.

Prinz, R. J., & Miller, G. E. (1996). Parental engagement in interventions for children at risk for conduct disorder. In R. D. Peters & R. J. McMahon (Eds.), *Preventing childhood disorders, substance abuse, and delinquency* (pp. 161–183). Thousand Oaks, CA: Sage.

Psychological Corporation. (1992). *Wechsler Individual Achievement Test, Comprehensive.* San Antonio, TX: Author.

Pumariega, A. J., & Glover, S. (1998). New developments in services delivery research for children, adolescents, and their families. In T. H. Ollendick & R. J. Prinz (Eds.), *Advances in clinical child psychology* (Vol. 20, pp. 303–343). New York: Plenum Press.

Quay, H. C. (1993). The psychology of undersocialized aggressive conduct disorder: A theoretical perspective. *Development and Psychopathology, 5,* 165–180.

Quay, H. C. (1997). Inhibition and attention deficit hyperactivity disorder. *Journal of Abnormal Child Psychology, 25,* 7–13.

Quay, H. C. (1999). Classification of the disruptive behavior disorders. In H. C. Quay & A. E. Hogan (Eds.), *Handbook of disruptive behavior disorders* (pp. 3–21). New York: Kluwer Academic/Plenum Press.

Quay, H. C., & Peterson, D. R. (1987). *Manual for the Revised Behavior Problem Checklist.* Odessa, FL: Psychological Assessment Resources.

Quinn, J. (1999). Where need meets opportunity: Youth development programs for early teens. *The Future of Children: When School Is Out, 9,* 96–116.

Raffaele, L. M., & Knoff, H. M. (1999). Improving home–school collaboration with disadvantaged families: Organizational principles, perspectives, and approaches. *School Psychology Review, 28,* 448–466.

Raine, A., Venables, P. H., & Mednick, S. A. (1997). Low resting heart rate at age 3 years predisposes to aggression at 11 years: Evidence from the Mauritius Child Heath Project. *Journal of the American Academy of Child and Adolescent Psychiatry, 36,* 1457–1464.

Raschke, D. (1981, December). Designing reinforcement surveys: Let the student choose the reward. *Teaching Exceptional Children,* pp. 92–96.

Rathvon, N. (1999). *Effective school interventions: Strategies for enhancing academic achievement and social competence.* New York: Guilford Press.

Reddy, L. A., & Pfeiffer, S. I. (1997). Effectiveness of treatment foster care with children and adolescents: A review of outcome studies. *Journal of the American Academy of Child and Adolescent Psychiatry, 36,* 581–588.

Reich, W. (2000). Diagnostic Interview for Children and Adolescents. *Journal of the American Academy of Child and Adolescent Psychiatry, 39,* 59–66.

Reid, J. B. (1993). Prevention of conduct disorder before and after school entry: Relating interventions to developmental findings. *Development and Psychopathology, 5,* 243–262.

Reid, J. B., & Eddy, J. M. (1997). The prevention of antisocial behavior: Some considerations in the search for effective interventions. In D. M. Stoff, J. Breiling, & J. D. Maser (Eds.), *Handbook of antisocial behavior* (pp. 343–356). New York: Wiley.

Reid, J. B., Eddy, J. M., Fetrow, R. A., & Stoolmiller, M. (1999). Description and immediate impacts of a preventative intervention for conduct problems. *American Journal of Community Psychology, 27,* 483–517.

Reid, R. (1995). Assessment of ADHD with culturally different groups: The use of behavioral rating scales. *School Psychology Review, 24,* 537–560.

Reid, R. (1996). Research in self-monitoring with students with learning disabilities: The present, the prospects, the pitfalls. *Journal of Learning Disabilities, 29,* 317–331.

Reid, R., DuPaul, G. J., Power, T. J., Anastopoulos, A. D., Rogers-Adkinson, D., Noll, M., & Riccio, C. (1998). Assessing culturally different students for attention deficit hyperactivity disorder using behavior rating scales. *Journal of Abnormal Child Psychology, 26,* 187–198.

Reid, R., Riccio, A., Kessler, R., DuPaul, G. J., Power, T. J., Anastopoulos, A. D., Rogers-Adkinson, D., & Noll, M. (2000). Gender and ethnic differences in ADHD as assessed by behavior ratings. *Journal of Emotional and Behavioral Disorders, 8,* 38–48.

Reschly, D. J. (1997). Utility of individual ability measures and public policy choices for the 21st century. *School Psychology Review, 26,* 234–241.

Reynolds, C. R., & Kamphaus, R. W. (1992). *Behavior Assessment System for Children (BASC).* Circle Pines, MN: American Guidance Service.

Reynolds, C. R., & Richmond, B. O. (1985). *Revised Children's Manifest Anxiety Scale (RCMAS).* Los Angeles: Western Psychological Services.

Reynolds, W. M. (1989). *Reynolds Child Depression Scale (RCDS).* Odessa, FL: Psychological Assessment Resources.

Rhodes, J. E., Grossman, J. B., & Resch, N. L. (2000). Agents of change: Pathways through which mentoring relationships influence adolescents' academic adjustment. *Child Development, 71,* 1662–1671.

Rhy, G. S., & Bear, G. G. (1997). Relational aggression and peer relations: Gender and developmental issues. *Merrill-Palmer Quarterly, 43,* 87–106.

Richters, J. E. (1992). Depressed mothers as informants about their children: A critical review of the evidence for distortion. *Psychological Bulletin, 112,* 485–499.

Rivera, V. R., & Kutash, K. (1994). *Components of a system of care: What does the research say?* Tampa: Florida Mental Health Institute, University of South Florida.

Roberts, M. W., Joe, V. C., & Rowe-Hallbert, A. (1992). Oppositional child behavior and parental locus of control. *Journal of Clinical Child Psychology, 21,* 170–177.

Roid, G. H., & Miller, L. (1996). *The Leiter International Performance Scale–Revised.* Wood Dale, IL: Stoelting.

Roland, E. (2000). Bullying in schools: Three national innovations in Norwegian schools in 15 years. *Aggressive Behavior, 26,* 135–143.

Rotter, J. B., & Rafferty, J. E. (1950). *Manual: The Rotter Incomplete Sentences Blank*. New York: Psychological Corporation.

Rubin, K. H., Chen, X., McDougall, P., Bowker, A., & McKinnon, J. (1995). The Waterloo Longitudinal Project: Predicting internalizing and externalizing problems in adolescence. *Development and Psychopathology, 7*, 751–764.

Rubin, K. H., Coplan, R. J., Fox, N. A., & Calkins, S. D. (1995). Emotionality, emotion regulation, and preschoolers' social adaptation. *Development and Psychopathology, 7*, 49–62.

Ruhl, K. L., & Berlinghoff, D. H. (1992). Research on improving behaviorally disordered students' academic performance: A review of the literature. *Behavioral Disorders, 17*, 178–190.

Russell, A., & Owens, L. (1999). Peer estimates of school-aged boys' and girls' aggression to same- and cross- sex targets. *Social Development, 8*, 364–379.

Sanders, M. R. (1999). Triple P—Positive Parenting Program: Towards an empirically validated multilevel parenting and family support strategy for prevention of behavior and emotional problems in children. *Clinical Child and Family Psychology Review, 2*, 71–90.

Sanders, M. R., Markie-Dadds, C., Tully, L. A., & Bor, W. (2000). The Triple P—Positive Parenting Program: A comparison of enhanced, standard, and self-directed behavioral family intervention for parents of children with early onset of conduct problems. *Journal of Consulting and Clinical Psychology, 68*, 624–640.

Sanders, M. R., & McFarland, M. (2000). Treatment of depressed mothers with disruptive children: A controlled evaluation of cognitive behavioral family intervention. *Behavior Therapy, 31*, 89–112.

Sattler, J. M. (1992). *Assessment of children* (3rd ed.). San Diego, CA: Author.

Scerbo, A. S., & Kolko, D. J. (1994). Salivary testosterone and cortisol in disruptive children: Relationship to aggressive, hyperactive, and internalizing behaviors. *Journal of the American Academy of Child and Adolescent Psychology, 33*, 1174–1184.

Schaal, B., Tremblay, R. E., Soussignan, R., & Susman, E. (1996). Male testosterone linked to high social dominance but low physical aggression in early adolescence. *Journal of the American Academy of Child and Adolescent Psychiatry, 34*, 1322–1330.

Schachar, R. (2000). The MTA study: Implications for medication management. *ADHD Report, 8*, 2–6.

Schachar, R., & Ickowicz, A. (1999). Pharmacological treatment of attention-deficit/hyperactivity disorder. In H. C. Quay & A. E. Hogan (Eds.), *Handbook of disruptive behavior disorders* (pp. 221–253). New York: Kluwer Academic/Plenum Press.

Schachar, R., & Tannock, R. (1995). Test of four hypotheses for the comorbidity of attention-deficit hyperactivity disorder and conduct disorder. *Journal of the American Academy of Child and Adolescent Psychiatry, 34*, 639–648.

Schoenwald, S. K., Brown, T. L., & Henggeler, S. W. (2000). Inside multisystemic therapy: Therapist, supervisor, and program practices. *Journal of Emotional and Behavioral Disorders, 8*, 113–127.

Schoenwald, S. K., & Henggeler, S. W. (1997). Combining effective treatment strategies with family-preservation models of service delivery. In R. J. Illback, C. T. Cobb, & H. M. Joseph Jr. (Eds.), *Integrated services for children and families:*

Opportunities for psychological practice (pp. 121–135). Washington, DC: American Psychological Association.

Schteingart, J. S., Molnar, J., Klein, T. P., Lowe, C. B., & Hartmann, A. H. (1995). Homelessness and child functioning in the context of risk and protective factors moderating child outcomes. *Journal of Clinical Child Psychology, 24,* 320–331.

Schulte, A. C., Osborne, S. S., & Erchul, W. P. (1998). Effective special education: A United States dilemma. *School Psychology Review, 27,* 66–76.

Schwartz, B. (1990). The creation and destruction of value. *American Psychologist, 45,* 7–15.

Schwartz, D., Dodge, K. A., Pettit, G., Bates, J. E., & Conduct Problems Prevention Research Group (2000). Friendship as a moderating factor in the pathway between early harsh home environment and later victimization in the peer group. *Developmental Psychology, 36,* 646–662.

Schwartz, D., & Proctor, L. J. (2000). Community violence exposure and children's social adjustment in the school peer group: The mediating roles of emotion regulation and social cognition. *Journal of Consulting and Clinical Psychology, 68,* 670–683.

Seguin, J. E., Pihl, R. O., Boulerice, B., Tremblay, R. E., & Harden, P. W. (1996). Pain sensitivity and stability of physical aggression in boys. *Journal of Child Psychology and Psychiatry, 37,* 823–834.

Seguin, J. R., Pihl, R. O., Harden, P. W., Tremblay, R. E., & Boulerice, B. (1995). Cognitive and neuropsychological characteristics of physically aggressive boys. *Journal of Abnormal Psychology, 104,* 614–625.

Seidman, L. J., Biederman, J., Faraone, S. V., Weber, W., Mennin, D., & Jones, J. (1997). A pilot study of neuropsychological function in girls with ADHD. *Journal of the American Academy of Child and Adolescent Psychiatry, 36,* 366–373.

Serketich, W. J., & Dumas, J. E. (1996). The effectiveness of behavioral parent training to modify antisocial behavior in children: A meta-analysis. *Behavior Therapy, 27,* 171–186.

Shaffer, D., Fisher, P., Lucas, C. P., Dulcan, M. K., & Schwab-Stone, M. E. (2000). NIMH Diagnostic Interview Schedule for Children Version IV: Description, differences from previous versions, and reliability of some common diagnoses. *Journal of the American Academy of Child and Adolescent Psychiatry, 39,* 28–38.

Shaffer, D., Gould, M. S., Brasic, J., Ambrosini, P., Fisher, P., Bird, H., & Aluwahlia, C. (1983). A Children's Global Assessment Scale (CGAS). *Archives of General Psychiatry, 40,* 1228–1231.

Shapiro, E. S., & Cole, C. L. (1994). *Behavior change in the classroom: Self-management interventions.* New York: Guilford Press.

Shaw, D. S., Owens, E. B., Giovannelli, J., & Winslow, E. B. (2001). Infant and toddler pathways to externalizing disorders. *Journal of the American Academy of Child and Adolescent Psychiatry, 40,* 36–43.

Shelton, K., Frick, P., & Wootton, J. (1996). Assessment of parenting practices in families of elementary school-age children. *Journal of Clinical Child Psychology, 25,* 317–329.

Shelton, T. L., Barkley, R. A., Crosswait, C., Moorehouse, M., Fletcher, K., Barrett, S., Jenkins, L., & Metevia, L. (1998). Psychiatric and psychological morbidity as a function of adaptive disability in preschool children with aggressive and hyperactive–impulsive–inattentive behavior. *Journal of Abnormal Child Psychology*, 26, 475–494.

Shelton, T. L., Barkley, R. A., Crosswait, C., Moorehouse, M., Fletcher, K., Barrett, S., Jenkins, L., & Metevia, L. (2000). Multi-method psycho-educational intervention for preschool children with disruptive behavior: Two-year posttreatment follow-up. *Journal of Abnormal Child Psychology*, 28, 253–266.

Sheridan, S. M., & Kratochwill, T. R. (1992). Behavioral parent–teacher consultation: Conceptual and research considerations. *Journal of School Psychology*, 30, 117–139.

Shields, A. M., & Cicchetti, D. (1998). Reactive aggression among maltreated children: The contributions of attention and emotion dysregulation. *Journal of Clinical Child Psychology*, 27, 381–395.

Shields, A. M., & Cicchetti, D. (2001). Parental maltreatment and emotion dysregulation as risk factors for bullying and victimization in middle childhood. *Journal of Clinical Child Psychology*, 30, 349–363.

Shields, A. M., Cicchetti, D., & Ryan, R. M. (1994). The development of emotional and behavioral self-regulation and social competence among maltreated school aged children. *Development and Psychopathology*, 6, 57–76.

Short, R. J. (1997). Education and training for integrated practice: Assumptions, components, and issues. In R. J. Illback, C. T. Cobb, & H. M. Joseph Jr. (Eds.), *Integrated services for children and families: Opportunities for psychological practice* (pp. 347–358). Washington, DC: American Psychological Association.

Silverthorn, P., & Frick, P. J. (1999). Developmental pathways to antisocial behavior: The delayed-onset pathway in girls. *Development and Psychopathology*, 11, 101–126.

Silverthorn, P., Frick, P. J., Kuper, K., & Ott, J. (1996). Attention deficit hyperactivity disorder and sex: A test of two etiological models to explain the male predominance. *Journal of Clinical Child Psychology*, 25, 52–59.

Simonoff, E., Pickles, A., Meyer, J., Silberg, J., & Maes, H. (1998). Genetic and environmental influences on subtypes of conduct disorder in boys. *Journal of Abnormal Child Psychology*, 26, 495–509.

Sinclair, M. F., Christenson, S. L., Evelo, D. L., & Hurley, C. M. (1998). Dropout prevention for youth with disabilities: Efficacy of a sustained school engagement procedure. *Exceptional Children*, 65, 7–21.

Skinner, C. H., Fletcher, P. A., & Henington, C. (1996). Increasing learning rates by increasing student response rates: A summary of research. *School Psychology Quarterly*, 11, 313–325.

Skinner, C. H., & Smith, E. S. (1992). Issues surrounding the use of self-management interventions for increasing academic performance. *School Psychology Review*, 21, 202–210.

Slavin, R. E. (1999). Comprehensive approaches to cooperative learning. *Theory into Practice*, 38, 74–79.

Smart, D., Sanson, A., & Prior, M. (1996). Connections between reading disability and behavior problems: Testing temporal and causal hypotheses. *Journal of Abnormal Child Psychology*, 24, 363–383.

Smith, D. J., Young, K. R., & West, R. P. (1992). The effect of a self-management procedure on the classroom and academic behavior of students with mild handicaps. *School Psychology Review*, 21, 59–72.

Smith, P. K., & Brain, P. (2000). Bullying in schools: Lessons from two decades of research. *Aggressive Behavior, 26,* 1–9.

Snyder, J., Horsch, E., & Childs, J. (1997). Peer relationships of young children: Affiliative choices and the shaping of aggressive behavior. *Journal of Clinical Child Psychology, 26,* 145–156.

Sobel, M. P., Ashbourne, D. R., Earn, B. M., & Cunningham, C. E. (1989). Parent's attributions for achieving compliance from attention-deficit disordered children. *Journal of Abnormal Child Psychology, 17,* 359–369.

Speltz, M. L., McClellan, J., Deklyen, M., & Jones, K. (1999). Preschool boys with oppositional defiant disorder: Clinical presentation and diagnostic change. *Journal of the American Academy of Child and Adolescent Psychiatry, 38,* 838–845.

Spencer, T., Biederman, J., Wilens, T., Harding, M., O'Donnell, D., & Griffen, S. (1996). Pharmacotherapy of attention-deficit hyperactivity disorder across the life cycle. *Journal of the American Academy of Child and Adolescent Psychiatry, 35,* 409–432.

Sroufe, L. A. (1997). Psychopathology as an outcome of development. *Development and Psychopathology, 9,* 251–268.

Sroufe, L. A., & Rutter, M. (1984). The domain of developmental psychopathology. *Child Development, 55,* 17–29.

Stage, S. A., & Quiroz, D. R. (1997). A meta-analysis of interventions to decrease disruptive classroom behavior in public education settings. *School Psychology Review, 26,* 333–368.

Stanger, C., Achenbach, T. M., & Verhulst, F. C. (1997). Accelerated longitudinal comparisons of aggressive vs. delinquent syndromes. *Development and Psychopathology, 9,* 43–58.

Stark, K. D., Sander, J. B., Yancy, M. G., Bronik, M. D., & Hoke, J. A. (2000). Treatment of depression in childhood and adolescence: Cognitive-behavioral procedures for the individual and family. In P. C. Kendall (Ed.), *Child and adolescent therapy: Cognitive-behavioral procedures* (2nd ed., pp. 173–234). New York: Guilford Press.

Stein, S., & Karno, M. (1994). Behavioral observation of anger and aggression. In M. Furlong & D. Smith (Eds.), *Anger, hostility, and aggression: Assessment, prevention and intervention strategies for youth* (pp. 245–283). Brandon, VT: Clinical Psychology Publishing.

Stevens, J., Quittner, A. L., & Abikoff, H. (1998). Factors influencing elementary school teachers' ratings of ADHD and ODD behaviors. *Journal of Clinical Child Psychology, 27,* 406–414.

Stipek, D. J., & Ryan, R. H. (1997). Economically disadvantaged preschoolers: Ready to learn but further to go. *Developmental Psychology, 33,* 711–723.

Stoolmiller, M., Eddy, J. M., & Reid, J. B. (2000). Detecting and describing preventive intervention effects in a universal school-based randomized trial targeting delinquent and violent behavior. *Journal of Consulting and Clinical Psychology, 68,* 296–306.

Stormshak, E. A., Bierman, K. L., & Conduct Problems Prevention Research Group (1998). The implications of different developmental patterns of disruptive behavior problem for school adjustment. *Development and Psychopathology, 10,* 451–468.

Stormshak, E. A., Bierman, K. L., McMahon, R. J., Lengua, L. J., & Conduct Problems Prevention Research Group (2000). Parent practices and child disruptive behavior problems in early elementary school. *Journal of Clinical Child Psychology, 29,* 17–29.

Strand, K., & Nowicki, S. (1999). Receptive nonverbal processing ability and locus of control orientation in children and adolescents with conduct disorders. *Behavioral Disorders, 24,* 102–108.

Strassberg, Z., Dodge, K. A., Pettit, G. S., & Bates, J. E. (1994). Spanking in the home and children's subsequent aggression toward kindergarten peers. *Development and Psychopathology, 6,* 445–462.

Straus, M. A., & Stewart, J. H. (1999). Corporal punishment by American parents: National data on prevalence, chronicity, severity and duration, in relation to child and family characteristics. *Clinical Child and Family Psychology Review, 2,* 55–70.

Striepling, S. H. (1997). The low-aggression classroom: A teacher's view. In A. P. Goldstein & J. C. Conoley (Eds.), *School violence intervention: A practical handbook* (pp. 23–45). New York: Guilford Press.

Stroul, B. A. (1995). Case management in a system of care. In B. J. Friesen & J. Poertner (Eds.), *From case management to service coordination for children with emotional, behavioral, or mental disorders: Building on family strengths* (pp. 3–25). Baltimore: Brookes.

Stroul, B. A., & Friedman, R. M. (1996). *A system of care for children and adolescents with severe emotional disturbance* (rev. ed.). Washington, DC: National Technical Assistance Center for Child Mental Health, Georgetown University Child Development Center.

Sugai, G., Horner, R. H., & Sprague, J. R. (1999). Functional-assessment-based behavior support planning: Research to practice to research. *Behavioral Disorders, 24,* 253–257.

Sugai, G., Sprague, J. R., Horner, R. H., & Walker, H. M. (2000). Preventing school violence: The use of office discipline referrals to assess and monitor school-wide discipline interventions. *Journal of Emotional and Behavioral Disorders, 8,* 94–101.

Sutherland, K. S., Wehby, J. H., & Copeland, S. R. (2000). Effect of varying rates of behavior-specific praise on the on-task behavior of students with EBD. *Journal of Emotional and Behavioral Disorders, 8,* 2–8.

Sutherland, K. S., Wehby, J. H., & Gunter, P. L. (2000). The effectiveness of cooperative learning with students with emotional and behavioral disorders: A literature review. *Behavioral Disorders, 25,* 225–238.

Sutton, C. T., & Broken Nose, M. A. (1996). American Indian families: An overview. In M. McGoldrick, J. Giordano, & J. K. Pearce (Eds.), *Ethnicity and family therapy* (pp. 31–44). New York: Guilford Press.

Swanson, H. L., & Hoskyn, M. (1998). Experimental intervention research on students with learning disabilities: A meta-analysis of treatment outcomes. *Review of Educational Research, 68,* 277–321.

Tafoya, N., & Del Vecchio, A. (1996). Back to the future: An examination of the Native American Holocaust. In M. McGoldrick, J. Giordano, & J. K. Pearce (Eds.), *Ethnicity and family therapy* (pp. 45–54). New York: Guilford Press.

Tannock, R. (1998). Attention deficit hyperactivity disorder: Advances in cognitive, neurobiological, and genetic research. *Journal of Child Psychology and Psychiatry, 39,* 65–99.

Tateyama-Sniezek, K. M. (1990). Cooperative learning: Does it improve the academic achievement of students with handicaps? *Exceptional Children, 56,* 426–437.

Taylor, T. K., & Biglan, A. (1998). Behavioral family interventions for improving child-rearing: A review of the literature for clinicians and policy makers. *Clinical Child and Family Psychology Review, 7,* 41–60.

Taylor, T. K., Eddy, J. M., & Biglan, A. (1999). Interpersonal skills training to reduce aggressive and delinquent behavior: Limited evidence and the need for an evidence-based system of care. *Clinical Child and Family Psychology Review, 2,* 169–182.

Tharp, R. G. (1989). Psychocultural variables and constants: Effects on teaching and learning in schools. *American Psychologist, 44,* 349–359.

Tharp, R. G. (1991). Cultural diversity and treatment of children. *Journal of Consulting and Clinical Psychology, 59,* 199–812.

Thompson, L. L., Riggs, P. D., Mikulich, S. K., & Crowley, T. J. (1996). Contribution of ADHD symptoms to substance problems and delinquency in conduct-disordered adolescents. *Journal of Abnormal Child Psychology, 24,* 325–347.

Thomson, G. O. B., Raab, G. M., Hepburn, W. S., Hunter, R., Fulton, M., & Laxen, D. P. H. (1989). Blood-lead levels and children's behavior: Results from the Edinburgh Lead Study. *Journal of Child Psychology and Psychiatry, 30,* 515–528.

Thorndike, R., Hagen, E., & Sattler, J. (1986). *The Stanford–Binet Intelligence Scale, fourth edition: Guide for administering and scoring.* Itasca, IL: Riverside.

Tolan, P. H., & Gorman-Smith, D. (1997). Treatment of juvenile delinquency: Between punishment and therapy. In D. M. Stoff, J. Breiling, & J. D. Maser (Eds.), *Handbook of antisocial behavior* (pp. 405–415). New York: Wiley.

Tolan, P. H., & Guerra, N. (1994). *What works in reducing adolescent violence?: An empirical review of the field.* Boulder, CO: Center for the Study and Prevention of Violence.

Tremblay, G. C., & Drabman, R. (1997). An intervention for childhood stealing. *Child and Family Behavior Therapy, 19,* 33–40.

Tremblay, R. E., LeMarquand, D., & Vitaro, F. (1999). The prevention of oppositional defiant disorder and conduct disorder. In H. C. Quay & A. E. Hogan (Eds.), *Handbook of disruptive behavior disorders* (pp. 525–555). New York: Kluwer Academic/Plenum Press.

Tremblay, R. E., Masse, L. C., Pagani, L., & Vitaro, F. (1996). From childhood physical aggression to adolescent maladjustment: The Montreal Prevention Experiment. In R. D. Peters & R. J. McMahon (Eds.), *Preventing childhood disorders, substance abuse, and delinquency* (pp.268–298). Thousand Oaks, CA: Sage.

Tremblay, R. E., Masse, L. C., Vitaro, F., & Dobkin, P. L. (1995). The impact of friends' deviant behavior on early onset delinquency: Longitudinal data from 6 to 13 years of age. *Development and Psychopathology, 7,* 649–667.

Tremblay, R. E., Pagani-Kurtz, L., Masse, L. C., Vitaro, F., & Pihl, R. O. (1995). A bimodal preventive intervention for disruptive kindergarten boys: Its impact through mid-adolescence. *Journal of Consulting and Clinical Psychology, 63,* 560–568.

Tuma, J. M. (1989a). Traditional therapies with children. In T. H. Ollendick & M. Hersen (Eds.), *Handbook of child psychopathology* (pp. 419–437). New York: Plenum Press.

Tuma, J. M. (1989b). Mental health services for children: The state of the art. *American Psychologist, 44*, 188–199.

Tutty, L. M. (1995). Theoretical and practical issues in selecting a measure of family functioning. *Research on Social Work Practice, 5*, 80–106.

Tynan, W. D., Schuman, W., & Lampert, N. (1999). Concurrent parent and child therapy groups for externalizing disorders: From the laboratory to the world of managed care. *Cognitive and Behavioral Practice, 6*, 3–9.

Urbain, E. S., & Kendall, P. C. (1980). Review of social-cognitive problem-solving interventions with children. *Psychological Bulletin, 80*, 109–143.

U.S. Department of Education and U.S. Department of Justice. (1998). *Safe and smart: Making after-school hours work for kids*. Washington, DC: Author.

U.S. Department of Health and Human Services. (1999). *Mental health: A report of the Surgeon General*. Rockville, MD: Author.

U.S. Department of Health and Human Services. (2001). *Youth violence: A report of the Surgeon General*. Rockville, MD: Author.

Vandell, D. L., & Shumow, L. (1999). After-school child care programs. *The Future of Children: When School Is Out, 9*, 64–80.

Vanden-Kierman, N., Ialongo, N. S., Pearson, J., & Kellam, S. (1995). Household family structure and children's aggressive behavior: A longitudinal study of urban elementary school children. *Journal of Abnormal Child Psychology, 23*, 553–568.

Vanyukov, M. M., Moss, H. B., Plail, J. A., Blackson, T., Mezzick, A. C., & Tarter, R. E. (1993). Antisocial symptoms in pre-adolescent boys and in their parents: Associations with cortisol. *Psychiatry Review, 46*, 9–17.

Verlinden, S., Hersen, M., & Thomas, J. (2000). Risk factors in school shootings. *Clinical Psychology Review, 20*, 3–56.

Villani, S. (2001). Impact of media on children and adolescents: A 10-year review of research. *Journal of the American Academy of Child and Adolescent Psychiatry, 40*, 392–401.

Vincent Roehling, P., & Robin, A. L. (1986). Development and validation of the Family Beliefs Inventory: A measure of unrealistic beliefs among parents and adolescents. *Journal of Consulting and Clinical Psychology, 54*, 693–697.

Vitaro, F., Brendgen, M., Pagani, L., Tremblay, R. E., & McDuff, P. (1999). Disruptive behavior, peer association, and conduct disorder: Testing the developmental links through early intervention. *Development and Psychopathology, 11*, 287–304.

Vitaro, F., Dobkin, P. L., Carbonneau, R., & Tremblay, R. E. (1996). Personal and familial characteristics of resilient sons of male alcoholics. *Addiction, 91*, 1161–1177.

Vitaro, F., Gendreau, P. L., Tremblay, R. E., & Oligny, P. (1998). Reactive and proactive aggression differentially predict later conduct problems. *Journal of Child Psychology and Psychiatry, 39*, 377–385.

Vitaro, F., & Tremblay, R. E. (1994). Impact of a prevention program on aggressive children's friendships and social adjustment. *Journal of Abnormal Child Psychology, 22*, 457–475.

Vitaro, F., Tremblay, R. E., Kerr, M., Pagani, L., & Bukowski, W. M. (1997). Disruptiveness, friends' characteristics, and delinquency in early adolescence: A test of two competing models of development. *Child Development, 68*, 676–689.

Vitiello, B., & Stoff, D. M. (1997). Subtypes of aggression and their relevance to child psychiatry. *Journal of the American Academy of Child and Adolescent Psychiatry, 36*, 307–315.

Wahler, R. G., & Dumas, J. E. (1989). Attentional problems in dysfunctional mother–child interactions: An interbehavioral model. *Psychological Bulletin, 105*, 116–130.

Wakschlag, L. S., & Hans, S. L. (1999). Relation of maternal responsiveness during infancy to the development of behavior problems in high-risk youths. *Developmental Psychology, 35*, 569–579.

Walker, H. M. (1979). *The acting-out child: Coping with classroom disruption.* Boston: Allyn & Bacon.

Walker, H. M., Colvin, G., & Ramsey, E. (1995). *Antisocial behavior in school: Strategies and best practices.* Pacific Grove, CA: Brooks/Cole.

Walker, H. M., Horner, R. H., Sugai, G., Bullis, M., Sprague, J. R., Bricker, D., & Kaufman, M. J. (1996). Integrated approaches to preventing antisocial behavior patterns among school-age children and youth. *Journal of Emotional and Behavioral Disorders, 4*, 194–209.

Walker, H. M., Kavanagh, K., Stiller, B., Golly, A., Severson, H. H., & Feil, E. G. (1998). First step to success: An early intervention approach for preventing school antisocial behavior. *Journal of Emotional and Behavioral Disorders, 6*, 66–80.

Walker, H. M., & McConnell, S. R. (1988). *The Walker–McConnell Scale of Social Competence and School Adjustment.* Austin, TX: PRO-ED.

Walker, H. M., & Sprague, J. R. (2001). Intervention strategies for diverting at-risk children and youth from destructive outcomes. *Report on Emotional and Behavioral Disorders in Youth, 1*, 5–18.

Walker, J. L., Lahey, B. B., Hynd, G. W., & Frame, C. L. (1987). Comparison of specific patterns of antisocial behavior in children with conduct disorder with or without coexisting hyperactivity. *Journal of Consulting and Clinical Psychology, 55*, 910–913.

Walker, K. E., Grossman, J. B., & Raley, R. (2000). *Extended service schools: Putting programming in place* [Online]. Available: www.ppv.org

Walsh, W. J., Isaacson, H. R., Rehman, F., & Hall, A. (1997). Elevated blood copper/zinc ratios in assaultive young males. *Physiology and Behavior, 62*, 327–329.

Wascbusch, D. A., Willoughby, M. T., & Pelham, W. E. (1998). Criterion validity and utility of reactive and proactive aggression: Comparisons to attention deficit hyperactivity disorder, oppositional defiant disorder, conduct disorder, and other measures of functioning. *Journal of Clinical Child Psychology, 27*, 396–405.

Waslick, B., Werry, J. S., & Greenhill, L. L. (1999). Pharmacotherapy and toxicology of oppositional defiant disorder and conduct disorder. In H. C. Quay & A. E. Hogan (Eds.), *Handbook of disruptive behavior disorders* (pp. 455–474). New York: Kluwer Academic/Plenum Press.

Webster-Stratton, C. (1984). Randomized trial of two parent-training programs for families with conduct-disordered children. *Journal of Consulting and Clinical Psychology, 52*, 666–678.

Webster-Stratton, C. (1990a). Stress: A potential disruptor of parent perceptions and family interactions. *Journal of Clinical Child Psychology, 19*, 302–312.

Webster-Stratton, C. (1990b). Enhancing the effectiveness of self-administered videotape parent training for families with conduct-problem children. *Journal of Abnormal Child Psychology, 18,* 479–492.

Webster-Stratton, C. (1992). *The incredible years: A trouble shooting guide for parents and children aged 3–8.* Toronto: Umbrella Press.

Webster-Stratton, C. (1994). Advancing videotape parent training: A comparison study. *Journal of Consulting and Clinical Psychology, 62,* 583–593.

Webster-Stratton, C. (1996a). Early-onset conduct problems: Does gender make a difference? *Journal of Consulting and Clinical Psychology, 64,* 554–551.

Webster-Stratton, C. (1996b). Early intervention with videotape modeling: Programs for families of children with oppositional defiant disorder or conduct disorder. In E. S. Hibbs & P. S. Jensen (Eds.), *Psychosocial treatments for child and adolescent disorders: Empirically based strategies for clinical practice* (pp. 435–474). Washington, DC: American Psychological Association.

Webster-Stratton, C. (1998a). Preventing conduct problems in Head Start children: Strengthening parenting competencies. *Journal of Consulting and Clinical Psychology, 66,* 715–730.

Webster-Stratton, C. (1998b). Parent training with low-income families: Promoting parental engagement through a collaborative approach. In J. R. Lutzker (Ed.), *Handbook of child abuse research and treatment* (pp. 183–210). New York: Plenum Press.

Webster-Stratton, C., & Hammond, M. (1988). Maternal depression and its relationship to life stress, perceptions of child behavior problems, parenting behaviors, and child conduct problems. *Journal of Abnormal Child Psychology, 16,* 299–315.

Webster-Stratton, C., & Hammond, M. (1990). Predictors of treatment outcome in parent training for families with conduct problem children. *Behavior Therapy, 21,* 319–337.

Webster-Stratton, C., & Hammond, M. (1997). Treating children with early-onset conduct problems: A comparison of child and parent training interventions. *Journal of Consulting and Clinical Psychology, 65,* 93–109.

Webster-Stratton, C., & Hammond, M. (1998). Conduct problems and level of social competence in Head Start children: Prevalence, pervasiveness, and associated risk factors. *Clinical Child and Family Psychology Review, 1,* 101–124.

Webster-Stratton, C., & Hammond, M. (1999). Marital conflict management skills, parenting style, and early-onset conduct problems: Processes and pathways. *Journal of Child Psychology and Psychiatry, 40,* 917–927.

Webster-Stratton, C. & Hooven, C. (in press). Parent training for child conduct problems. In A. S. Bellack & M. Hersen (Eds.), *Comprehensive clinical psychology.* New York: Pergamon Press.

Webster-Stratton, C., Kolpacoff, M., & Hollinsworth, T. (1988). Self-administered videotape therapy for families with conduct problem children: Comparison with two cost-effective treatments and a control group. *Journal of Consulting and Clinical Psychology, 56,* 558–566.

Webster-Stratton, C., & Lindsay, D. W. (1999). Social competence and conduct problems in young children: Issues in assessment. *Journal of Clinical Child Psychology, 28,* 25–43.

Webster-Stratton, C., Reid, M. J., & Hammond, M. (2001). Preventing conduct problems, promoting social competence: A parent and teacher training partnership in Head Start. *Journal of Clinical Child Psychology, 30,* 283–302.

Wechsler, D. (1991). *Wechsler Intelligence Scale for Children* (3rd ed.). New York: Psychological Corporation.

Wehby, J. H., Symons, F. J., Canale, J. A., & Go, F. J. (1998). Teaching practices in classrooms for students with emotional and behavioral disorders: Discrepancies between recommendations and observations. *Behavioral Disorders, 24,* 51–56.

Weiss, B., & Catron, T. (1994). Specificity of the comorbidity of aggression and depression in children. *Journal of Abnormal Child Psychology, 22,* 389–401.

Weiss, B., Catron, T., & Harris, V. (2000). A 2-year follow-up of the effectiveness of traditional child psychotherapy. *Journal of Consulting and Clinical Psychology, 68,* 1094–1101.

Weiss, B., Catron, T., Harris, V., & Phung, T. M. (1999). The effectiveness of traditional child psychotherapy. *Journal of Consulting and Clinical Psychology, 67,* 82–94.

Weiss, B., Dodge, K. A., Bates, J. E., & Pettit, G. S. (1992). Some consequences of early harsh discipline: Child aggression and a maladaptive social information processing style. *Child Development, 63,* 1321–1335.

Weissman, M. M., Warner, V., Wickramaratne, P. J., & Kandel, B. B. (1999). Maternal smoking during pregnancy and psychopathology in offspring followed to adulthood. *Journal of the American Academy of Child and Adolescent Psychiatry, 38,* 892–899.

Weist, M. D. (1997). Expanded school mental health services: A national movement in progress. In T. H. Ollendick & R. J. Prinz (Eds.), *Advances in clinical child psychology* (pp. 319–352). New York: Plenum Press.

Weisz, J. R., Donenberg, G. R., Han, S. S., & Weiss, B. (1995). Bridging the gap between lab and clinic in child and adolescent psychotherapy. *Journal of Consulting and Clinical Psychology, 63,* 688–701.

Weisz, J. R., Han, S. S., & Valeri, S. M. (1997). More of what?: Issues raised by the Fort Bragg study. *American Psychologist, 52,* 541–545.

Weisz, J. R., Huey, S. J., & Weersing, V. R. (1998). Psychotherapy outcome research with children and adolescents: The state of the art. In T. H. Ollendick & R. J. Prinz (Eds.), *Advances in clinical child psychology* (Vol. 20, pp. 49–91). New York: Plenum Press.

Weisz, J. R., Weiss, B., Han, S. S., Granger, D. A., & Morton, T. (1995). Effects of psychotherapy with children and adolescents revisited: A meta-analysis of treatment outcome studies. *Psychological Bulletin, 117,* 450–468.

Wekerle, C., & Wolfe, D. A. (1996). Child maltreatment. In E. Mash & R. A. Barkley (Eds.), *Childhood psychopathology* (pp. 492–537). New York: Guilford Press.

Welch, A. B. (1999). Increasing academic engagement of students with ADHD. *ADHD Report, 7,* 1–5.

Wells, K. C., & Egan, J. (1988). Social learning and systems family therapy for childhood oppositional disorder: Comparative treatment outcome. *Comprehensive Psychiatry, 29,* 138–146.

Werthamer-Larsson, L., Kellam, S. G., & Wheeler, L. (1991). Effects of first-grade classroom environment on shy behavior, aggressive behavior, and concentration problems. *American Journal of Community Psychology, 19,* 585–602.

Wheeler Maedgen, J., & Carlson, C. L. (2000). Social functioning and emotional regulation in the attention deficit hyperactivity disorder subtypes. *Journal of Clinical Child Psychology, 29,* 30–42.

White, J. L., Moffitt, T. E., & Silva. P. A. (1989). A prospective replication of the protective effects of IQ in subjects at high risk for juvenile delinquency. *Journal of Consulting and Clinical Psychology, 57,* 719–724.

Whitehurst, G. J., Falco, F. L., Lonigan, C. J., Fischel, J. E., DeBaryshe, B. D., Valdez-Menchaca, M. C., & Caulfield, M. (1988). Accelerating language development through picture book reading. *Developmental Psychology, 24,* 552–559.

Wilens, T. E. (1999). *Straight talk about psychiatric medications for kids.* New York: Guilford Press.

Wilkinson, G. S. (1993). *The Wide Range Achievement Test: Administration manual.* Wilmington, DE: Wide Range.

Wolfe, D. A. (1999). *Child abuse: Implications for child development and psychopathology* (2nd ed.). Thousand Oaks, CA: Sage.

Woodcock, R. W., McGrew, K. S., & Mather, N. (2001). *Woodcock–Johnson III.* Itasca, IL: Riverside Publishing.

Woolston, J. L. (1996). Psychiatric inpatient services. In M. Lewis (Ed.), *Child and adolescent psychiatry: A comprehensive textbook* (pp. 890–894). Baltimore: Williams & Wilkins.

Wootton, J. M., Frick, P. J., Shelton, K. K., & Silverthorn, P. (1997). Ineffective parenting and childhood conduct problems: The moderating role of callous-unemotional traits. *Journal of Consulting and Clinical Psychology, 65,* 301–308.

Wyman, P. A., Cowen, E. L., Work, W. C., Hoyt-Meyers, L., Magnus, K. B., & Fagen, D. B. (1999). Caregiving and developmental factors differentiating young at-risk urban children showing resilient versus stress-affected outcomes: A replication and extension. *Child Development, 70,* 645–659.

Wyman, P. A., Cowen, E. L., Work, W. C., & Parker, G. R. (1991). Developmental and family milieu correlates of resilience in urban children who have experienced major life stress. *American Journal of Community Psychology, 19,* 405–426.

Yoshikawa, H. (1994). Prevention as cumulative protection: Effects of early family support and education on chronic delinquency and its risks. *Psychological Bulletin, 115,* 28–54.

Youngstrom, E., Izard, C., & Ackerman, B. (1999). Dysphoria-related bias in maternal ratings of children. *Journal of Consulting and Clinical Psychology, 67,* 905–916.

Youngstrom, E., & Loeber, R., & Stouthamer-Loeber, M. (2000). Patterns and correlates of agreement between parent, teacher, and male adolescent ratings of externalizing and internalizing problems. *Journal of Consulting and Clinical Psychology, 68,* 1038–1050.

Zametkin, A. J., & Rapoport, J. L. (1987). Neurobiology of attention deficit disorder with hyperactivity: Where have we come in 50 years? *Journal of the American Academy of Child and Adolescent Psychiatry, 26,* 676–686.

Zangwill, W. M. (1983). An evaluation of a parent training program. *Child and Family Behavior Therapy, 5,* 1–6.

Zentall, S. (1995). Modifying classroom tasks and environments. In S. Goldstein, *Understanding and managing children's classroom behavior* (pp. 73–94). New York: Wiley.

Zigler, E. F., Finn-Stevenson, M., & Stern, B. M. (1997). Supporting children and families in the schools: The school of the 21st century. *American Journal of Orthopsychiatry, 67,* 396–407.

Zigler, E., Taussig, C., & Black, K. (1992). Early childhood intervention: A promising preventive for juvenile delinquency. *American Psychologist*, *47*, 997–1006.

Zins, J. E., & Erchul, W. P. (1995). Best practices in school consultation. In A. Thomas & J. Grimes (Eds.), *Best practices in school psychology–III* (pp. 609–623). Washington, DC: National Association of School Psychologists.

Zoccolilo, M. (1993). Gender and the development of conduct disorder. *Development and Psychopathology*, *5*, 65–78.

Index